Recent Advances in
HAEMATOLOGY

A. V. HOFFBRAND MA DM FRCP FRCPath
Professor of Haematology and Honorary Consultant, Royal Free Hospital and School of Medicine, London, UK

Recent Advances in
HAEMATOLOGY

EDITED BY
A. V. HOFFBRAND

NUMBER FIVE

CHURCHILL LIVINGSTONE
EDINBURGH LONDON MELBOURNE AND NEW YORK 1988

CHURCHILL LIVINGSTONE
Medical Division of Longman Group UK Limited

Distributed in the United States of America by
Churchill Livingstone Inc., 1560 Broadway, New York,
N.Y. 10036, and by associated companies, branches
and representatives throughout the world.

© Longman Group UK Limited 1988

First edition 1988

ISBN 0 443 03997 6
ISSN 0143–697X

Printed in Great Britain at The Bath Press, Avon

Preface

The fifth volume of Recent Advances in Haematology attempts to cover the areas of the field where major increases in knowledge have occurred in the three years since the fourth volume appeared. A substantial proportion of these advances have been achieved by the application of the techniques of molecular biology to the study of blood diseases and many of the chapters reflect these scientific achievements. We are fortunate to include among the contributors to this volume, haematologists of different interests who have themselves carried out outstanding original research which has resulted in some of this increased knowledge. Progress not only in understanding the nature of genetic and acquired blood disease at a molecular level is described, but also the practical applications of this knowledge both in ante-natal diagnosis and in therapy.

New information appears with frightening speed and it has been difficult in many sections to draw the line where no more information could be added. It is hoped, however, that all these reviews will encompass major changes up to the middle of 1988.

Several of the authors have written previously in this series and the editor is grateful to them for agreeing to a further demand on time and energy. I also wish to thank the new contributors, all of whom have put in a tremendous effort to gather together a vast amount of recently published literature and summarise this in a lucid and authoritative fashion. In a book of this size, it has been impossible to be totally comprehensive and the editor apologises if his choice of subjects has resulted in important omissions.

It is a pleasure to thank not only the contributors but also Charlotte Dew and Megan Evans for excellent secretarial help and the staff of Churchill Livingstone for their major role in ensuring the editor and authors delivered the book to time and in helping in every possible way to assemble what we hope will be a widely read volume.

London, 1988   A.V.H.

Contributors

STYLIANOS E. ANTONARAKIS PhD
Associate Professor of Pediatrics, Genetics Unit, Department of Pediatrics, The Johns Hopkins University School of Medicine, Baltimore, Maryland, USA

M. K. BRENNER
Department of Haematology, Royal Free Hospital, London, UK

G. G. BROWNLEE PhD FRS
E.P. Abraham Professor of Chemical Pathology, University of Oxford, Oxford, UK

DÉSIRÉ COLLEN MD PhD
Professor of Medicine, Center for Thrombosis and Vascular Research, Katholieke Universiteit Leuven, Leuven, Belgium; Visiting Professor, Harvard Medical School; Professor of Biochemistry and Medicine, University of Vermont, Vermont, USA

CARLO M. CROCE MD
Associate Director and Institute Professor, The Wistar Institute of Anatomy and Biology, Philadelphia, Pennsylvania, USA

BRIAN G. M. DURIE MD
Professor of Medicine and Director of Clinical Hematology, The Arizona Cancer Center College of Medicine, Tucson, USA

KENNETH FOON MD
Chief, Division of Clinical Immunology, State University of New York at Buffalo, New York, USA

R. P. GALE MD PhD FACP
Associate Professor of Medicine, Division of Hematology and Oncology, UCLA School of Medicine, Los Angeles, California, USA

HERMAN K. GOLD MD
Division of Cardiology, Massachusetts General Hospital, Harvard Medical School, Boston, Massachusetts, USA

JOHN M. GOLDMAN DM FRCP FRCPath
Professor of Leukaemia Biology, Royal Postgraduate Medical School; Honorary Consultant Physician, Hammersmith Hospital, London, UK

JUDITH S. GREENGARD PhD
Research Fellow, Scripps Clinic and Research Foundation, La Jolla, California, USA

JOHN H. GRIFFIN PhD
Associate Member, Scripps Clinic and Research Foundation, La Jolla, California, USA

HENRIK GRIESSER MD
Research Fellow, Ontario Cancer Institute, Toronto, Canada

JEROME E. GROOPMAN MD
Chief, Division of Hematology and Oncology, New England Deaconess Hospital; Associate Professor of Medicine, Harvard Medical School, Boston, Massachusetts, USA

FRANK G. HALUSKA
Graduate Student, The Wistar Institute, Philadelphia, USA

A. VICTOR HOFFBRAND MA DM FRCP FRCPath
Professor of Haematology and Honorary Consultant, Royal Free Hospital, London, UK

B. VAUGHAN-HUDSON MPBS PhD
Research Associate, British National Lymphoma Investigation, Department of Oncology, UCMHMS, London, UK

MASACHARU ISOBE PhD
Associate Scientist, The Wistar Institute, Philadelphia, Pennsylvania, USA

HAIG H. KAZAZIAN, Jr MD
Professor of Pediatrics, Genetics Unit, Department of Pediatrics, The Johns Hopkins University School of Medicine, Baltimore, Maryland, USA

GEORGE J. KONTOGHIORGHES BSc PhD
Lecturer, Royal Free Hospital and School of Medicine, London, UK

DAVID LINCH MB BChir FRCP
Reader in Haematology, University College and Middlesex School of Medicine, London, UK

TAK W. MAK PhD
Professor, Departments of Medical Biophysics and Immunology, University of Toronto, Toronto, Canada

A. R. MIRE-SLUIS
Research Assistant, Department of Haematology, Royal Free Hospital, Pond Street, London, UK

H. GRANT PRENTICE MB FRCP FRC Path
Director of the Bone Marrow Transplant Programme; Senior Lecturer and Honorary
Consultant, Department of Haematology, Royal Free Hospital, London, UK

MARCIANO D. REIS MD
Research Fellow, Ontario Cancer Institute, Toronto, Canada

GIANDOMENICO RUSSO MD
The Wistar Institute, Philadelphia, Pennysylvania, USA

COLIN A. SIEFF MRCPath
Assistant Professor of Pediatrics, Division of Pediatric Oncology, The Children's
Hospital and Dana-Farber Cancer Institute, Department of Pediatrics, Harvard
Medical School, Boston, Massachusetts, USA

DAVID C. STUMP MD
Assistant Professor of Medicine and Biochemistry, University of Vermont, College
of Medicine, Burlington, Vermont, USA

S. L. THEIN MRCP MRCPath
Wellcome Senior Research Fellow in Clinical Science, Honorary Consultant in
Haematology, Nuffield Department of Clinical Medicine, John Radcliffe Hospital,
Oxford, UK

DAVID J. WEATHERALL MD FRCP FRS
Nuffield Professor of Clinical Medicine, University of Oxford; Honorary Director,
MRC Molecular Haematology Unit, University of Oxford, Oxford, UK

R. GITENDRA WICKREMASINGHE BSc PhD
Honorary Lecturer, Department of Haematology, Royal Free Hospital, London, UK

Contents

1. Haemopoietic growth factors: in vitro and in vivo studies   *C. A. Sieff*   1

2. Biochemical mechanisms of transduction of signals for proliferation and differentiation in normal and malignant haemopoietic cells
R. G. Wickremasinghe   A. R. Mire-Sluis   A. V. Hoffbrand   19

3. The thalassaemias   *S. L. Thein   D. J. Weatherall*   43

4. Prospects for effective and oral chelation in transfusional iron overload   *G. J. Kontoghiorghes   A. V. Hoffbrand*   75

5. Gene rearrangements in leukemias and lymphomas   *M. D. Reis   H. Griesser   T. W. Mak*   99

6. Molecular basis of B- and T-cell neoplasia   *G. Russo   F. G. Haluska   M. Isobe   C. M. Croce*   121

7. Chronic myeloid leukaemia: pathogenesis and management
J. M. Goldman   131

8. Recent advances in bone marrow transplantation in the treatment of leukaemia   *H. G. Prentice   M. K. Brenner*   153

9. Chronic lymphocytic leukemia and related diseases   *K. A. Foon   R. P. Gale*   179

10. The management of Hodgkin's disease and the non-Hodgkin's lymphomas   *D. C. Linch   B. Vaughan-Hudson*   211

11. Hemophilia A in man: molecular defects in the factor VIII gene
S. E. Antonarakis   H. H. Kazazian   243

12. Haemophilia B: a review of patient defects, diagnosis with gene probes and prospects for gene therapy   *G. G. Brownlee*   251

13. Thrombolytic therapy   *D. Collen   D. C. Stump   H. K. Gold*   265

14. Protein C pathways   *J. S. Greengard   J. H. Griffin*   275

15. Acquired immunodeficiency syndrome   *J. E. Groopman*   291

16. Plasma cell disorders: recent advances in the biology and treatment
    B. G. M. Durie   305

Index   329

1. Haemopoietic growth factors: in vitro and in vivo studies

C. A. Sieff

INTRODUCTION

Every minute of adult life, the human bone marrow produces approximately 2 000 000 erythrocytes and 300 000 white blood cells. While circulating cell numbers are maintained within quite narrow limits, in the face of infection or bleeding this prodigious rate of production can be rapidly amplified. How is haemopoiesis maintained, and what are the mechanisms that regulate this constant supply of blood cells and the extraordinary expansion that is required to meet increased demand?

It is established that haemopoiesis is sustained throughout life by pluripotent stem cells with capacities for both self-renewal and differentiation. Recent evidence (Lemischka 1986) supports Kay's hypothesis (1965) that a relatively small number of clones are actively proliferating and differentiating, and that the continuity of supply is maintained during life by clonal succession. Stem cells, by a poorly understood stochastic mechanism, give rise to lineage-restricted progenitor cells that in turn proliferate and develop to produce the mature cells of the different blood cell lineages.

The proliferation, differentiation and survival of immature haemopoietic progenitor cells is sustained by a family of glycoproteins, the haemopoietic growth factors (HGFs) (Table 1.1). In addition to their effect on immature cells, these factors also influence

Table 1.1 HGFs. *Key:* n, polymorphonuclear neutrophils; m, monocytes; eo, eosinophils; CHO, carbohydrate.

Factor	Chromosome	RNA (kb)	Protein (kDa)			Biological Activities	
			Core	CHO linkage	Glyco-sylated	Progenitors	Mature cells
IL-3	5q 23–31	1.0	14–15	N(2), O	20–26	All CFC	eo
GM-CSF	5q 23–31	1.0	14–15	N(2), O	14–35	All CFC	n, m, eo
G-CSF	17q 11.2–21	1.6	18–19	O	19–20	CFU-G	n
M-CSF	5q 33.1	4.0	26	N	35–45 ($\times$2)	CFU-M	m
		1.6	16	N	20–25 ($\times$2)		
ep	7q 11–22	1.6	18	N(3), O	34–39	BFU-E CFU-E	—

the survival and function of mature cells. The HGFs are also known collectively as the colony-stimulating factors (CSFs), a term derived from the in vitro observation that they stimulate progenitor cells to form colonies of recognizable maturing cells; prefixes are used to denote the cell type in the mature colonies, e.g. G-CSF, granulocyte-CSF (Metcalf 1984). The term CSF is more restrictive, however, because it does not cover several factors that lack colony-stimulating activity on their own but have synergistic properties when added to cultures in combination with other factors (see p. 10).

1

During the past 5 years, the genes for five murine and human CSFs have been cloned, and this in turn led to the production and purification of the respective recombinant proteins. This breakthrough in molecular haematology has allowed intensive investigations of the actions of purified CSFs, their cellular origins, and their regulatory mechanisms, while the availability of large quantities of highly purified CSFs such as granulocyte-macrophage CSF (GM-CSF), G-CSF and erythropoietin (ep), has led to preclinical and clinical evaluation of their effectiveness in vivo.

While the molecular biology, structure, cellular sources, regulation of production and therapeutic uses of CSFs form the focus of this review, it should be borne in mind that normal adult haemopoiesis occurs only in the microenvironment of the bone marrow (Wolf 1979). The role of this microenvironment is not well understood. Sustained in vitro haemopoiesis requires an adherent stromal cell layer (Dexter et al 1977) that consists of fibroblastoid cells, adipocytes, 'blanket cells', macrophages and possibly endothelial cells as well (Dexter et al 1984). These cells secrete components of a complex extracellular matrix that include fibronectin, laminin, collagen, and glycosaminoglycans (Zuckerman & Wicha 1983, Gallagher et al 1983). The precise roles of the constituents of this microenvironment are not known. The cellular components have been shown to synthesize CSFs (Heard et al 1982, Shadduck et al 1983b) and factors that affect stem cell cycling (Toksoz et al 1980). Furthermore, synthesis of proteins such as fibronectin and haemonectin may provide essential substrates to which developing erythroid and myeloid progenitors adhere during maturation (Tsai et al 1986b, 1987, Campbell et al 1987a), while glycosaminoglycans may bind secreted GM-CSF (Gordon et al 1987). Both the cells that secrete CSFs and many components of the extracellular matrix are common to almost every organ. Thus, a major question concerns the nature of the specificity of the bone marrow microenvironment for haemopoietic stem and progenitor cells. The recent report of a myeloid lineage-specific adhesion protein that can be extracted only from bone marrow extracellular matrix is therefore of interest. The protein, called haemonectin, is not present in spleen or kidney (Campbell et al 1987a). A fuller understanding of the functional properties of the cells of the haemopoietic microenvironment will be necessary before the recently acquired knowledge concerning the HGFs can be integrated into a more complete picture of the process of blood cell production and its regulation.

TYPES OF HAEMOPOIETIC GROWTH FACTORS

The colony stimulating factors

The development of semisolid colony-forming assays for progenitor cells of all the haemopoietic lineages provided the means to distinguish several colony stimulating activities that were present both in media conditioned by different murine and human cell types and in human urine. Separative protein chemistry applied to large volumes of starting material led to the purification of murine macrophage CSF (M-CSF), GM-CSF, G-CSF and interleukin 3 (IL-3) or multi-CSF (for a review see Metcalf 1984). Human urine yielded M-CSF (Stanley et al 1975) and erythropoietin (ep) (Miyake et al 1977) while a human bladder carcinoma cell line (HBT 5637) was used to purify human G-CSF (Welte et al 1985).

In general, IL-3 and GM-CSF stimulate the survival, proliferation, and differentiation of a broad range of progenitors, including cells with stem cell properties. In contrast, G-CSF, M-CSF, and ep are lineage-restricted and stimulate the proliferation and differentiation of more mature granulocyte, monocyte and erythroid progenitor cells, respectively. Both sets of factors influence mature cell function, and the pattern of responsive cells for each CSF broadly coincides with the lineages of the less mature cells affected by each factor.

Other HGFs

Interleukin 1 alpha (IL-1α) has recently been shown to be identical to a factor called haemopoietin 1 that Jubinsky & Stanley (1985, Stanley et al 1986) purified from HBT 5637 cell line CM (Mochizuki et al 1987). This protein, termed synergistic factor by Bradley & Hodgson (1979), does not stimulate colony formation alone; it acts synergistically with M-CSF to induce the formation of large macrophage colonies from primitive colony forming cells with high proliferative potential that are enriched in bone marrow obtained from 5-fluoruroacil treated mice. The data from these investigators suggest that primitive cells responsive to IL-1 and M-CSF proliferate and differentiate into cells responsive to IL-3 and M-CSF, and subsequently to cells responsive to M-CSF alone (Bartelmez & Stanley 1985, McNiece et al 1986). The synergistic effects of IL-1 are evident when bone marrow cells are plated at low density (500 cells per 35 mm plate), suggesting that its action is direct. IL-1 α and β, however, are now known to be potent inducers of GM-CSF, G-CSF, and IL-6 production by mesenchymal cells (see below), and it is possible that the IL-1 effects are mediated indirectly by induction of known or as yet unidentified HGFs.

Several other interleukins may act synergistically with the CSFs on haemopoietic progenitors. Interleukin 4 (B cell stimulatory factor 1) is a murine B lymphocyte proliferation and activation factor that is also a growth factor for mast cells and T lymphocytes (Noma et al 1986). Recent evidence suggests that it may act as a co-stimulant with ep, G-CSF and possibly M-CSF to increase erythroid, granulocyte and macrophage colony numbers; paradoxically, it may inhibit IL-3 effects on less mature progenitors (Rennick et al 1987). Although the human homologue has been cloned (Yokota et al 1986), its actions on haemopoietic progenitors have not been reported.

Murine interleukin 5 (eosinophil differentiation factor or B cell growth factor II) induces eosinophil differentiation and acts as a proliferative and differentiating stimulus for B cells. The human gene was recently cloned, and the recombinant protein stimulates the development of eosinophil colonies from human bone marrow (Campbell et al 1987b).

Interleukin 6 (interferon β_2, B cell differentiation factor) induces B cells to mature into antibody secreting cells. The human gene has been cloned (Hirano et al 1986) and the expressed protein has intriguing properties. Like IL-3, it acts as a permissive factor for blast cell colony proliferation in cultures of murine marrow from 5-fluorouracil treated mice. However, in combination with IL-3, it reduces the time period during which the blast cells begin to divide to form colonies, suggesting that it influences stem cell cycling (Ikebuchi et al 1987).

MOLECULAR BIOLOGY, STRUCTURE AND RECEPTOR BINDING

Several recent reviews have detailed the steps in the isolation of the human CSF genes (Clark & Kamen 1987, Metcalf 1986, Sieff et al 1987a). Some general comments

follow together with a brief summary. Two approaches were taken to identify comple-
mentary DNAs (cDNAs) for these genes. The first was the classic route by which
the G-CSF, M-CSF and ep proteins were purified, part of their amino acid sequence
determined, and oligonucleotide probes constructed to screen appropriate cDNA
libraries (Welte et al 1985, Kawasaki et al 1985, Jacobs et al 1985). The CSFs are
present in minute concentrations in most starting materials, however, and for several
CSFs purification has been very difficult. The second approach obviated the obstacle
of CSF purification: GM-CSF and IL-3 cDNA libraries were constructed from suitable
cell lines; the cDNAs were then introduced into vectors and directly expressed in
mammalian cell lines. Because of the potency of these CSFs, the gene products of
cDNA pools could then be screened in sensitive bioassays.

G-CSF

Two G-CSF cDNA clones were isolated from different tumour cell lines. The first
clone encodes a 207 amino acid protein, of which 177 amino acids comprise mature
G-CSF, while 30 hydrophobic amino acids determine the probable leader sequence
(Nagata et al 1986b). The second clone is identical apart from a deletion of three
amino acids at position 36–38, which results in a 174 amino acid protein (Souza
et al 1986). Sequence analysis of a genomic clone that expresses both proteins indicates
that alternative use of two donor splice sites nine nucleotides apart at the 5′ end
of intron 2 is responsible for the production of two mRNAs (Nagata et al 1986a).
The predicted molecular masses of the two proteins are 19 and 18.6 kilodaltons (kDa),
respectively, while purified native G-CSF has a molecular mass of 19.6 kDA. This
difference is due to O-glycosylation; no N-glycosylation sites exist. Differences in
bioactivity of the two proteins may exist, but it is not yet known whether two analogous
forms of native G-CSF are produced.

M-CSF

Because of two alternative splice sites and extensive post-translational modification,
the biosynthesis of M-CSF is much more complex (Fig. 1.1). The first reported cDNA,
isolated from a library made from a phorbol myristate acetate stimulated pancreatic
tumour cell line, encodes a 1.6 kb mRNA (Kawasaki et al 1985). This is translated
into a 26 kDa precursor that undergoes amino-terminus (32 residue leader sequence)
and carboxyl-terminus processing to yield a mature subunit of approximately 145
amino acids (16 kDa). Recently, analysis of a cDNA that represents the more common
4 kb mRNA shows that this form of message results from alternative splicing during
transcription; this leads to an in frame insertion of 894 nucleotides (Wong et al 1987).
The transcript also has a larger 3′ non-coding region that, unlike the untranslated
region of the shorter mRNA, contains an AU rich region that is associated with
RNA instability (Shaw & Kamen 1986). This mRNA produces a primary translation
product of 61 kDa that contains an extra 298 residues. Identical amino-terminal processing (32 amino acids) and more extensive carboxyl-terminus processing (294 residues) yields a mature protein of 223 amino acids (26 kDa). Both the 16 kDa and
26 kDa forms of M-CSF are N-glycosylated to yield monomers of 20–25 kDa and
35–45 kDa respectively. M-CSF is the only CSF that exists as a dimer, and the
monomers thus yield two forms of CSF, 40–50 kDa and 70–90 kDa glycoproteins,
respectively. Native M-CSFs of both sizes have been purified (Stanley & Heard 1977,

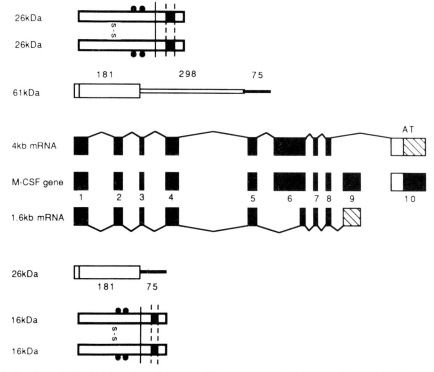

Fig. 1.1 Biosynthesis of M-CSF. Two different mRNAs are transcribed from the 10 exon M-CSF gene, which spans some 20 kb. The 5' portion of both the 4 kb and 1.6 kb mRNAs are identical and are derived from the first 5 exons; they encode the first 181 amino acids of both primary translation products. The 4 kb message results from the use of a splice site at the 5' end of exon 6 which results in an 894 base pair insertion that is translated into 298 amino acids of the primary translation product. The 1.6 kb mRNA uses an alternative splice site toward the 3' end of exon 6 and the primary translation product therefore does not contain this insertion. The 3' coding regions of both mRNAs are also identical, encoded from the 3' end of exon 6 to exon 8. The 3' untranslated portions are different: the 4 kb message version is encoded by exon 10 (crosshatched, 5' end not determined (open box)) and contains an adenine and thymidine stretch that is absent from the exon 9 encoded untranslated region of the shorter mRNA.

The carboxy-termini of both proteins contains a hydrophobic region that indicates transmembrane insertion (solid boxes bounded by dashed lines). Both the 5' (32 amino acid leader sequence) and 3' ends of the primary translation products are processed (vertical solid lines) resulting in core proteins of 26 kDa and 16 kDa. N-linked glycosylation and dimerization lead to the final molecular weights of 70–90 kDa and 40–50 kDa. (Wong et al 1987, Ladner et al 1987, Rettenmier et al 1987)

Stanley et al 1975, Motoyoshi et al 1982). However, it is not yet clear whether the smaller protein, purified from human urine, results from biosynthesis of the 1.6 kb mRNA or from proteolysis of the large molecule. The common 75 amino acid carboxyl-termini contain a 23 amino acid hydrophobic region that suggests transmembrane insertion. This is consistent with studies that suggest that membrane and secretory forms of M-CSF may exist (Cifone & Defendi 1974, Stanley et al 1976, Rettenmier et al 1987).

Erythropoietin
The ep molecule was first purified to apparent homogeneity from the urine of patients with aplastic anemia (Miyake et al 1977). Analysis of cDNA clones isolated from

a fetal liver cDNA library show that a reading frame of 579 nucleotides encodes a 27 amino acid hydrophobic leader sequence followed by the 166 amino acid mature protein (Jacobs et al 1985). The N-terminus of the mature protein was located by comparison with the sequence of purified human urinary ep originally determined by Goldwasser and his colleagues (Lai et al 1986). The molecular weight of natural ep is 34–39 kDa and the deduced MW of the recombinant polypeptide backbone is 18.4 kDa; the difference in MW is due to glycosylation; there are three sites of N-linked glycosylation at amino acids 24, 38, and 83, and the molecule is also O-glycosylated. There are four cysteine residues, and at least two must be involved in disulphide bonds since biological activity is lost on reduction.

GM-CSF

Clones containing cDNAs for GM-CSF were isolated by constructing a cDNA library from the Mo T-lymphoblast cell line in an expression vector, and directly screening transfected monkey COS cells for transient expression of GM-CSF (Wong et al 1985). The DNA sequence contains a single open reading frame of 432 nucleotides encoding a 144 amino acid precursor protein. In an analogous fashion to other secreted proteins, 17 amino acids are cleaved from the amino-terminal sequence to yield a mature protein of 127 amino acids. Purification of both natural and recombinant human GM-CSF to homogeneity yields identical proteins which are heterogeneous when analysed by sodium dodecyl sulfate-polyacrylamide gel electrophoresis (SDS-PAGE), migrating with an apparent molecular mass of 14–35 kDa (Wong et al 1985). This is due to variable glycosylation; the sequence contains two potential N-linkage (asparagine) glycosylation sites, and 0, 1 or 2 asparagines may be occupied by oligosaccharides (Donahue 1986b). The degree of occupancy appears to affect function. The most heavily glycosylated form of the molecule is not as active in vitro but is cleared much more slowly in vivo from the circulation than the non-glycosylated form. This may have important implications in the choice of bacteria (non-glycosylated) or mammalian/yeast cells (glycosylated) as expression systems for producing recombinant CSF for therapy.

IL-3

The cDNA clone for primate IL-3 was recently isolated by expression screening of a library made from a gibbon T-lymphoblast cell line (Yang et al 1986a). This cDNA clone was used to obtain the human gene, and analysis of the gibbon and human recombinant proteins show that they differ in only 11 positions. The human gene shows homology with murine IL-3: the genes have similar structures (5 exons) and show nucleotide homology that is greater in the 5′ and 3′ non-coding regions (59%) than in the coding regions (49%); the proteins are 29% homologous. The 456 nucleotide human IL-3 open reading frame encodes a 152 amino acid precursor that is N-terminally modified to yield a 133 amino acid mature protein that has one internal disulphide bridge.

Although human IL-3 and GM-CSF are quite distinct in that they show no gene structural or sequence homologies, there are a number of similarities. Like GM-CSF, IL-3 has two potential N-linked glycosylation sites, and polyacrylamide gel analysis of the recombinant protein expressed in mammalian cells shows a rather similar broad range of molecular weights (14–28 kDa). More intriguing are the the in situ hybridization and somatic cell hybrid analyses that map the IL-3 and GM-CSF genes close together on the long arm of chromosome 5 (5q 23–32) (Huebner et al 1985, LeBeau et al 1987a,b) (Fig. 1.2). The 5' non-coding regions contain similar eukaryotic promoter

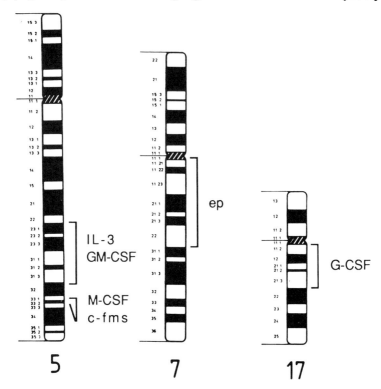

Fig. 1.2 Chromosomal location of the human CSF genes and the receptor for M-CSF (c-fms) as determined by somatic cell hybrid analysis and in situ hybridisation (see text for references).

elements (Miyatake et al 1985, Yang et al, 1986a), and the 3' non-coding regions both contain a sequence rich in adenine-thymidine base pairs that has been implicated as an important determinant of RNA instability; this sequence may be related to expression of inducible genes (Shaw & Kamen 1986). Lastly, the genes appear to be coordinately regulated in T lymphocytes. Despite these similarities, it is interesting to note that only T lymphocytes produce both CSFs; other mesenchymal cells that produce GM-CSF do not produce IL-3 (see below).

Gene localization

The gene for M-CSF and its receptor c-fms have been mapped to 5q 33.1 (Fig. 1.2) (LeBeau 1987b, Pettenati et al 1987); both endothelial cell growth factor and the receptor for platelet derived growth factor (PDGF) have also been mapped to this region. G-CSF and ep have been mapped to chromosomes 17 and 7, respectively (Simmers et al 1987, Watkins et al 1986, Law et al 1986). A proportion of patients with either refractory anaemia or acute myeloblastic leukaemia have an interstitial deletion of the long arm of chromosome 5 (5q$^-$): these cases appear always to show a critical deletion of bands 5q 21–32. IL-3 and GM-CSF are deleted in every case, while M-CSF and c-fms are usually deleted as well. How this deletion bears on the pathogenesis of the myeloproliferative disorder in these patients is unknown. Abnormal function of one of the HGFs or growth factor receptors is one possibility; alternatively, loss of one allele of an as yet unidentified suppressor gene is also possible.

Membrane receptors

Membrane receptors for all five murine HGFs have been characterized using iodinated purified natural or recombinant preparations (Palaszynski & Ihle 1984, Park et al 1986a, 1986c, Walker & Burgess 1985, Nicola & Metcalf 1984, 1985, Guilbert & Stanley 1980, Morgan & Stanley 1984, Byrne et al 1981, Shadduck et al 1983a, Sawyer et al 1987). Consistent with the lack of structural homology among the growth factors is the existence of distinct receptors for each factor, which range in size from 50–160 kDa. Distribution of receptors is restricted to undifferentiated and maturing cells of the appropriate target cell lineages. Since granulocytes and macrophages respond to more than one factor, overlap in receptor expression occurs. The number of IL-3, GM-CSF, G-CSF and ep receptors per cell is strikingly low (~1000 sites per cell), while those for M-CSF are about one log higher. In all cases affinity of receptor for ligand is high (10^{12}–10^9 M^{-1} range). Stimulation of target cells can occur at concentrations of factor orders of magnitude lower than the equilibrium constant at which 50% of receptors are occupied, and therefore it is apparent that low receptor occupancy is sufficient to produce biological effects. The interaction of M-CSF with its receptor on bone marrow macrophages has been studied and shows that at 37°C, these cells internalize labelled CSF (Guilbert & Stanley 1986). Recent evidence shows that the major mechanism of clearance of M-CSF in mice occurs through binding and internalization of circulating M-CSF by liver and splenic macrophages (Bartocci et al 1987). Although the four murine CSFs do not cross compete for binding at 0°C, at 21° or 37°C IL-3 inhibits binding of the other three CSFs, and GM-CSF inhibits binding of G-CSF and M-CSF to bone marrow cells (Walker et al 1985). Metcalf and colleagues have suggested that this hierarchical down modulation results in activation of the modulated receptor without binding ligand, and the model provides an intriguing explanation for the correlation between the pattern of down regulation and the biological activity of the different murine CSFs.

Little published information exists concerning human growth factor receptors (Gasson et al 1986, Park et al 1986b). Low numbers of GM-CSF receptors are expressed by mature polymorphonuclear neutrophils and by the myeloid leukemic cell lines KG1 and HL60. Reported affinity constants range from 1.5×10^{12} to 10^9 M^{-1} and only one class of binding sites has been reported, in contrast to one of the murine GM-CSF binding studies in which both high and low affinity classes of receptors were reported (Walker & Burgess 1985).

Recent evidence (Sherr et al 1985) suggests strongly that the M-CSF receptor and the proto-oncogene product c-fms are closely related and probably identical proteins: both proteins are of similar size (165 000 daltons) and exhibit tyrosine kinase activity; an antibody to c-fms precipitates a protein that is phosphorylated on tyrosine in the presence of purified M-CSF, and ^{125}I M-CSF can be recovered from immunoprecipitates of receptor-membrane extracts. These data are of considerable interest and provide new evidence linking oncogenes and growth factors: v erb B encodes a protein that is a truncated form of the epidermal growth factor receptor (Downward et al

1984), and c-sis codes for a polypeptide chain of platelet derived growth factor (Waterfield et al 1983). v-fms is the oncogene of the McDonough strain of feline sarcoma virus, and expression at the cell surface is required for transformation (Roussel et al 1984). The virus was first isolated from a feline fibrosarcoma (McDonough et al 1971), and fibroblast cell lines are transformed with the highest efficiency (Sherr et al 1985); it has not been implicated in naturally occurring haemopoietic neoplasms in vivo. However, bone marrow infected with helper-free virus containing v-fms can be engrafted into irradiated mice. Spleen cells that contain the integrated provirus can be transplanted into irradiated secondary recipients, and some of these animals develop erythroleukaemias or B cell lymphomas (Heard et al 1987). Since fibroblasts secrete M-CSF (Tushinski et al 1982), and the v-fms product appears to contain an almost complete extracellular domain, it is possible that transformation of fibroblasts depends on ligand binding and transduction of a signal through a functional receptor in a cell that does not normally require M-CSF for growth. However, simian virus 40 immortalized macrophages that are M-CSF dependent do not secrete or express M-CSF. They can be rendered M-CSF independent after introduction of the v-fms gene (Wheeler et al 1986). The carboxyl-terminal end of v-fms differs from c-fms in that 40 amino acids of c-fms are replaced by 11 unrelated residues in the v-fms product (Coussens et al 1986). This change results in constitutive autophosphorylation of the v-fms, in contrast to the c-fms product, in which autophosphorylation is enhanced by M-CSF. This suggests that the factor independence induced by v-fms expression in macrophages is due to unregulated kinase activity that provides growth stimulation in the absence of ligand.

Cellular sources and regulation of production of the CSFs

While all murine tissues contain extractable haematopoietic growth factors, it is likely that synthesis of the four major CSFs is restricted to cells common to all organs: fibroblasts, endothelial cells, lymphocytes and macrophages (Metcalf 1984 for a full review). Similarly, many human organs are capable of synthesizing CSFs, and bioactivity assays on medium conditioned by purified cell populations have likewise documented CSF production by T lymphocytes (Cline & Golde 1974, Nathan et al 1978, Mangan et al 1982), monocytes (Chervenick & LoBuglio 1972, Golde & Cline 1972, Zuckerman 1981, Reid et al 1981), endothelial cells (Knudson & Mortenson 1975, Quesenberry & Gimbrone 1980, Ascencao et al 1984), and fibroblasts (Tsai et al 1986a, Zucali et al 1986). Two points are worth noting: one, the bioactivity experiments do not clearly distinguish the factors from each other because of overlapping spectra of activity, and two, these cell types are more easily purified than many tissue constituents; an answer to the question of whether other cells synthesize growth factors therefore will depend on antibody studies or on the use of in situ RNA hybridization techniques with radioactive probes to the different factors. RNA extracted from purified cell populations can be assayed by the Northern technique. Phytohaemagglutinin-stimulated blood mononuclear cells (comprising monocytes and lymphocytes) contain GM-CSF mRNA. Furthermore, phorbol-ester stimulated T cell clones and T cell/natural killer cell fractions isolated from mononuclear cell preparations are the only source of RNA that are positive with IL-3 cDNA or RNA probes (Niemeyer et al 1987). Recently, we and others have probed endothelial, fibroblast and monocyte mRNA with labelled cDNAs to the CSFs. Primary umbilical vein endothelial cells

(Broudy et al 1986a, Munker et al 1986, Sieff et al 1987b) and lung, skin, and fetal liver fibroblasts (Munker et al 1986, Yang et al 1986b) accumulate detectable GM-CSF mRNA after induction with interleukin 1 (IL-1) and/or tumour necrosis factor (TNF). Monocyte synthesis of G-CSF appears to depend on induction with endotoxin. While in our hands, uninduced cells of all three types appear to contain M-CSF mRNA, other investigators report that phorbol myristate acetate, γ-interferon or GM-CSF induce M-CSF accumulation in monocytes (Horiguchi 1986, 1987, Rambaldi et al 1987, Ralph et al 1986), while IL-1 and TNF have the same effect in endothelial cells (Seelentag et al 1987). Since monocytes produce IL-1 in response to endotoxin (Dinarello 1984), this cell type may perform a central role in inducing increased haemopoiesis during stress, both by producing growth factors, and perhaps more importantly by producing IL-1 and TNF. Together with antigen, IL-1 may induce circulating T lymphocytes to produce both GM-CSF and IL-3. Removal of T lymphocytes from bone marrow before allogeneic bone marrow transplantation in order to prevent graft versus host disease therefore could be depleting the marrow of a cell critical for proliferation of the transplanted pluripotent stem cells. Monocyte-derived IL-1 and/or TNF may also induce 'fixed' bone marrow stromal cell populations to produce GM-CSF and G-CSF as well (Broudy et al 1986b). This is consistent with published evidence demonstrating the ability of 'monokines' present in monocyte conditioned medium to induce endothelial (Bagby et al 1983a, Zuckerman et al 1985), fibroblast (Bagby et al 1983b, Zucali et al 1986) and T lymphocyte (Bagby et al 1981) production of burst-promoting and colony-stimulating activities.

Biological activities
Murine IL-3 stimulates a broad spectrum of cells including pluripotent stem cells, granulocyte and/or macrophage colony-forming cells or units (CFU-GM, CFU-G, CFU-M), erythroid burst-forming units (BFU-E), eosinophil CFU (CFU-Eo), megakaryocyte CFU (CFU-Meg) and mast cells. As its name implies, GM-CSF was initially shown to be more restricted as a stimulus of the proliferation and development of CFU-GM. However, murine studies with purified or recombinant factor have shown that it also stimulates the initial proliferation of other progenitors such as BFU-E as well (Metcalf 1984). The other murine factors, G-CSF, M-CSF and ep are more restricted and predominantly stimulate granulocyte, monocyte and mature erythroid colony forming units (CFU-G, CFU-M, and CFU-E), respectively (Metcalf & Nicola 1983, Metcalf & Stanley 1971, Adamson et al 1978).

With the possible exception of GM-CSF, the activities of the human CSFs are similar to those of the corresponding murine factors. However, because of the lack of an assay for human pluripotent stem cells that is analogous to the murine CFU-S spleen colony assay, it is difficult to compare results in the two species. Both IL-3 and GM-CSF affect a similar broad spectrum of human progenitor cells. This includes progenitors that mature into colonies containing granulocytes, erythrocytes, macrophages, and megakaryocytes (CFU-GEMM) and BFU-E, provided ep is added to the cultures to induce terminal differentiation of erythroid cells (Sieff et al 1985, 1986, 1987a, Donahue et al 1985, Emerson et al 1985, Tomonaga et al 1986, Strife et al 1987, Metcalf et al 1986b). IL-3 is a more potent stimulus of BFU-E than is GM-CSF (Sieff et al 1987a). In full serum cultures, IL-3 and GM-CSF alone stimulate the formation of colonies derived from CFU-GM, CFU-G, CFU-M, CFU-Eo and

CFU-Meg. Preliminary data from serum free cultures suggest that in the presence of IL-3 or GM-CSF alone, myeloid colony-formation is much reduced, and that optimal CFU-G or CFU-M proliferation requires the addition of G-CSF or M-CSF, respectively, to the cultures (Sonoda et al 1987, Sieff, in preparation). Even in serum replete conditions, IL-3 acts additively or synergistically with G-CSF to induce more granulocyte colony formation than is observed with either factor alone (Sieff 1987a). The serum free studies may have important implications for the use of combinations of CSFs in vivo, and it is apparent that the use of such culture conditions may provide further insight into the in vitro activities of the different factors.

In addition to their effects on progenitor differentiation, the CSFs also induce a variety of functional changes in mature cells. GM-CSF inhibits polymorphonuclear neutrophil migration under agarose (Gasson et al 1984), is a potent activator of neutrophils, eosinophils, and macrophages (Weisbert et al 1985, Grabstein et al 1986), induces antibody dependent cytotoxicity (ADCC) for human target cells (Vadas et al 1983a,b), and increases neutrophil phagocytic activity (Metcalf et al 1986a). Some of these functional changes may be related to GM-CSF induced increase in the cell surface expression of a family of antigens that function as cell adhesion molecules (Arnaout et al 1986). The increase in antigen expression is rapid and is associated with increased aggregation of neutrophils; both are maximal at the migration inhibitory concentration of 500 pM, and granulocyte-granulocyte adhesion can be inhibited by an antigen-specific monoclonal antibody. Indirect support for the association of increased cell surface expression of adhesion molecules with functional activation of mature cells comes from the observation that IL-3 does not alter neutrophil antigen expression (Arnaout & Sieff, unpublished) and also does not affect neutrophil ADCC or superoxide production; in contrast, it acts as a potent stimulus of eosinophil ADCC, superoxide production and phagocytosis (Lopez et al 1987).

G-CSF acts as a potent stimulus of neutrophil superoxide production, ADCC, and phagocytosis (Lopez et al 1983), while M-CSF activates mature macrophages (Hamilton et al 1980) and enhances macrophage cytotoxicity (P. Mufson, personal communication).

It is apparent then that with the exception of IL-3, the actions of the CSFs on mature cells parallels their spectrum of activity on immature progenitors. Murine IL-3, in contrast to human IL-3, does activate neutrophil function. Murine neutrophils express the IL-3 receptor (Nicola & Metcalf 1986) and it is possible that human neutrophils have lost the receptor for IL-3.

In vivo effects

Correction or amelioration of marrow failure syndromes by administration of haematopoietic growth factors has been and continues to be the major practical goal of research in haematopoiesis. The goal could not be achieved, however, until recombinant DNA technology provided sufficient amounts of the hormones to permit interpretable investigations.

The discovery, cloning and expression of the gene for murine multi-CSF or IL-3 presented the first opportunity to evaluate haemopoietic growth factors in an unambiguous fashion (Fung et al 1984, Yokota et al 1984). Sublethally irradiated mice were infused for 7 days with recombinant IL-3 or with control protein (Kindler et al 1986). The spleens of the IL-3 treated marrow recipients were much larger than those of the controls, were more cellular and contained more progenitors. The increase in progenitor cells affected erythroid and myeloid lineages. In contrast, bone marrow cellularity was unaffected and progenitor content was reduced. Metcalf et al (1986b) injected mice with purified bacterially synthesized IL-3 by the intraperitoneal route and obtained similar results. In addition, 10 fold increases in blood eosinophil and 2 to 3 fold increases in neutrophil and monocyte levels were observed. The intraperitoneal injections also resulted in 6 to 15 fold increase in peritoneal phagocytes with an increase in macrophage phagocytic activity.

These experiments clearly demonstrate that murine IL-3 influences the replication and growth potential of primitive haemopoietic progenitors, and strongly suggest that whatever effect such hormones have on blood counts are related to their influences on progenitor function rather than to their effects on peripheral blood cell kinetics. They also suggest that the function of mature cells can be altered in vivo, an effect that would be expected to decrease rather than increase numbers of circulating phagocytes.

The first indications that the human haemopoietic growth factor, GM-CSF, could broadly stimulate haemopoiesis in vivo resulted from the studies of Donahue et al (1986a). These workers infused cynomolgous macaques with COS cell produced GM-CSF and markedly stimulated haemopoiesis in the recipients. In preliminary studies, Donahue and co-workers demonstrated that human recombinant GM-CSF induced colony formation by a broad array of simian progenitor cells. They showed that the human hormone stimulated simian BFU-E, CFU-GM, and CFU-GEMM to form progenitor derived colonies at nanomolar concentrations. Recombinant GM-CSF, metabolically labelled with ^{35}S methionine, was purified, injected into simian recipients, and the rate of disappearance of radioactivity from the blood determined. The disappearance curve was complex, suggesting a multi-compartment turnover model, but the overall initial half-time of 15–20 minutes clearly demonstrated that infusion of the hormone at a concentration sufficient to maintain a functional blood level could be achieved. The effects of such infusions into normal *Macaca fasicularis* were striking. Large increments in all classes of leucocytes including eosinophils and lymphocytes as well as reticulocytes, were observed during the hormone infusion. When the hormone treatment was terminated, the blood counts rapidly fell toward normal. A particularly striking reticulocytosis was observed in an animal with an acquired type D retroviral infection that was associated with secondary pancytopenia and an elevated erythropoietin level. This 'preclinical' trial in a severely ill monkey encouraged the conclusion that GM-CSF might play an important therapeutic role in various cytopenias such as those observed in viral infections, including AIDS, or in autologous or allogeneic marrow transplantation.

To investigate the potential role of human recombinant GM-CSF in marrow transplantation, Nienhuis and co-workers (1987) infused autologous marrow into rhesus monkeys (*Macaca mulatta*) 2 hours after the animals had received 1200 rads of total body irradiation at 12 rads per minute. In this model, a granulocyte nadir is achieved in about 5 days, and recovery of granulocytes to a total count of $1.0 \times 10^9/l$ does not occur until day 17 or later. In the experiments designed by Nienhuis et al, human recombinant GM-CSF was administered at a daily dose of 50 units/min/kg continuously from 10–19 days prior to radiation and/or from 9–17 days beginning 2 or 3 days after irradiation. Both dosage schedules produced the same final results, though the blood counts of the animals that received the hormone prior to radiation were much higher at the onset of radiation than those who received the hormone only after radiation. In five separate studies, granulocytes recovered to a level greater than $1 \times 10^9/l$ in 9 days rather than the minimum of 17 days observed in 2 untreated controls. In four of the five experiments, platelets recovered more rapidly as well.

Human G-CSF has also undergone simian preclinical trials. Welte et al (1987) treated cynomolgous monkeys with two daily subcutaneous injections of purified G-CSF for 14–28 days. A dose-related increase in polymorphonuclear neutrophils was observed, the plateau being reached after 1 week of treatment. At the intermediate dose of $10\,\mu g/kg/day$, total white blood cell counts of 40–$50 \times 10^9/l$ were observed. Neutrophil function was also enhanced. Encouraging results were also achieved in two cyclophosphamide treated animals that received G-CSF either from 6 days before until 21 days after the cyclophosphamide treatment, or for 14 days from day three after cyclophosphamide. In both monkeys, the neutrophil count increased dramatically by day 6–7 after cyclophosphamide, reaching levels of $50 \times 10^9/l$ by the tenth day. The control animal remained pancytopenic for 3–4 weeks after treatment.

A phase I/II GM-CSF trial in 16 patients with acquired immunodeficiency syndrome (AIDS) and leukopenia has now been completed (Groopman et al 1987). 48 hours after a test bolus dose, patients received a 14-day continuous intravenous infusion of GM-CSF at doses that ranged from 1.3×10^3 to 2×10^4 U/kg/day (0.5–$8\,\mu g/kg$ day). Dose-dependent increases in circulating neutrophils, monocytes and eosinophils were observed. The peak leucocyte count ranged from $4.5 \times 10^9/l$ at the lowest, to $48 \times 10^9/l$ at the highest dose. No serious toxic effects occurred. Low grade fever, myalgia, and flushing were noted in some patients and mild phlebitis was associated with administration of the drug through a peripheral vein. No phlebitis or clinical thrombosis occurred when the drug was administered by central venous catheter.

Vadhan-Raj et al (1987) have carried out a phase I trial of GM-CSF in 8 patients with myelodysplasia. GM-CSF was given by continuous intravenous infusion for 14 days and then again after a 2-week rest period. Doses of 30–$500\,\mu g$ per square metre body-surface area were used. Peripheral blood leucocytes rose 5–70-fold, with granulocytes 5–373-fold in all 8 patients. Monocytes eosinophils and lymphocytes increased in all patients, 3 had a rise in platelet count (2–10-fold) and 2 of 3 patients no longer needed red cell and platelet transfusions. Marrow cellularity increased, the proportion of blast cells decreased in the marrows of patients with excess blasts and no patient developed overt leukaemia during the period of follow-up (up to 32 weeks). Bone pain was the main side-effect, and it was associated with high white cell counts. Clearly the use of GM-CSF in this condition needs very careful long-term studies since GM-CSF may stimulate proliferation of leukaemic myeloblasts.

Using a yeast-derived recombinant human GM-CSF, Devereux et al (1987) have found that there is a transient leucopenia due to sequestration of white cells in the lungs. This occurred at the start of each infusion in three patients with advanced malignant disease (but without pulmonary infection). The fall in neutrophil and monocyte counts recovered in 60–120 minutes.

Brand et al (1988) have reported on the effect of recombinant GM-CSF on haemopoietic reconstitution following high dose chemotherapy and autologous bone marrow transplantation. They treated 19 patients with either metastatic breast cancer or melanoma with an ablative course of chemotherapy followed 3 days later by autologous marrow cells. GM-CSF was then given by continuous intravenous infusion for 14 days beginning 3 hours after bone marrow infusion. The doses ranged from 2–32 µg/kg/day. Recovery of blood counts was compared to 29 age, diagnosis and treatment-matched historical controls. White blood cell recovery was accelerated in the GM-CSF treated group. No effects on platelet or reticulocyte recovery were demonstrated. The white count recovery was dose related and little toxicity was observed between 2 and 16 µg/kg/day. Oedema, weight gain or myalgias occurred in patients given 32 µg/kg.

Preliminary information from a phase I/II study of recombinant G-CSF in cancer patients showed a dose related increase in neutrophils when the factor was given before the first course of chemotherapy (Gabrilove et al 1987). When the G-CSF was evaluated after the first course of chemotherapy, a 3-fold higher white blood cell count was observed on day 14 in patients who received G-CSF compared with patients not receiving the factor; furthermore, the neutrophil count did not fall below $1 \times 10^9/l$ in the G-CSF treated group, and more of them were able to receive the next course of chemotherapy on schedule.

Morstyn et al (1988) have administered G-CSF to patients with advanced cancer receiving melphalan. 12 patients were treated in groups of 3, each of which received either 0.3, 1, 3 or 10 µg/kg of G-CSF intravenously on days 1–5 and days 10–18 of a protocol in which a cytopenic dose of melphalan was given on day 9. Serum levels of G-CSF fell in a biphasic manner with a 'half life' of 5–10 and 100 minutes. No comparison was offered between treated and untreated patients, but the neutropenia after melphalan was partially abolished at doses as low as 1 and 3 µg/kg and the subcutaneous route of administration produced higher neutrophil levels than did the intravenous route.

Human trials of recombinant erythropoietin have clearly documented that it is effective in reducing or eliminating the red cell transfusion requirement of patients with end-stage renal disease (Winearls et al 1986, Eschbach et al 1987). A dose-related rise in haematocrit was observed. An increase in blood pressure in 4 of 25 patients, and increases in serum creatinine and potassium levels in most patients were the only significant toxic effects noted.

CONCLUSION

It is interesting to reflect that the rapid acquisition of information that resulted from the application of molecular approaches to the study of haemopoiesis virtually all occurred during the past 3–4 years. It is important to realize, however, that the impact of molecular approaches on the ability to investigate the structure and function of the CSFs occurred because well-defined culture systems were available for in vitro studies, and these set the direction for the in vivo work. This has occurred to a large extent where collaborations have been established between molecular biologists working in the biotechnology field and academic institutes with long-standing interests in the biology of haemopoiesis.

It is likely that the CSFs will find a place in the management of bone marrow hypoplasia secondary to radiation and/or chemotherapy associated with bone marrow transplantation, or with the treatment of malignant disease. Caution will need to be exercised here, since the blast cells from many patients with acute myeloblastic leukaemia are responsive to CSFs in culture (Griffin et al 1986). It will be necessary to establish that malignant cells from other tissues or tumours do not express receptors for the CSFs. The recent observation that cells of the placenta express M-CSF receptors and that M-CSF is produced by uterine cells may be pertinent in this regard (Pollard et al 1987).

Primary bone marrow failure (aplastic anaemia, neutropenias, and congenital cytopenias) will provide more of a challenge. Because acquired aplastic anaemia is heterogeneous with respect to aetiology, clinical severity at onset, and probable pathogenesis as well, it is likely that responsiveness to the CSFs may vary; one could predict that the severe forms of the disease with absent stem cells would be less likely to respond, while moderate forms may be more responsive.

It is likely that combinations of CSFs will prove more efficacious than single factors. In an important study, Donahue et al (1987) have shown that primates treated with the combination of 20 µg/kg/d of rhIL-3 from day 1 through 7, and 2 µg/kg/d of rhGM-CSF from day 8 exhibit prompt and marked changes in all classes of phagocytes, lymphocytes, reticulocytes, and platelets. That dose of GM-CSF has little or no effect when given alone, and that dose of IL-3 alone only variably and slightly stimulates reticulocytes and platelet counts or phagocytic counts in the primate species that they studied. When the GM-CSF preceded the IL-3 dose, there was no effect. The observation suggests that IL-3 is capable of acting on an immature population of progenitors which in turn can be stimulated to proliferate and terminally differentiate in the presence of a second low dose of haemopoietic growth factor such as GM-CSF.

The rapid rate of progress will almost certainly slow as the initial phase I/II clinical studies lead to larger randomized trials of CSF efficacy. It is to be hoped that the next few years will clearly establish the indications for CSF use and bring the recombinant CSFs from the molecular biology laboratories to the bedside.

REFERENCES

Adamson J W, Torok-Storb B, Lin N 1978 Blood Cells 4: 89–103
Arnaout M A, Wang E A, Clark S C, Sieff C A 1986 Journal of Clinical Investigation 78: 597–601
Ascencao J L, Vercellotti G M, Jacob H S, Zanjani E D 1984 Blood 63: 553–558
Bagby G C, Rigas V D, Bennett R M, Vandenbark A A, Garewal H S 1981 Journal of Clinical Investigation 68: 56–63
Bagby G C, McCall E, Bergstrom K A, Burger D 1983a Blood 62: 663–668
Bagby G C, McCall E, Layman D L 1983b Journal of Clinical Investigation 71: 340–344
Bartelmez S H, Stanley E R 1985 Journal of Cellular Physiology 122: 370–378
Bartocci A, Mastrogiannis D S, Migliorati G, Stockert R J, Wolkoff A W 1987 Proceedings of the National Academy of Science USA 84: 6179–6183
Bentley S A, Foidart J-M 1981 Blood 56: 1006
Bradley T K, Hodgson G S 1979 Blood 54: 1446
Brandt S J, Peters W P, Atwater S K et al 1988 NEJM 318: 869–876
Broudy V C, Kaushansky K, Segal G M, Harland J M, Adamson J W 1986a Proceedings of the National Academy of Science USA 83: 7467–7471
Broudy V C, Zuckerman K S, Jetmalani S, Fitchen J H, Bagby G C 1986b Blood 68: 530–534
Byrne P V, Guilbert L J, Stanley E R 1981 Journal of Cellular Biology 91: 848–853
Campbell A D, Long M W, Wicha M S 1987a Nature 329:744–746
Campbell H D, Tucker W Q J, Hort Y et al 1987b Proceedings of the National Academy of Sciences 84: 6629–6633
Castro-Malaspina H, Saletan S, Gay R E, Oettgen B, Gay S, Moore M A S 1981 Blood 58: supplement 1, 339
Chervenick P A, LoBuglio A F 1972 Science 178: 164–166

Cifone M, Defendi V 1974 Nature 252: 151
Clark S C, Kamen R 1987 Science 236: 1229–1237
Cline M J, Golde D W 1974 Nature 248: 703–704
Coussens L, Van Beveren C, Smith D et al 1986 Nature 320: 277–280
Deverieux S, Linch D C, Campos Costa D, Spittle M F, Jelliffe A M 1987 Lancet ii: 1523–1524
Dexter T M, Allen T D, Lajtha L G 1977 Journal of Cellular Physiology 91: 335–344
Dexter T M, Spooncer F, Simmons P, Allen T D 1984 In: Wright D G, Greenberger J S (eds) Long-term bone marrow culture. Liss: New York. Kroc Foundation Series, vol 18, pp 57–96
Dinarello C A 1984 NEJM 311: 1413–1418
Donahue R E, Emerson S G, Wang E A, Wong G G, Clark S C, Nathan D G 1985 Blood 66: 1479–1481
Donahue R E, Wang E A, Stone D et al 1986a Nature 321: 872–875
Donahue R E, Wang E A, Kaufman R J et al 1986b Cold Spring Harbor Symposium Quantitative Biology 51: 685
Donahue R E, Seehra J, Norton C et al 1987 Blood 70: 133a
Downward J, Yarden Y, Mayes E et al 1984 Nature 307: 521–527
Emerson S G, Sieff C A, Wang E A, Wong G G, Clark S C, Nathan D G 1985 Journal of Clinical Investigation 76: 1286–1290
Eschbach J W, Egrie J C, Downing M R, Browne J K, Adamson J W 1987 New England Journal of Medicine 316: 73–78
Fung M C, Hapel A J, Ymer S et al 1984 Nature 307: 233–236
Gabrilove J, Jakubowski A, Soher H et al 1987 1988 New England Journal of Medicine 318: 1414–1422
Gallagher J J, Spooncer E P, Dexter T M 1983 Journal of Cellular Science 632: 1565–1571
Gasson J C, Weisbart R H, Kaufman S E, Weisbart R H, Tomonaga M, Golde D W 1984 Science 1984; 226: 1339–1342
Gasson J C, Kaufman S E, Weisbart R H, Tomonaga, Golde D W 1986 Proceedings of the National Academy of Sciences USA 83: 669–673
Golde D W, Cline M J 1972 Journal of Clinical Investigation 51: 2981–2983
Gordon M Y, Riley G P, Watt S M, Greaves M F 1987 Nature 326: 403–405
Grabstein K H, Urdal D, Tushinski R J et al 1986 Science 232: 506–508
Griffin J D, Young D, Herrman F, Wiper D, Wagner K, Sabbath K D 1986 Blood 67: 1448–1453
Groopman J E, Mitsuyasu R T, DeLeo M J et al 1987 New England Journal of Medicine 317: 593–598
Guilbert L J, Stanley E R 1980 Journal of Cellular Biology 85: 153–159
Guilbert L J, Stanley L J 1986 Journal of Biological Chemistry 261: 4024–4032
Hamilton J A, Stanley E R, Burgess A W, Shadduck R K 1980 Journal of Cellular Physiology 103: 435–445
Heard J-M, Fichelson S, Varat B 1982 Blood 59: 761–767
Heard J-M, Roussel M F, Rettenmier C W, Sherr C J 1987 Cell 51: 663–673
Hirano T, Yasukawa K, Harada H et al 1986 Nature 324: 73–76
Horiguchi J, Warren M K, Ralph P, Kufe D 1986 Biochemical and Biophysical Research Communication 141: 924
Horiguchi J, Warren M K, Kufe D 1987 Blood 69: 1259–1261
Huebner K, Isobe M, Croce C M, Golde D W, Kaufman S E, Gasson J C 1985 Science 230: 1282–1285
Ikebuchi K, Wong G G, Clark S C, Ihle J N, Hirai Y, Ogawa M 1987 Blood 70: supplement 1, 173a, abstract 549
Jacobs K, Shoemaker C, Rudersdorf R, Neil S D et al 1985 Nature 313: 806–810
Jubinsky P T, Stanley E R 1985 Proceedings of the National Academy of Sciences USA 82: 2764–2768
Kawasaki E S, Ladner M B, Wang A M et al 1985 Science 230: 291–296
Kay H E M 1965 Lancet 2: 418–419
Keating A, Singer J W, Killen P D et al 1982 Nature 298: 280
Kindler J, Thorens B, De Kossodo S et al 1986 Proceedings of the National Academy of Sciences USA 83: 1001–1005
Knudson S, Mortenson B T 1975 Blood 46: 937–943
Ladner M B, Martin G A, Noble J A et al 1987 EMBO Journal 6: 2693–2698
Lai P-H, Everett R, Wang F-F, Arakawa T, Goldwasser E 1986 Journal of Biological Chemistry 261: 3116–3121
Law M L, Cai G-Y, Lin F-K 1986 Proceedings of the National Academy of Sciences 83: 6920–6924
LeBeau M M, Epstein N D, O'Brien S J et al 1987a Proceedings of the National Academy of Sciences USA 84: 5913–5917
LeBeau M M, Westbrook C A, Diaz M O et al 1987b Science 231: 984–987
Lemischka I R, Raulet D H, Mulligan R C 1986 Cell 45: 917–927
Lopez A F, Nicola N A, Burgess A W et al 1983 Journal of Immunology 131: 2983–2988
Lopez A F, To L B, Yang Y-C et al 1987 Proceedings of the National Academy of Sciences USA 84: 2761–2765

McDonough S K, Larsen S, Brodey R S, Stock N D, Hardy W D J 1971 Cancer Research 31: 953–956
McNiece I K, Bradley T R, Kriegler A B, Hodgson G S 1986 Experimental Hematology 14: 856–860
Mangan K F, Chikkappa G, Sieler L Z, Scharfman W B, Parkingson D R 1982 Blood 59: 990–996
Metcalf D 1984 The hemopoietic growth factors. Elsevier, Amsterdam
Metcalf D 1986 Blood 67: 257–267
Metcalf D, Nicola N A 1983 Journal of Cellular Physiology 116: 198–206
Metcalf D, Stanley E R 1971 British Journal of Haematology 21: 481–492
Metcalf D, Begley C G, Johnson G R 1986a Blood 67: 37–45
Metcalf D, Begley C G, Johnson G R, Nicola N A, Lopez A F, Williamson D J 1986b Blood 68: 46–57
Miyake T, Kung CK-H, Goldwasser E 1977 Journal of Biological Chemistry 252: 5558–5564
Miyatake S, Otsuka T, Yokota T, Lee F, Arci K 1985 EMBO Journal 4: 2561–2568
Mochizuki D Y, Eisenman J R, Conlon P J, Larsen A D, Tushinski R J 1987 Proceedings of the National
    Academy of Sciences USA 84: 5267–5271
Morgan C J, Stanley E R 1984 Biochemical and Biophysical Research Communications 119: 35–41
Morstyn G, Souza L M, Keech J et al 1988 Lancet i: 667–672
Motoyoshi K, Suda T, Kusumoto K, Takaku F, Miura Y 1982 Blood 60: 1378–1386
Munker R, Gasson J, Ogawa M, Koeffler H P 1986 Nature 323: 79–82
Nagata S, Tsuchiya M, Asano S et al 1986a EMBO Journal 5: 575–581
Nagata S, Tsuchiya M, Asano S et al 1986b Nature 319: 415–418
Nathan D G, Chess L, Hillman D G et al 1978 Journal of Experimental Medicine 147: 324–339
Nicola N A, Metcalf D 1984 Proceedings of the National Academy of Sciences USA 81: 3765–3769
Nicola N A, Metcalf D 1985 Journal of Cellular Physiology 124: 313–321
Nicola N A, Metcalf D 1986 Journal of Cellular Physiology 128: 180–188
Niemeyer C M, Sieff C A, Mathey-Prevot B, Bierer B E, Clark S, Nathan D G 1987 Blood 70:
    supplement 1, 182a, abstract 582
Nienhuis A W, Donahue R, Karlsson S et al 1987 Journal of Clinical Investigation 80: 573–577
Noma Y, Sideras P, Naito T et al 1986 Nature 319: 640–646
Palaszynski E W, Ihle J N 1984 Journal of Immunology 132: 1872–1878
Park L W, Friend D, Gillis S, Urdal D L 1986a Journal of Biological Chemistry 261: 4177–4183
Park L W, Friend D, Gillis S, Urdal D L 1986b Journal of Experimental Medicine 164: 251–262
Park L W, Friend D, Gillis S, Urdal D L 1986c Journal of Biological Chemistry 261: 205–210
Pettenati M J, LeBeau M M, Lemons R S et al 1987 Proceedings of the National Academy of Sciences
    USA 84: 2970–2974
Pollard J W, Bartocci A, Arceci R, Orlofsky A, Ladner M B, Stanley E R 1987 Nature 330: 484–486
Quesenberry P J, Gimbrone M A 1980 Blood 56: 1060–1067
Ralph P, Warren M K, Lee M T et al 1986 Blood 68: 633–639
Rambaldi A, Young D C, Griffin J D 1987 Blood 69: 1409–1413
Reid C P L, Batista L C, Chanarin I 1981 British Journal of Haematology 48: 155–164
Rennick D, Yang C, Muller-Sieburg C et al 1987 Proceedings of the National Academy of Sciences USA
    84: 6889–6893
Rettenmier C W, Roussel M F, Ashman R A, Ralph P, Price K, Sherr C J 1987 Molecular and Cellular
    Biology 7: 2378–2387
Roussel M F, Rettenmier C W, Look A T, Sherr C J 1984 Molecular and Cellular Biology 4: 1999–2009
Sawyer S T, Krantz S B, Luna J 1987 Proceedings of the National Academy of Sciences USA 84:
    3690–3694
Seelentag W K, Mermod J-J, Montesano R, Vassalli P 1987 EMBO Journal 6: 2261–2265
Shadduck R K, Pigoli G, Caramatti C et al 1983a Blood 62: 1197–1202
Shadduck R K, Waheed A, Greenberger J S, Dexter T M 1983b Journal of Cellular Physiology 114: 88–92
Shaw G, Kamen R 1986 Cell 46: 659–667
Sherr C J, Rettenmier C W, Sacca R, Roussel M F, Look A T, Stanley E R 1985 Cell 41: 665–676
Sieff C A 1986 Journal of Clinical Investigation 79: 1549–1557
Sieff C A, Emerson S G, Donahue R E et al 1985 Science 230: 1171–1173
Sieff C A, Emerson S G, Mufson A, Gesner T G, Nathan D G 1986 Journal of Clinical Investigation
    77: 74–81
Sieff C A, Niemeyer C M, Nathan D G et al 1987a Journal of Clinical Investigation 80: 818–823
Sieff C A, Tsai S, Faller D V 1987b Journal of Clinical Investigation 79: 48–51
Simmers R N, Webber L M, Shannon F et al 1987 Blood 70: 330–332
Sonoda Y, Yang Y-C, Wong G G, Clark S C, Ogawa M 1987 1988 Proceedings of the National Academy
    of Sciences USA 85: 4360–4364
Souza L M, Boone T C, Gabrilove J et al 1986 Science 232: 61–65
Stanley E R, Heard P M 1977 Journal of Biological Chemistry 252: 4305–4312
Stanley E R, Hansen G, Woodcock J, Metcalf D 1975 Federation Proceedings 34: 2272–2278

Stanley E R, Cifone M, Heard P M, Defendi V 1976 Journal of Experimental Medicine 143: 631–647
Stanley E R, Bartocci A, Patinkin D, Rosendaal M, Bradley T R 1986 Cell 45: 667–674
Strife A, Lambek C, Wisniewski D et al 1987 Blood 69: 1508–1523
Toksoz D, Dexter T M, Lord B I, Wright E G, Lajtha L G 1980 Blood 55: 931–936
Tomonaga M, Golde D W, Gasson J C 1986 Blood 67: 31–36
Tsai S, Emerson S G, Sieff C A, Nathan D G 1986a Journal of Cellular Physiology 127: 137–145
Tsai S, Sieff C A, Nathan D G 1986b Blood 67: 1418–1426
Tsai S, Patel V, Beaumont E, Lodish H F, Nathan D G, Sieff C A 1987 Blood 69: 1587–1594
Tushinski R J, Oliver I T, Guilbert L J, Tynan P W, Warner J R, Stanley E R 1982 Cell 28: 71–81
Vadas M A, Nicola N A, Metcalf D 1983a Journal of Immunology 130: 795–799
Vadas M A, Varigos A G, Nicola N et al 1983b Blood 61: 1232–1241
Vadhan-Raj S, Keating M, LeMaistre A et al 1987 New England Journal of Medicine 317: 1545–1552
Walker F, Burgess A W 1985 EMBO Journal 4: 933–939
Walker F, Nicola N A, Metcalf D, Burgess A W 1985 Cell 43: 269–276
Waterfield M D, Scrace G T, Whittle N et al 1983 Nature 304: 35–39
Watkins P C, Eddy R, Hoffman N et al 1986 Cytogenetic Cellular Genetics 42: 214–218
Weisbart R H, Golde D W, Clark S C, Wong G G, Gasson J C 1985 Nature 314: 361–363
Welte K, Platzer E, Lu L, Gabrilove J L, Levi E, Mertelsmann R, Moore M A S 1985 Proceedings of the National Academy of Sciences USA 82: 1526–1530
Welte K, Bonilla M A, Gillio A P et al 1987 Journal of Experimental Medicine 165: 941–948
Wheeler E F, Rettenmeier C W, Look A T, Sherr C J 1986 Nature 324: 377–380
Winearls C G, Oliver D O, Pippard M J, Reid C, Downing M R, Cotes P M 1986 Lancet ii: 1175–1178
Wolf N S 1979 Clinical Haematology 8: 469–500
Wong G G, Witek J S, Temple P A et al 1985 Science 228: 810–815
Wong G G, Temple P A, Leary A C et al 1987 Science 235: 1504–1509
Yang Y-C, Ciarletta A B, Temple P A et al 1986a Cell 47: 3–10
Yang Y-C, Tsai S, Wong G G, Clark S C 1986b Journal of Cellular Physiology 134: 292–296
Yokota T, Lee T, Rennick D et al 1984 Proceedings of the National Academy of Sciences USA 81: 1070–1074
Yokota T, Otsuka, Mosmann T et al 1986 Proceedings of the National Academy of Sciences USA 83: 5894–5898
Zucali J R, Dinarello C A, Oblondi D A, Gross M A, Anderson L, Weiner R S 1986 Journal of Clinical Investigation 77: 1857–1863
Zuckerman K S 1981 Journal of Clinical Investigation 67: 702–709
Zuckerman K S, Wicha M S 1983 Blood 61: 540–547
Zuckerman K S, Bagby G C, McCall E et al 1985 Journal of Clinical Investigation 75: 722–725

2. Biochemical mechanisms of transduction of signals for proliferation and differentiation in normal and malignant haemopoietic cells

R. G. Wickremasinghe   A. R. Mire-Sluis   A. V. Hoffbrand

INTRODUCTION

Knowledge of the mechanisms involved in the regulation of proliferation and differentiation of normal cells by external growth factors or hormones is a pre-requisite for the understanding of aberrant regulatory processes which drive uncontrolled proliferation of leukaemic cells. The combined application of biological, biochemical and genetic techniques, together with the powerful new approaches afforded by recombinant DNA technology has led to considerable progress in unravelling the details of the intracellular events triggered by growth factor binding to cultured cells, especially fibroblasts. However, despite the availability of cloned haemopoietic growth factors, progress in studying these mechanisms in haemopoietic cells has been slow, largely due to the difficulties in obtaining large numbers of suitable progenitor cells for study. Nonetheless, a fragmentary picture is beginning to emerge, and it appears that mechanisms similar to those described in other cell types may also operate in haemopoietic cells. This data will be the subject of this review, which will also summarise information on the aberrant versions of normal regulatory mechanisms which may drive malignant proliferation. Since certain common motifs recur in many different growth regulatory systems, we will first describe the general principles of growth signal transduction as gleaned from studies on fibroblasts and other non-haemopoietic cells.

GENERAL MECHANISMS OF GROWTH SIGNAL TRANSDUCTION

Cultured fibroblasts deprived of serum cease proliferation and enter a state of quiescence, the G_0 phase. The quiescent cells require the co-operative action of polypeptide growth factors to traverse the cell cycle. Platelet-derived growth factor (PDGF) induces a state of 'competence', which permits the cell to respond to epidermal growth factor (EGF) and traverse the G_1 phase. Once the DNA synthetic S phase commences, the cell is no longer dependent on growth factors. A general principle of all growth factor signalling mechanisms is that binding of the factor to a cell surface receptor triggers the generation of biochemical second messengers within the cell. These second messengers then trigger cascades of biochemical events which culminate in initiation of DNA synthesis and in mitosis. The key element in transducing the PDGF growth signal to the cell interior is the PDGF receptor, a transmembrane glycoprotein with a PDGF-binding domain orientated to the cell exterior and linked by a single membrane-spanning α-helix to an intracellular domain (Fig. 2.1) (Heldin et al 1985). The latter domain possesses a tyrosine protein kinase (TPK) activity which transfers a phosphate group from ATP to tyrosine residues in either the receptor itself or in target proteins. Binding of PDGF to the PDGF binding domain of the receptor

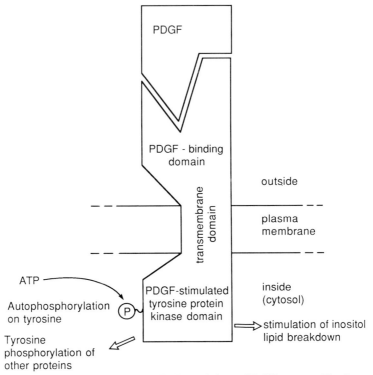

Fig. 2.1   Signal transduction via the platelet-derived growth factor (PDGF) receptor. *Key:* P, protein-bound phosphate moiety.

stimulates the tyrosine kinase domain to phosphorylate itself on a tyrosine residue (Heldin et al 1985). This autophosphorylation reaction activates the receptor TPK to phosphorylate other substrates. Since the phosphorylation of proteins is a well known mechanism for rapid and reversible regulation of their enzymic activity, it is presumed that tyrosine phosphorylation of other enzymes may activate processes which contribute to transduction of the growth signal (Heldin & Westermark 1984). Although several substrates of the PDGF and EGF receptor TPKs have been identified there is no direct proof of their roles in signal transduction. However, protein phosphorylation on tyrosine is probably a key element in the regulation of proliferation since TPK activity is a common feature of many growth factor receptors, including the receptors for EGF and insulin and also of the protein products of one-half of the known retroviral oncogenes. The importance of tyrosine phosphorylation in stimulation of cell proliferation is also emphasised by the observation that addition of sodium vanadate, an inhibitor of tyrosine protein phosphatases to culture media, increases the levels of tyrosine phosphorylated proteins in fibroblasts and simultaneously stimulates their proliferation (Klarlund 1985). A number of TPKs which are not transmembrane receptors have also been described. The normal roles of these non-receptor TPKs are not known.

Signal transduction by generation of inositol lipid-derived second messengers
The binding of PDGF to its receptor also activates further biochemical pathways. Phosphatidylinositol (PI) is a rare membrane lipid. PI and its derivatives PI-monophos-

phate (PIP) and PI-bisphosphate (PIP_2) undergo a turnover cycle of sequential phosphorylations and cleavage of PIP_2 with consequent generation of two second messengers, the neutral lipid diacylglycerol (DAG) and the water-soluble inositol trisphosphate (IP_3) (Nishizuka 1986). Sequential breakdown of IP_3 to IP_2, IP and inositol, and the consequent resynthesis of PI completes the inositol lipid cycle (Fig. 2.2). The key growth-factor stimulated step appears to be the cleavage of PIP_2 to yield DAG and IP_3. This step is catalysed by a specific phospholipase, phosphatidylinositol bisphosphate phosphodiesterase (PIP_2-PDE) whose activity is stimulated by the binding of PDGF to its receptor (Habenicht et al 1981).

A family of proteins called G proteins (guanine nucleotide binding proteins) are implicated in the coupling of receptors, including growth factor receptors, to PIP_2-PDE (Fig. 2.3) (Wakelam et al 1986). In the resting stage G proteins contain bound GDP. Upon stimulation of the receptor, a conformation change is induced in the G protein, which stimulates exchange of the bound GDP for a GTP molecule (Fig. 2.3). In this activated, GTP-bound form, the G protein stimulates PIP_2-PDE to generate DAG and IP_3 from PIP_2. A GTPase activity intrinsic to the G protein hydrolyses the bound GTP to GDP, thereby returning the G protein to its resting state. While G proteins themselves are tightly associated with the plasma membrane by virtue of a covalently bound fatty acid moiety, a soluble GTPase activating protein (GAP) additionally appears to be required for the maximal expression of GTPase activity by at least some G proteins (Trahey & McCormick 1987). Mutations which destroy its GTPase activity or impair its interaction with the GAP protein render the G protein incapable of undergoing the deactivation step, and may lead to continued proliferation due to factor-independent stimulation of PIP_2-PDE. The ras family of oncogenes appears to be derived by single point mutations from normal ras genes (proto-oncogenes) encoding G proteins, and are thought to contribute to the neoplastic characteristics of a wide variety of cancers, including leukaemias (see later).

However, the lipid turnover cycle may also be regulated at steps other than the PIP_2-PDE reaction. Cells expressing oncogenes with TPK activity have altered patterns of PI metabolism, suggesting that their PI and PIP kinases (Fig. 2.2) may be activated, with the consequent excess generation of PIP_2, the precursor of DAG and IP_3 (Jackowski et al 1986). It has been proposed, therefore, that phosphorylation and activation of the lipid kinases by TPKs may be a further link between receptors and the inositol lipid cycle (Macara 1985).

Recent work has demonstrated the presence in cells treated with PDGF of an 85 kDa protein which is phosphorylated on tyrosine residues and which may also express PI kinase activity (Kaplan et al 1987). This is consistent with the possibility that PDGF stimulation of the PDGF receptor kinase may result in phosphorylation and so activation of a PI kinase, thereby contributing to the enhanced turnover of inositol lipids in PDGF treated cells.

A further intriguing link between tyrosine kinases and the PI cycle has been revealed by the observation that the protein product of crk, the oncogene of CT10 retrovirus, contains three domains bearing strong structural homology to regions in the non-catalytic domains of PI-specific PDE and also of the TPK oncogenes encoded by the src family (Mayer et al 1988). Although the crk oncogene does not appear to contain a TPK domain, cells expressing this oncogene contain greatly elevated levels of proteins phosphorylated on tyrosine. One possible explanation is that the

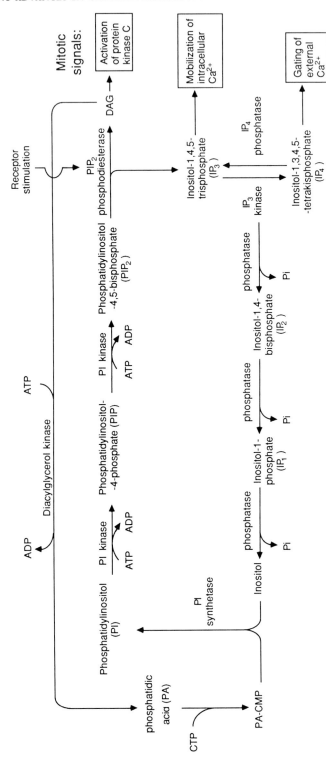

Fig. 2.2   The inositol lipid turnover cycle. *Key:* DAG, diacylglycerol; P$_i$, inorganic phosphate; PA-CMP, phosphatidic acid bound to cytidine monophosphate.

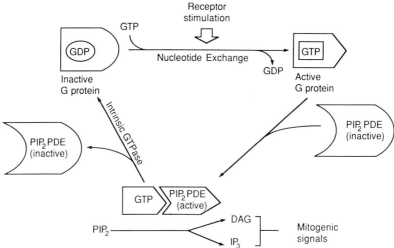

Fig. 2.3 The G protein activation, deactivation cycle. *Key:* GTP, guanosine triphosphate; GDP, guanosine diphosphate; PIP$_2$-PDE, phosphatidylinositol-4,5-bisphosphate-specific phosphodiesterase.

logous domains represent sites for interaction of negative and/or positive regulatory molecules, and that overexpression of these domains in crk-expressing cells leads to the neutralization of negative regulatory proteins which would otherwise inhibit expression of TPK activity (Mayer et al 1988).

The second messenger roles of DAG and IP$_3$

DAG is hydrophobic and remains in the plasma membrane. It functions as an allosteric activator of protein kinase C (PKC), an enzyme which phosphorylates proteins on serine and threonine residues, and requires phospholipid and Ca^{2+} ions as well as DAG for activity (Nishizuka 1986). The cellular targets of PKC in cells stimulated by growth factors or phorbol esters such as 12-0-tetradecanoylphorbol-13-acetate (TPA) which activates PKC directly include an 80 kDa protein of unknown function (Rozengurt et al 1983a). PKC activation by growth factors also results in an elevation of intracellular pH, which is thought to be permissive for mitogenesis.

By contrast, IP$_3$ is a water-soluble second messenger, which binds to specific sites on the endoplasmic reticulum and triggers release of intracellular Ca^{2+} stores (Nishizuka 1986). The resultant increase in cytoplasmic Ca^{2+} is thought to activate protein kinases dependent on Ca^{2+}-calmodulin and also to synergise with DAG in the activation of PKC. Although no key substrates of Ca^{2+}-dependent phosphorylation have been identified, the importance of Ca^{2+} in mitogenesis is also emphasised by the ability of Ca^{2+} ionophores to synergise with other growth stimuli (Truneh et al 1985).

Inositol tetrakisphosphate (IP$_4$), which is derived by the phosphorylation of IP$_3$ (Fig. 2.2) also plays a key role in regulation of Ca^{2+} levels. IP$_4$ appears to trigger the entry of Ca^{2+} from the cell exterior into the cytoplasm (Irvine & Moor 1986).

Growth-factor stimulated expression of cellular proto-oncogenes

The increased expression of the cellular proto-oncogenes c-fos and c-myc are among the earliest nuclear events identified following stimulation of cells with PDGF (Greenberg & Ziff 1984, Kelly et al 1983) and various other growth stimuli. In general, c-fos expression is rapid and transient, and peaks within minutes post-stimulation.

By contrast, c-myc expression peaks at about 1 hour following stimulation and declines prior to initiation of DNA synthesis. Despite the sequential expression of c-fos and c-myc, inhibitors of protein synthesis do not inhibit expression of either gene and it is thought that c-myc expression is not a consequence of a build-up of c-fos protein.

The products of both c-fos and c-myc proto-oncogenes are DNA binding proteins and are located largely within the nucleus. The fos gene product may function by interacting with regulatory elements of specific genes and thereby regulate their expression (Franza et al 1988). The c-myc gene product participates directly in DNA replication (Studzinski et al 1986). The importance of the products of both the c-fos and c-myc genes in cell cycle progression is suggested by observations that anti-sense polynucleotides to the transcripts of either gene will inhibit progression through the cell cycle (Holt et al 1986, Heikkila et al 1987).

The links between the early membrane-associated events described previously and the expression of c-fos and c-myc remain elusive. However, growth factors, TPA, calcium ionophores, or cyclic AMP can stimulate expression of these genes in certain cells (Greenberg & Ziff 1984, Tsuda et al 1986, Grausz et al 1986), suggesting that phosphorylation and activation of a regulatory protein which then binds to regulatory regions in DNA may be responsible for growth factor stimulated expression of c-fos and c-myc. Short DNA sequences which can confer TPA inducibility to heterologous genes have been described (Chiu et al 1987) implying that activation of PKC through which TPA presumably acts can regulate the activity of these enhancer elements. This action may be mediated via post-translational modification of protein factors which bind these enhancers. A DNA element which confers serum inducibility to the c-fos gene also serves as a binding site for a protein factor (Treisman 1986). However, the mechanism of serum inducibility is unclear, and may involve modification of proteins other than the protein factor itself, which subsequently influence the interaction of the protein factor with its cognate DNA element.

The role of receptor internalisation

Much emphasis has been placed on the early events stimulated by growth factor binding to receptors. However, PDGF receptors which have bound their ligand are internalised by endocytosis (Heldin et al 1985). Internalised receptors may have a continuing role in promoting cell cycle traverse. Thus, methylamine inhibits processing of internalised EGF receptors by preventing acidification within the endocytotic vesicles. Methylamine treatment of fibroblasts does not inhibit early EGF induced events such as c-myc and c-fos expression, but prevents commitment to mitosis (Matrisian et al 1987). The precise biochemical roles of internalised receptors have not been defined. However, internalised EGF receptor has been shown to be associated with a DNA topoisomerase, an enzyme which uses ATP-derived energy to unwind DNA and which may play a role in regulating gene expression by rendering DNA accessible to the transcription apparatus.

Cyclic AMP

The role of cyclic AMP in regulation of proliferation has long been controversial (Boynton & Whitfield 1983). In some systems, e.g. Swiss 3T3 fibroblasts, PDGF stimulates cAMP production. Agents which elevate cellular cAMP levels are co-mitogenic with growth factors in these cells. However, in most cell types, addition of cyclic AMP elevating agents to culture media inhibits cell division. Boynton & Whitfield (1983) have pointed out the difficulties of interpreting such experiments. In particular, the continuous elevation of cAMP may be deleterious to cell cycle progression, whereas transient programmed increases at specific points of the cycle may play a role in mitogenesis.

Other mechanisms in growth signalling
The cytoskeleton of fibroblasts undergoes a transient disruption and reformation following treatment with growth factors (Bockus & Stiles 1984) and drugs which disrupt the microtubule system can actually trigger proliferation (Crossin & Carney 1981). The cytoskeleton may also be involved in propagation of initial growth signals. Cytoskeletal proteins are substrates for phosphorylation by oncogene-encoded and growth factor receptor TPKs (Hunter & Cooper 1985). However, the biochemical roles of the cytoskeleton in growth signal transduction remain elusive.

HAEMOPOIETIC GROWTH FACTORS

The survival, self-renewal, proliferation and differentiation of haemopoietic stem cells, committed progenitors and also the functions of mature blood cells are under the regulation of a set of glycoprotein growth factors. The nomenclature, biology and potential clinical uses of these factors is covered in Chapter 1. The target cell ranges and the structures of their cell-surface receptors (where known) are summarised in Table 2.1.

Biochemical mechanisms of growth signal transduction in lymphocytes
Among haemopoietic cells, lymphocytes have been the best studied and it appears that similar elements are involved in growth regulation of these cells and in fibroblasts. Mitogenic stimulation of resting T lymphocytes requires two consecutive signals. The first involves perturbation of the clonotypic T cell antigen receptor (TCR) complex. This signal triggers expression of receptors for interleukin-2 (IL2). Binding of IL2 to its receptor triggers proliferation (Cantrell & Smith 1984). Recent work shows that stimulation of the TCR complex alone triggers a single, IL2-independent round of cell division with further proliferation being dependent on IL2 (Mire-Sluis et al 1987b). The mechanisms of signal transduction employed by the TCR and by the IL2 receptor will be discussed below.

The T cell antigen receptor (TCR) structure
The idiotype-specific portion of the TCR (T_i) which recognises specific antigen in association with products of the major histocompatibility complex, consists of two protein chains α(49 kDa) and β(43 kDa) which are linked by disulphide bonds. Each subunit contributes to the binding site, which is orientated toward the exterior of the cell. The α and β chains each contain a single hydrophobic membrane-spanning domain which links the extracellular regions to short cytoplasmic regions (Fig. 2.4) In early thymocytes a second receptor composed of T_γ and T_δ chains may function instead of the TCR of more mature thymocytes and T cells. Associated with T_i is the CD3 complex, which consists of at least three membrane-bound protein subunits (Fig. 2.4). The CD3 complex is not clone-specific, but is nevertheless important

Table 2.1 Growth factor and mitogen receptors of haemopoietic cells and lymphocytes. The information summarised here refers to the murine growth factors and receptors, since the most complete information is available in this system. CSF-1 is the human equivalent of murine M-CSF. (See text for details and references)

Factor or mitogen	Receptor distribution	Receptor	Possible biochemical function(s) of receptor
IL3 (=multi-CSF)	Wide spectrum of haemopoietic lineages	60–70 kDa	?
GM-CSF	Neutrophil, eosinophil, monocyte progenitors	130 kDa	? Potentially large enough to include kinase domain
M-CSF (=CSF-1)	Restricted to monocyte/macrophage lineage	165 kDa	Ligand-stimulated tyrosine protein kinase; probably encoded by c-fms gene
G-CSF	Restricted to granulocytic lineage	150 kDa	? Potentially large enough to include a kinase domain
Erythropoietin	Restricted to erythroid progenitors	60 kDa	?
Antigen	B lymphocytes	Membrane bound immunoglobulin	No intrinsic protein kinase activity
Antigen in complex with products of major histocompatibility complex	T lymphocytes	T cell antigen receptor; α chain 49 kDa, β chain 43 kDa	No intrinsic protein kinase activity
Interleukin-2	Activated B and T lymphocytes	Two chains of 55 and 75 kDa respectively	55 kDa chain lacks intrinsic kinase activity. Not known for 75 kDa chain
Interleukin-4	Activated B and T lymphocytes		

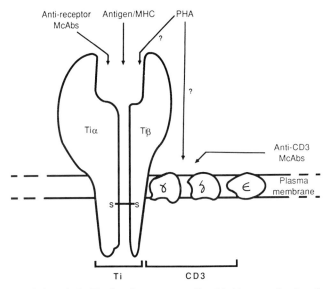

Fig. 2.4 Mitotic stimulation via the T cell antigen receptor. *Key:* McAb, monoclonal antibody; MHC, product of the major histocompatibility complex; PHA, phytohaemagglutinin; Tiα, Tiβ, α and β subunits of the T cell antigen receptor; γ, δ, ε, subunits of the T$_i$-associated CD3 complex.

in transducing the proliferative signal. In contrast to the PDGF receptor, the cytoplasmic domain of the T$_i$ and CD3 components of the TCR are too small to contain TPK activity. Nevertheless, stimulation of protein phosphorylation appears to be important in transducing growth signals from the TCR complex (see below).

In the intact animal, T lymphocytes are activated by the binding of antigen-MHC, presented on the surface of antigen-presenting cells to the T$_i$ moiety of specific T cell clones. Research on biochemical mechanisms of signal transduction has been greatly facilitated by the use of lectins such as phytohaemagglutinin (PHA) which bind to either T$_i$ or CD3 and specific monoclonal antibodies (McAbs) which bind T$_i$ or CD3.

Biochemical consequences of stimulation of the T cell antigen receptor
The earliest event described following stimulation of the T$_i$/CD3 complex with antigen (Patel et al 1987), lectins (Hasegawa-Sasaki & Sasaki 1983, Wickremasinghe et al 1987) or anti-T$_i$/CD3 McAbs (Imboden & Stobo 1985) is the increased turnover of inositol lipids. The precise mechanism by which perturbation of T$_i$/T$_3$ triggers PI turnover is unclear, but a number of studies suggest that activation of a G protein by perturbation of T$_i$/CD3 leads in turn to the stimulation of the PIP$_2$-PDE which catalyses breakdown of inositol-containing lipids (Sasaki & Hasegawa-Sasaki 1987, Mire-Sluis et al 1987a).

Activation of PKC and increase in Ca^{2+}
The generation of IP$_3$ by inositol lipid breakdown and an increase in cytoplasmic Ca^{2+} levels follows mitogenic stimulation of T lymphocytes. The initial, rapid increase

in Ca^{2+} appears to be a consequence of liberation of Ca^{2+} from intracellular stores whereas the subsequent, more prolonged elevation of Ca^{2+} is probably a consequence of the opening of Ca^{2+} channels in the plasma membrane (Gelfand et al 1987). There is also a rapid, transient translocation of PKC to the lymphocyte membrane following PHA stimulation (Farrar & Ruscetti 1986, Mire et al 1986a). The important targets of the activated PKC with respect to growth signalling are unclear. However, direct activation of T cell PKC by TPA or stimulation of the antigen receptor results in phosphorylation of subunits of the CD3 complex (Cantrell et al 1985, Samelson et al 1986).

Although the components of $T_i/CD3$ do not include a TPK, tyrosine phosphorylation of a soluble 66 kDa protein (Wedner & Bass 1986) and of a 42 kDa protein (Mire et al 1986b) have been reported following PHA stimulation of normal human T cells. The latter protein was partially associated with the detergent resistant fraction of the cell, suggesting that its phosphorylation may serve to link events at the membrane to the cytoskeleton. The mechanism of activation of tyrosine phosphorylation following stimulation and phosphorylation of $T_i/CD3$ is unclear. Tyrosine phosphorylation of the 42 kDa protein is stimulated by TPA as well as by PHA and anti-CD3 McAbs, suggesting that activation of PKC is the common pathway which leads to the activation of tyrosine phosphorylation (Mire et al 1986b).

Membrane fractions from normal T cells do contain TPKs. The best characterised is a 56 kDa enzyme (pp56[lck]) (Marth et al 1985) with strong structural homology to the product of the c-src gene, the cellular homologue of v-src, the oncogene of Rous sarcoma virus. Membrane-bound TPKs with molecular weights of 40 kDa and 70 kDa have been detected by their ability to phosphorylate exogenous tyrosine-containing peptides (Hall et al 1987). These kinases are down-regulated following mitogen-stimulation of T cells suggesting, by analogy with other growth factor receptor systems a role in the early stages of signal transduction. By contrast pp56[lck] is not down-regulated (Hall et al 1987).

The pathways downstream from activation of PKC, TPKs and of Ca^{2+}-dependent processes are unclear, but are likely to consist of multiple parallel cascades of events occurring throughout the long (1–2 day) G_1 phase. It appears, however, that the combined activation of PKC and the elevation of intracellular Ca^{2+} are sufficient early events to trigger all the processes required for commitment to S phase (Truneh et al 1985).

Mitogen-induced elevation of mRNA encoding c-fos and c-myc
Mitogen stimulation of T (and B) lymphocytes leads to increased levels of the mRNAs encoding c-fos and c-myc. The rise in c-fos mRNA is detectable by 10 min following stimulation, and declines to pre-stimulation levels by 2–3 h (Moore et al 1986). By contrast, the c-myc mRNA level rises more slowly, with maximal levels at 2–10 h with a subsequent decline, though the elevation persists even after initiation of DNA synthesis at 24 h. Inhibition of translation of c-myc mRNA into protein by antisense oligodeoxynucleotides does not prevent transit of PHA-stimulated T cells through G_1, but blocks their entry into S phase, also suggesting a role for the c-myc product in the S phase itself rather than in pre-replicative events (Heikkila et al 1987).

The mechanism by which early mitogen-stimulated events at the lymphocyte membrane result in changes in expression of proto-oncogenes are unclear. Either Ca^{2+}

ionophores or TPA stimulate increased expression of c-fos and c-myc mRNA and the two agents together synergise strongly (Pantaleo et al 1987). Since neither agent alone is mitogenic (Truneh et al 1985) the increased expression of these oncogenes alone cannot be sufficient for G_1 traverse and entry into S phase.

Biochemical mechanisms of IL2 signal transduction

Further proliferation of T lymphocytes activated via the T_i/CD3 structure is dependent on binding of IL2, which is itself produced by a subset of T cells in response to binding the cytokine IL1. IL2 may also be an important growth factor during early T cell ontogeny, since thymocytes which lack a T cell receptor secrete and respond to IL2 (De la Hera et al 1987).

Structure of the IL2 receptor

The cell surface receptor for IL2 consists of two glycoproteins of 75 and 55 kDa which are not covalently linked (Dukovich et al 1987). Each polypeptide can bind IL2 with low affinity, but the mitogenic action of IL2 requires the formation of a high affinity ternary complex involving IL2 and both receptor components.

The components of the IL2 receptor are not known to express protein kinase activity. However, binding of IL2 to its receptor triggers the phosphorylation of proteins on serine and/or threonine residues. Serine/threonine phosphorylation (but not tyrosine phosphorylation) of 85 kDa (Mire et al 1985) and 63 and 67 kDa proteins (Ishii et al 1987) following IL2 treatment of human T lymphocytes or HTLV-1 infected cell lines has been reported. IL2 stimulates the transient generation of cyclic AMP (Wickremasinghe et al 1987) and cyclic AMP, as well as IL2, triggers phosphorylation of the 85 kDa protein. Thus, stimulation of a cAMP-dependent kinase may be part of the cellular response to IL2 binding. A G protein may link IL2 receptors to adenylate cyclase since reagents which stimulate G proteins directly could also cause increases in cAMP levels and phosphorylation of the 85 kDa protein (A.R.M-S, A.V.H. and R.G.W., submitted). No evidence was found for a role of inositol lipid breakdown or translocation of PKC from cytosol to membrane in IL2 signal transduction (Gelfand et al 1987, Wickremasinghe et al 1987). Unknown signals other than cyclic AMP generation are, however, probably of importance in IL2 signalling. Signals dependent on internalisation of the IL2-IL2 receptor ternary complex may play a role since only the high affinity form of the receptor can be internalised (Fuji et al 1986). A significant proportion of internalised IL2 is found in the nucleus and it is possible that nuclear IL2-receptor complexes may influence genetic events. Mechanisms for the further transduction of the IL2 signal are also largely unknown, but probably include stimulated expression of cellular oncogenes such as c-myc (Broome et al 1987).

In summary, the mitogenic response to IL2 appears to involve protein phosphorylation on serine and threonine residues, although the precise pathways involved are not clear. Although phosphorylation of proteins on tyrosine residues has not been detected, the involvement of TPKs cannot be ruled out at present.

Biochemical mechanisms of signalling via the M-CSF receptor

The receptor for M-CSF (=CSF-1) has recently been shown to be encoded by the c-fms gene, the normal cellular counterpart of the oncogene v-fms. This has facilitated analysis of the structure and function of this receptor (Sherr et al 1985).

The M-CSF receptor contains a ligand stimulated TPK activity. The v-fms product differs from the normal M-CSF receptor only in the C-terminal 40 amino acids which endows it with a constitutive (i.e. M-CSF independent) TPK activity. Replacement of the missing 40 C-terminal amino acids of v-fms with c-fms sequences results in a protein which is no longer tumorigenic (Browning et al 1986).

Circumstantial evidence suggests that the TPK activity of the M-CSF receptor is important in growth signalling. Simian virus 40 infection immortalises macrophages, which grow in culture but are dependent on the addition of M-CSF. Introduction of the v-fms gene renders them independent of M-CSF (Wheeler et al 1986) implying that the M-CSF-stimulated TPK activity of the normal M-CSF receptor may be of importance in growth signal transduction. Furthermore, replacement of tyrosine 969 in the carboxy terminus of the M-CSF receptor (whose phosphorylation is thought to negatively regulate kinase activity) with phenylalanine activates the ability of the M-CSF receptor to transform fibroblasts (Roussel et al 1987).

Mechanisms other than tyrosine protein phosphorylation may also be of importance in growth signal transduction by the M-CSF receptor. M-CSF bound to its receptor is internalised rapidly by macrophages, with a half-life of a few minutes, and the internalised complex may play a continuing role in signalling.

Inositol lipid metabolism in signalling via the M-CSF receptor

Cells infected with viruses containing the v-fms gene exhibit enhanced turnover of inositol lipids and in vitro measurements suggest that this is due to increased activity of a guanine-nucleotide stimulated PIP_2-PDE (Jackowski et al 1986). Cells infected with viruses containing the v-fes oncogene, whose product also exhibits TPK activity, show a similar elevation of PI turnover and of guanine-nucleotide stimulated PIP_2-PDE. Elevation of PIP_2-PDE in v-fms- and v-fes-expressing cells correlates well with the relative TPK activities of their protein products, suggesting that the TPK activity of these proteins stimulates the PIP_2-PDE activity (Jackowski et al 1986) but it is also possible that the increased PIP_2-PDE is due to the induction by retrovirus infection of other cellular gene products. M-CSF induces expression of the c-fos gene in macrophages, probably via the induction of PKC, although cyclic AMP elevation also has this effect (Bravo et al 1986).

The levels of M-CSF receptor expressed at the surface of myeloid cells increases during differentiation, with mature macrophages expressing higher numbers (about 50 000 per cell) than earlier progenitors and it appears likely that M-CSF affects the survival and functioning of mature cells as well as the proliferation and differentiation of more primitive progenitors.

Mechanisms of growth signal transduction by IL3, GM-CSF, G-CSF and erythropoietin

The cell surface receptors for these growth factors have been identified and partially characterised by growth factor binding and cross-linking studies. The G-CSF (150 kDa) (Nicola & Peterson 1986) and the GM-CSF (130 kDa) receptors (Park et al 1986) are potentially large enough to include an intracytoplasmic kinase domain. However, the receptor for IL3 is of a smaller size (65–70 kDa) (Park et al 1986).

There is evidence that ligand binding to all these receptors stimulates protein phosphorylation events.

IL3

Treatment of IL3 dependent murine FDCP-1 cells with IL3 triggered the translocation of PKC from the cytosolic to the membrane fraction (Farrar et al 1985, Whetton et al 1987). Furthermore IL3 treatment of FDCP-1 cells stimulates phosphorylation of a 68 kDa cytosolic protein (p68) on threonine residues and this action is mimicked by DAG addition, also suggesting a role for PKC in this event (Evans et al 1986). PKC activation by TPA can partially replace the requirement for IL3 for the survival and proliferation of multipotent IL3 dependent murine progenitors, by mimicking the IL3 stimulated maintenance of glucose transport and ATP production (Whetton et al 1986). Binding of IL3 to cell surface receptors has also been shown to stimulate phosphorylation of a 67–69 kDa membrane protein on tyrosine and serine residues (Sorensen et al 1987). Although this protein has a molecular weight similar to that of the IL3 receptor, there is at present no direct evidence to suggest that it is the receptor. Phosphorylation of a 33 kDa protein in response to IL3 binding to IL3-dependent murine cell lines has also been reported (Garland 1988). A protein of the same molecular weight was constitutively phosphorylated in an IL3-independent, malignant subclone, but no firm evidence was presented that this protein was identical to the IL3-responsive substrate of the factor-dependent parent.

G-CSF, GM-CSF

Less is known about how G-CSF and GM-CSF signals are transmitted. Treatment of appropriate murine cell lines with G-CSF also caused the phosphorylation of a p68 on threonine residues (S. W. Evans et al 1987), and this phosphorylation event was also mimicked by DAG, implying the role of PKC in transduction of the G-CSF signal also. By contrast, GM-CSF did not stimulate p68 phosphorylation in a factor-responsive cell line, suggesting a different mechanism of signal transduction (S. W. Evans et al 1987).

Treatment of permeabilised HL60 human promyelocytic leukaemia cell line with agents which trigger differentiation to either granulocytes (G-CSF, GM-CSF) or to monocytes (tumour necrosis factor, γ interferon) stimulated very rapid (less than 2 minutes) phosphorylation of a 75 kDa protein on tyrosine and serine residues (Evans et al 1988). TPA did not elicit this phosphorylation, suggesting that PKC was not required at this stage of signal transduction. G-CSF, DMSO or agents which elevate cAMP, all of which induce granulocytic differentiation of HL60 cells, stimulated phosphorylation of a 22 kDa protein on serine residues only (Yamamoto et al 1988). This phosphorylation represents a later event than the p75 phosphorylation described above.

Erythropoietin

Little is known about signal transduction mechanisms utilised by erythropoietin. Treatment of erythroid cell membranes with this growth factor abolishes the phosphorylation on serine residues of a 43 kDa protein (Choi et al 1987). Tentative evidence suggests that this is due to inhibition of a kinase rather than the activation of a phosphatase. In erythroid cells transformed by Friend virus, erythropoietin stimulates Ca^{2+} flux (Sawyer & Krantz 1984).

Conclusion

It appears that growth factors acting on primitive haemopoietic progenitors may utilise similar biochemical mechanisms for the transduction of signals as those in fibroblasts and T lymphocytes. The stimulation of inositol lipid breakdown and the stimulation of phosphorylation of specific proteins by PKC, TPKs and by Ca^{2++}-dependent kinases will probably be established as common motifs in the regulation of proliferation of all cell types.

Signalling mechanisms in differentiation

In addition to stimulating the proliferation of progenitor cells haemopoietic growth factors trigger the differentiation of their target cells and are also required for the functioning of mature blood cells (see Ch. 1). Similar mechanisms (e.g. Ca^{2+} elevation, PKC activation and the expression of cellular proto-oncogenes) may operate both in triggering of proliferation and in the induction of differentiation accompanied by a withdrawal from the proliferative cycle. While this may appear at first sight paradoxical, these observations may reflect the use of common signalling mechanisms for different purposes in different cells or even in the same cells at different stages of development.

ABERRANT PROLIFERATION REGULATION MECHANISMS IN LEUKAEMIA

In principle, aberrations in genes encoding any of the components of the growth factor regulated pathways (proto-oncogenes) can lead to uncontrolled stimulation of cell proliferation and result in the transformation of a normal cell into a neoplastic one. Examples of relationships between proto-oncogenes and oncogenes are summarised in Table 2.2 and some of these are discussed further in the text. First, unregulated production of a growth factor by a cell which responds to it can lead to autocrine growth stimulation of that cell and its progeny. Second, a growth factor receptor or a non-receptor TPK which has constitutive rather than growth factor stimulated activity as a result of genetic alteration will trigger proliferation independent of growth factor control. Third, genetic alterations which lead to unregulated triggering of the intramembrane or intracellular biochemical growth control pathways (e.g. aberrant G proteins or de-regulated expression of c-myc or c-fos) will contribute to transformation. The normal growth factor stimulation of haemopoietic cells triggers not only proliferation but also differentiation of progenitors into non-dividing mature blood cells (see Ch. 1). Therefore, in order to convert a normal progenitor in a fully transformed cell it is necessary to impose a block on differentiation as well as to stimulate proliferation. This requirement is reflected in the multi-stage nature of leukaemogenesis, with activation of more than one proto-oncogene being required to produce complete malignant transformation. Model studies in which active oncogenes were introduced into haemopoietic progenitor cells have been instructive in understanding the leukaemogenic process, and will be summarised below.

Table 2.2 Relation of genes encoding components of growth regulatory pathways (proto-oncogenes) to altered genes implicated in neoplastic transformation (oncogenes). For further details and references see text and Heldin & Westermark (1984)

Identity and/or function of proto-oncogene product	Cellular location	Oncogene	Occurrence
A. *Growth factors* Platelet-derived growth factor	Extracellular	v-sis	Simian sarcoma virus
B. Growth factor receptors with *tyrosine kinase activity* EGF receptor M-CSF receptor	Transmembrane proteins	v-erbB v-fms	Avian erythroblastosis virus Feline sarcoma virus
C. *Non-receptor tyrosine kinase* (functions unknown)	Inner face of plasma membrane or cytosol	v-src v-abl phl-abl fusion genes encoding: p210$^{phl\text{-}abl}$ p190$^{phl\text{-}abl}$	Rous sarcoma virus Abelson murine leukaemia virus CGL ALL, Ph$^+$ AML
D. Guanine nucleotide-binding proteins (p21s) (may couple receptors to inositol lipid breakdown)	Inner face of plasma membrane	v-H-ras, v-K ras Oncogenically activated c-H-ras, c-K-ras, N-ras	Murine sarcoma viruses Leukaemias and other tumours; myelodysplasias
E. Proteins which mediate growth factor or hormonal regulation of nuclear events	Nucleus	v-myc v-fos Transcriptionally activated c-myc v-erbA (modified thyroid hormone receptor)	Avian myelocytomatosis virus FBJ murine osteosarcoma virus Burkitt's lymphoma Avian erythroblastosis virus

The consequences of introduction of activated oncogenes into haemopoietic cells

v-erbB is a truncated form of the epidermal growth factor receptor, which has lost its factor binding domain as well as its extreme carboxy-terminus (Downward et al 1984) and displays an unregulated TPK activity. The v-erbA gene is an altered form of the thyroid hormone receptor which displays hormone-independent ability to bind to chromatin (Greene et al 1986) and presumably to stimulate unregulated gene transcription. Infection of avian erythroid progenitors with avian erythroblastosis virus (AEV) carrying both v-erbA and v-erbB produces an erythroleukaemia that is independent of erythropoietin for in vitro growth (Beug et al 1982). Introduction of v-erbB alone results in cells which are not tightly blocked in differentiation and are able to proliferate to a limited extent only. While introduction of v-erbA alone does not transform cells, co-infection with v-erbB and v-erbA results in cells which are completely blocked in differentiation and fully transformed (Frykberg et al 1983). The v-erbA oncogene can also co-operate with other oncogenes with deregulated TPK activity (e.g. v-src, v-fps, v-sea) to produce a fully transformed phenotype. The v-H ras oncogene, an activated version of a G protein, can also co-operate with v-erbA in this experimental system. Again, introduction of v-src or v-fps in the absence of v-erbA transforms avian erythroid cells into lines with a limited lifespan of 20–30 generations and which can differentiate spontaneously.

A similar two-step transformation mechanism is a feature of the myeloid leukaemia caused by Friend murine leukaemia virus (FrMuLV) in mice. Stage I cells produced by infection with FrMuLV, can proliferate in diseased animals but are neither transplantable to syngeneic animals nor capable of in vitro growth in the absence of added growth factors, whereas stage II cells can do so. Stage I cells will, however, grow in vitro in the presence of multi-CSF (IL3). Superinfection of stage I cells with Abelson murine leukaemia virus, which contains the TPK oncogene v-abl, abrogates the growth factor requirement and simultaneously renders the cells leukaemogenic in secondary hosts (Oliff et al 1985). This suggests that stage I cells are blocked in differentiation but still dependent on exogenous growth factors. A second genetic event relieves factor dependence and results in a fully transformed cell.

In principle the abrogation of growth factor dependence by oncogenes of the TPK family could result either from the switching on of autocrine factor production or by the TPK activity of the oncogene product substituting for signals arising from the occupied receptor. Experimental observations suggest that both mechanisms may be operative. Chicken myeloid cells transformed by the oncogenes v-myb or v-myc require chicken myelomonocytic growth factor (cMGF) for growth in vitro. Superinfection with retroviruses containing the v-src, v-fps, v-yes or v-ros oncogenes (all of which encode TPKs) permit growth independent of added cMGF. Since antisera against cMGF block proliferation of the superinfected cells, it was suggested that factor independence resulted from autocrine secretion and utilisation of cMGF (Adkins et al 1984). Similarly, direct introduction of the GM-CSF gene into factor-dependent murine FDCP-1 cells using a retroviral vector results in autocrine GM-CSF production, autocrine growth and leukaemogenicity. However, by contrast to the above study, single GM-CSF-expressing FDC-P1 cells can proliferate in culture and antisera against GM-CSF do not block proliferation (Lang et al 1985), suggesting the intriguing possibility that the factor might interact with its receptor within an intracellular compartment.

Oncogenes other than those encoding TPKs can also confer autocrine growth properties. Avian macrophages transformed by the v-myc oncogene proliferate in vitro, presumably due to the unregulated production of v-myc protein, whose normal cellular homologue (c-myc) is induced by growth factor treatment (Table 2.2). However, these transformed macrophages require cMGF for growth, and this replacement is abolished by the simultaneous expression of the v-mos oncogene, whose product has serine/threonine kinase activity (Graf et al 1986). Factor independence was due to autocrine production of cMGF.

Myeloid cell lines established from normal bone marrow and dependent on multi-CSF or GM-CSF for in vitro growth are transformed to factor independence by retrovirus-mediated introduction of the v-abl oncogene (Cook et al 1985). Hybridisation analysis of mRNA or bioassay of supernatants failed to demonstrate autocrine growth factor production and antisera against multi-CSF do not block proliferation. It seems probable, therefore, that in these studies the v-abl oncogene product is directly activating biochemical pathways which are normally triggered by growth factor binding.

The relevance of these studies to human leukaemia is not established. Primary human myeloid leukaemias invariably require growth factors for clonal growth in vitro, but lose this requirement on prolonged culture or following serial transplantation. A degree of autocrine growth in vivo is not ruled out by these in vitro observations, since factors such as cell density in the in vivo environment may well influence the ability of leukaemic cells to build up sufficient levels of autocrine factors which influence their proliferation. Murine bone marrow progenitor cells propagated in vitro in the presence of growth factors are not leukaemogenic. Variants which secrete and utilise their own growth factors are tumorigenic. Notably, these cells still require exogenous growth factors for proliferation at low cell density, presumably due to their inability to condition the medium at high dilution (Schrader & Crapper 1983).

De-regulated tyrosine kinases in human leukaemia

Chronic granulocytic leukaemia (CGL) (see also Ch. 7)

The reciprocal translation between chromosome 9 and chromosome 22, generates an abnormal chromosome (Philadelphia chromosome, Ph'), which is a feature of about 90% of CGL cases (see Ch. 7 for details). As a result of the translocation the c-abl gene is moved from its normal position on chromosome 9 onto chromosome 22. The normal c-abl locus on chromosome 9 encodes a TPK of 145 kDa (Table 2.2). This p145 has no transmembrane region and is thus unlikely to be a growth factor receptor. The Philadelphia translocation results in the fusion of part of the c-abl gene with part of a gene known as the BCR or PHL gene on chromosome 22 (Heisterkamp et al 1985). The translocation breakpoints within the BCR gene in different CGL patients are almost without exception clustered in a 5.8 kilobase region, referred to as the breakpoint cluster region (bcr). This translocation results in the expression of a chimaeric 210 kDa bcr-abl-encoded protein with enhanced TPK activity.

It appears likely that enhanced tyrosine phosphorylation of key substrates may contribute to the neoplastic phenotype but this is not established. Fresh CGL leukaemic cells and cell lines established from patients with CGL contain a nearly identical spectrum of tyrosine phosphorylated proteins with a wide MW range (Naldini et al 1986, Huhn et al 1987). Two cell lines established from lymphoid or myeloid blast crises of CGL also contain tyrosine-phosphorylated proteins of identical MWs (J. P. M. Evans et al 1987a). However, there is no direct evidence that all or any of these proteins are substrates of the 210 kDa bcr-abl TPK, nor is it known which if any of these proteins plays a role in maintenance of the neoplastic state. Fresh chronic phase CGL cells contain only low amounts of TPK substrates. This was attributed to the down-regulation of expression of the p210 bcr-abl kinase during differentiation of the abnormal CGL progenitors, and is consistent with the complete lack of detectable TK substrates in mature granulocytes (Evans et al 1987b). Mouse fibroblasts expressing v-abl contain nuclear proteins phosphorylated on tyrosine residues, and which bind mouse DNA in preference to bacterial DNA (Bell et al 1987). It is possible, but unproven, that these proteins act as regulators of gene expression.

About 10% of CGL patients have no cytogenetically detectable Philadelphia chromosome. However, 5 out of 12 such patients were found to have a rearranged bcr (Ph⁻ bcr⁺) and were morphologically indistinguishable from Ph⁺ CGL. The remaining 7 were reclassified as atypical chronic myeloid leukaemia (CML) (6 patients) or chronic myelomonocytic leukaemia (CMML) (1 patient) (Wiedemann et al 1988). While cells from 11 cases of bcr⁻ CGL had no detectable 210 kDa TPK, 3 Ph⁺ bcr⁺ cases and 4 Ph⁻ bcr⁺ were positive for this protein. Two CGL patients with variant (t(10;22),t(11,22)) and 2 with complex (t(9;11;22),t(9;14;22)) translocations had bcr rearrangements indicating that a chimaeric bcr-abl gene may also be present in these cases (Browett et al 1988b). Therefore, bcr⁺ CGL is associated with p210 expression, regardless of whether the Philadelphia chromosome is detectable cytogenetically. Furthermore, Ph⁻ bcr⁻ CGL in one study was distinguished from Ph⁺ bcr⁺ and Ph⁻ bcr⁺ CML by careful clinical and morphological evaluation (Wiedemann et al 1988).

A chromosomally identical t(9:22) variant translocation in a proportion of Ph⁺ acute lymphoblastic leukaemia (ALL) cases results from a breakpoint on chromosome 22 which is upstream from the bcr region (bcr⁻) but within the BCR gene. This results in the expression of a different chimaeric abl related protein of enhanced TPK activity and molecular weight 190 kDa (Kurzrock et al 1987a, Chan et al 1987) (see also Ch. 7). It has been suggested that Ph⁺ bcr⁺ p210 ALL may represent blast transformation of CGL and that Ph⁺ bcr⁻ p190 ALL de novo ALL (Chan et al 1987). However, Secker-Walker et al (1988) found no differences in clinical, cytogenetic or blast cell features between bcr⁺ and bcr⁻ cases of Ph⁺ ALL. A single patient with the rare Ph⁺ AML has also been shown to express a 190 kDa chimaeric abl protein indistinguishable from that seen in Ph⁺ ALL (Kurzrock et al 1987b).

AML, ALL, CLL (Acute myeloid, acute lymphoblastic, chronic lymphocytic leukaemia)
Cells from patients with AML, ALL or CLL contain a similar set of high M.W. (100–200 kDa) proteins phosphorylated on tyrosine residues (J. P. M. Evans et al 1987b). These proteins have MWs similar to tyrosine phosphorylated proteins present in mitogen-stimulated T lymphocytes but absent in non-activated T-cells which show lower MW substrates (40–60 kDa) only. Furthermore, normal bone marrow cells also contain substrates restricted to the 40–60 kDa range. It is unclear whether any of these substrates are involved in driving de-regulated proliferation of the leukaemia cells or are simply markers of the proliferation or differentiation state of the cell. It is also unknown whether these substrates detected in the leukaemic cells are

phosphorylated by structurally aberrant activated TPKs or by normal TPKs activated in turn by aberrant upstream regulatory elements. Clearly, the identification of the substrates of TPKs and their characterisation at the biochemical level are important future areas for investigation.

The M-CSF receptor gene in leukaemia

The gene encoding the M-CSF receptor is located on the long arm of chromosone 5 (5q 33–34). Deletions of the region are associated with refractory anaemia, myelo-dysplastic syndrome and therapy-related AML. In some instances the loss of the receptor gene has been demonstrated directly by hybridisation to c-fms gene probes and genes for IL3 and GM-CSF are also lost from chromosome 5 in all cases (Le Beau et al 1986). The contribution of this aberration to the disease phenotype, however, remains to be established. One possibility is that the M-CSF signal stimulates differen-tiation as well as proliferation and therefore cells with reduced M-CSF receptor expres-sion may be blocked in differentiation. However, the role of the remaining M-CSF gene on the normal allele remains to be elucidated.

Mouse myeloblastic leukaemias induced by infection with Friend murine leukaemia virus often contain the viral genome inserted adjacent to the c-fms gene, resulting in enhanced expression of c-fms (Gisselbrecht et al 1987). This is consistent with leukaemic cell proliferation being driven by the abnormal level of c-fms expression, although it is not known whether the tumour cells also produce CSF-1 (the murine equivalent of M-CSF) in an autocrine fashion.

The activation of ras genes in leukaemia

Some activated oncogenes may be detected by introduction of DNA from tumour cells into established cultures of rodent fibroblasts, and assaying for the ability of the introduced DNA to confer a transformed phenotype to the recipient cells (transfec-tion assay). The majority of activated oncogenes detected in this way belong to a closely related family, the ras family (reviewed by Barbacid 1987). The family consists of three members, designated H-ras, K-ras and N-ras, and activated versions of the first two have also been detected as the transforming genes of the Harvey and Kirsten murine sarcoma viruses. All three ras genes encode proteins of 21 kDa (p21), which can bind guanine nucleotides thus resembling other known G proteins in their proper-ties (Table 2.2). The p21 proteins are attached to the inner surface of the plasma membrane by virtue of covalent binding to a palmitic acid residue at the carboxy terminus. Recent evidence suggests that the product of the normal (i.e. non-oncogenic) allele of N-ras acts as a G protein coupling the stimulation of the bombesin receptor to the generation of second messengers via hydrolysis of inositol phospholipids (Wake-lam et al 1986).

Activation of ras is due to a single point mutation, usually resulting in the substitu-tion of amino acids at positions 12, 13, 59 or 61 (Barbacid 1987). These mutations drastically reduce the GTPase activity of the p21s presumably leading to a prolonged trapping of the p21 in the activated form, hence causing prolonged or excessive signal-ling (Fig. 2.3). The transformation of murine fibroblasts by ras oncogenes leads to changes in inositol lipid metabolism consistent with activation of PIP_2-PDE and result-ing in increased levels of DAG and inositol phosphates (Fleischman et al 1986). Micro-injection of the p21 protein encoded by the H-ras oncogene into Xenopus oocytes rapidly stimulated the breakdown of inositol phospholipids, whereas the product of the normal (non-mutant) H-ras allele did not (Lacal et al 1987) suggesting that p21 proteins with impaired GTPase activity could stimulate PIP_2 breakdown independently of external stimulation.

As mentioned earlier a soluble GTPase activator protein (GAP) has recently been shown to markedly stimulate the GTPase activity of normal ras proteins (Trahey & McCormick 1987). GAP does not stimulate the GTPase activity of oncogenic ras p21 (Cales et al 1988). Site-directed mutagenesis of amino acids in the region 35–40 also destroy the ability of GAP to stimulate the GTPase of normal p21ras (Cales et al 1988). Mutations in this region also destroy the transforming potential of oncogenic p21 ras, while leaving its membrane localization and GTP binding capacity unaltered. Taken together these data suggest that GAP may serve as the target or effector for both normal and oncogenic p21 ras and that amino acids 35–40 of p21 ras interact with GAP. However, the alternative possibility that GAP may act upstream of ras by coupling growth factor receptors to the ras protein cannot be eliminated at present (Sigal 1988).

Of a number of myeloid leukaemia cell lines tested, three contained activated ras genes as detected by transfection assay. The HL60 (myelocytic leukaemia) and Rc2a (myelomonocytic leukaemia) and KG-1 (acute myeloid leukaemia) lines contained activated N-ras alleles (Janssen et al 1985). DMSO-induced granulocytic differentiation of HL60 cells was associated with a decrease in inositol lipid-derived second messengers which preceded cessation of proliferation, suggesting that abnormal production of these substances, possibly triggered by activation of PIP_2-PDE by the mutant N-ras protein, may have contributed to the autonomous proliferation of the cell line (Porfiri et al 1988).

ras gene activation is often an early, but not necessarily the first, event in neoplastic transformation. However, additional genetic events are required for the expression of a fully malignant phenotype. Bone marrow cells from 3 of 8 patients studied with myelodysplastic syndrome (MDS) had N-ras alleles with mutations in codon 13, and all 3 patients developed leukaemia within 1 year (Hirai et al 1987). In another study 10 of 58 patients with MDS were found to contain N-ras genes mutated at codons 12 or 13. Patients with mutations had significantly worse prognoses, with shorter survival times, than patients without detectable mutant N-ras genes (Padua et al 1987). In the same study, a patient with chronic myelomonocytic leukaemia had detectable levels of mutant N-ras, which became undetectable following evolution to AML, possibly suggesting that the AML arose from a different progenitor cell to that affected in the earlier chronic phase. Layton et al (1988) report a lower incidence of ras mutations (3/34) in MDS and found it to have no prognostic significance.

ras genes are frequently activated in AML (Eva et al 1983). Bos et al (1985) found that leukaemic cells from 5 of 6 AML patients studied contained N-ras genes which were oncogenically activated by mutation at codon 13. Peripheral blood cells from one of these patients in remission did not contain the mutation.

In a recent study using the sensitive polymerase chain reaction method, Farr et al (1988) found that 14 out of 52 (27%) of AML cell DNAs contained activated N-ras genes. The mutation was undetectable in the peripheral blood from 2 of these patients in remission. Surprisingly, DNA taken at relapse from 4 patients whose presentation samples contained activated N-ras genes were negative for these alleles, suggesting that the relapse originated in persistent preleukaemic clones which did not harbour activated N-ras genes. It is thus unlikely that N-ras activation was the initiating leukaemogenic event, at least in these 4 patients, but was instead part of the clonal evolution of the disease.

Activation of ras genes is less frequent in ALL than AML, but also appears to involve N-ras (Eva et al 1983). In a recent survey of 48 cases of CLL, no instances of activation of the K-ras oncogene were detected, whereas K-ras activation in both AML (1/11) and ALL (1/7) were seen in the same study (Browett et al 1988a).

The genetic changes underlying the transition from chronic phase CGL to blast crisis have not been defined. In a recent study activated ras genes were surprisingly detected in leukaemic cells from 1 of 6 patients in blast crisis (2 H-ras, 1 N-ras), and in 1 of 6 cases in chronic phase (Liu et al 1988). The higher incidence of ras gene activation in blast crisis suggests that ras gene activation may accompany blast transformation in some cases of CGL, but that it may be an early event in others. An activated oncogene of unknown origin was also detected in single examples of chronic phase and of blast crisis CGL (Liu et al 1988). The findings of Liu et al (1988) need confirmation.

The c-myc gene in Burkitt's lymphoma

The t(8;14) chromosomal translocation in Burkitt's lymphoma results in the juxtaposition of the c-myc gene and the immunoglobulin heavy chain locus. Molecular details of this translocation are described by Russo et al (Ch. 6). The translocation probably disrupts the normal growth factor-regulated expression of this gene (Kelly et al 1983) and allows its constitutive expression due to the operation of B lymphocyte-specific enhancer elements in the immunoglobulin locus, whose normal function is to drive transcription of the heavy chain genes. Transgenic mice, all of whose cells contained an enhancer-c-myc construction introduced at the fertilised egg stage developed B lymphoid malignancies, consistent with B cell-specific expression of the myc gene driven by the juxtaposed enhancer element (Adams et al 1985). However, these tumours were clonal, whereas all the B cells contained the enhancer-c-myc construct, indicating that increased c-myc expression alone did not result in neoplasia. In fact, young transgenic mice containing the construct have an expanded, non-malignant polyclonal B cell population, suggesting that further genetic events were required for the evolution of the malignant state (Langdon et al 1986).

CONCLUDING REMARKS

This review has focused on the biochemical mechanisms involved in the transduction of proliferative signals in normal haemopoietic cells. Model experiments involving the introduction of activated oncogenes into progenitor cells have also been described and show that aberrant versions of the proteins involved in normal growth control can perturb regulation and result in a malignant phenotype. Activation of oncogenes in naturally occurring human leukaemia has also been studied and some well-defined examples have been detailed in this and other chapters.

ACKNOWLEDGEMENTS

We thank the Cancer Research Campaign of Great Britain and the Kay Kendall Leukaemia Fund for financial support. We are grateful to Mrs Megan Evans for invaluable assistance in preparation of the manuscript.

REFERENCES

Adams J M, Harris A W, Pinkert C A et al 1985 Nature 318: 533–538
Adkins B, Leutz A, Graf T 1984 Cell 39: 439–445
Barbacid M 1987 Annual Review of Biochemistry 56: 779–827
Bell J C, Mahadevan L C, Colledge W H, Frackleton A R, Sargent M G, Foulkes J G 1987 Nature 325: 552–554
Bertics P J, Gill G N 1985 Journal of Biological Chemistry 266: 14642–14647
Beug H, Palmieri S, Freudenstein C, Zentgraf H, Graf T 1982 Cell 28: 907–919
Bockus B J, Stiles C D 1984 Experimental Cell Research 153: 186–197
Bos J L, Toksoz D, Marshall C J et al 1985 Nature 315: 726–730
Boynton A L, Whitfield J F 1983 Advances in Cyclic Nucleotide Research 15: 193–294
Bravo R, Neuberg M, Burckhardt J, Almendral J, Wallich R, Muller R 1986 Cell 48: 251–260
Broome H E, Reed J C, Godillot E P, Hoover R G 1987 Molecular and Cellular Biology 7: 2988–2993
Browett P J, Ganeshaguru K, Hoffbrand A V, Norton J D 1988a Leukemia Research 12: 25–31
Browett P J, Cooke H M, Secker-Walker L M, Norton J D 1988b British Journal of Haematology (in press)
Browning P J, Bunn H F, Cline A, Shuman M, Nienhuis A W 1986 Proceedings of the National Academy of Sciences USA 83: 7800–7804
Cales C, Hancock J F, Marshall C J, Hall A 1988 Nature 332: 548–551
Cantrell D A, Smith K A 1984 Science 224: 1312–1316
Cantrell D A, Davies A A, Crumpton M J 1985 Proceedings of the National Academy of Sciences USA 82: 8158–8162
Chan L C, Karhi K K, Rayter S I et al 1987 Nature 325: 635–637
Chiu R, Imagawa M, Imbra R J, Bockoven J R, Karin M 1987 Nature 329: 648–651
Choi H-S, Wojchowski D M, Sytkowski A J 1987 Journal of Biological Chemistry 262: 2933–2936
Cook W D, Metcalf D, Nicola N A, Burgess A W, Walker F 1985 Cell 41: 677–683
Crossin K L, Carney D H 1981 Cell 23: 61–71
De la Hera A, Toribio M L, Marcos M A R, Marquez C, Martinez A C 1987 European Journal of Immunology 17: 683–687
Downward J, Yarden Y, Mayes E et al 1984 Nature 307: 521–527
Dukovich M, Wano Y, Bich Thuy L et al 1987 Nature 327: 518–522
Eva A, Tronick S, Gol R A, Pierce J H, Aaronson S A 1983 Proceedings of the National Academy of Sciences USA 80: 4926–4930
Evans J P M, Wickremasinghe R G, Hoffbrand A V 1987a Leukemia 1: 524–525
Evans J P M, Wickremasinghe R G, Hoffbrand A V 1987b Leukemia 1: 782–785
Evans J P M, Mire-Sluis A R, Hoffbrand A V, Wickremasinghe R G 1988 British Journal of Haematology (in press) (Abstract)
Evans S W, Rennick D, Farrar W L 1986 Blood 68: 906–913
Evans S W, Rennick D, Farrar W L 1987 Biochemical Journal 244: 683–691
Farr C J, Saiki R K, Erlich H A, McCormick F, Marshall C J 1988 Proceedings of the National Academy of Sciences USA 85: 1629–1633
Farrar W L, Thomas T P, Anderson W B 1985 Nature 315: 235–237
Farrar W L, Ruscetti F W 1986 Journal of Immunology 136: 1266–1273
Fleischman L F, Chahwala S B, Cantley L 1986 Science 231: 407–410
Franza B R, Rauscher F J, Josephs S F, Curran T 1988 Science 239: 1150–1153
Frykberg L, Palmieri S, Beug H, Graf T, Hayman M J, Vennstrom B 1983 Cell 32: 227–238
Fuji M, Sugamura K, Sano K, Nakai M, Sugita K, Hinuma Y 1986 Journal of Experimental Medicine 163: 550–562
Garland J M 1988 Leukemia 2: 94–102
Gelfand E W, Mills G B, Cheung R K, Lee J W W, Grinstein S 1987 Immunological Reviews 95: 59–87
Gisselbrecht S, Fischelson S, Sola B et al 1987 Nature 329: 259–261
Graf T, Weiszaecker F V, Grieser S et al 1986 Cell 45: 357–364
Grausz J D, Fradelizi D, Dautry F, Monier R, Lehn P 1986 European Journal of Immunology 16: 1217–1221
Greenberg M E, Ziff E B 1984 Nature 311: 433–438
Greene S, Walter P, Kumar V et al 1986 Nature 320: 134–139
Habenicht A J R, Glomset J A, King W C, Nist C, Mitchell C D, Ross R 1981 Journal of Biological Chemistry 256: 12329–12335
Hall B, Hoffbrand A V, Wickremasinghe R G 1987 FEBS Letters 223: 6–10
Hasegawa-Sasaki H, Sasaki T 1983 Biochimica et Biophysica Acta 754: 305–314
Heikkila R, Schwab G, Wickstrom E et al 1987 Nature 328: 445–449
Heisterkamp N, Stam K, Groffen J, deKlein A, Grosveld G 1985 Nature 315: 758–761
Heldin C-H, Westermark B 1984 Cell 37: 9–20

Heldin C-H, Betsholtz C, Johnsson A et al 1985 Journal of Cell Science Supplement 3: 65–76
Hirai M, Kobayishi Y, Mano H et al 1987 Nature 327: 430–432
Holt J T, Venkat Gopal T, Moulton A D, Nienhuis A W 1986 Proceedings of the National Academy of Sciences USA 83: 4794–4798
Huhn R D, Posner M R, Rayter S I, Foulkes J G, Frackleton A R 1987 Proceedings of the National Academy of Sciences USA 84: 4468–4412
Hunter T, Cooper J A 1985 Reviews in Biochemistry 54: 897–930
Imboden J B, Stobo J D 1985 Journal of Experimental Medicine 161: 446–456
Irvine R F, Moor R M 1986 Biochemical Journal 240: 917–920
Ishii T, Kohno M, Nakamura H, Hinuma Y, Sugamura K 1987 Biochemical Journal 242: 211–219
Jackowski S, Rettenmeier C W, Sherr C J, Rock C O 1986 Journal of Biological Chemistry 261: 4978–4985
Janssen J W G, Steenvoorden A C M, Collard J G, Nusse R 1985 Cancer Research 45: 3262–3267
Kaplan D R, Whitman M, Schaffhausen B 1987 Cell 50: 1021–1029
Kelly K, Cochran B H, Stiles C D, Leder P 1983 Cell 35: 603–610
Klarlund J 1985 Cell 41: 707–717
Kurzrock R, Shtalrid M, Romero P et al 1987a Nature 325: 631–635
Kurzrock R, Shtalrid M, Talpaz M, Kloetzer W S, Gutterman J U 1987b Blood 70: 1584–1588
Lacal J C, De La Pena P, Moscat J, Garcia-Barreno P, Anderson P S, Aaronson S A 1987 Science 238: 533–536
Lang R A, Metcalf D, Gough N M, Dunn A R, Gonda T J 1985 Cell 43: 531–541
Langdon W Y, Harris A W, Cory S, Adams J M 1986 Cell 47: 11–18
Layton D M, Lyons J, Janssen J W G, Bartram C R, Mufti G J 1988 British Journal of Haematology 69: 121(a)
Le Beau M M, Westbrook C A, Diaz M O et al 1986 Science 231: 984–987
Liu E, Hjelle B, Bishop J M 1988 Proceedings of the National Academy of Sciences USA 85: 1952–1956
Macara I G 1985 American Journal of Physiology 248: C3–C11
Marth J D, Peet R, Krebs E G, Perlmutter R M 1985 Cell 43: 393–404
Matrisian L M, Rodland K D, Magun B D 1987 Journal of Biological Chemistry 262: 6908–6913
Mayer B J, Hamaguchi M, Hanafusa H 1988 Nature 332: 272–275
Mire A R, Wickremasinghe R G, Michalevicz R, Hoffbrand A V 1985 Biochimica et Biophysica Acta 847: 159–163
Mire A R, Wickremasinghe R G, Hoffbrand A V 1986a Biochemical and Biophysical Research Communications 137: 128–134
Mire A R, Wickremasinghe R G, Hoffbrand A V 1986b FEBS Letters 206: 53–58
Mire-Sluis A R, Hoffbrand A V, Wickremasinghe R G 1987a Biochemical and Biophysical Research Communications 148: 1223–1231
Mire-Sluis A R, Wickremasinghe R G, Hoffbrand A V, Timms A M, Francis G E 1987b Immunology 60: 7–12
Moore J P, Todd J A, Hesketh T R, Metcalfe J C 1986 Journal of Biological Chemistry 261: 8158–8162
Naldini L, Stacchini A, Cirillo D M, Aglietta M, Gavosto F, Comoglio P M 1986 Molecular and Cellular Biology 6: 1803–1822
Nicola N A, Peterson L 1986 Journal of Biological Chemistry 261: 12384–12389
Nishizuka Y 1986 Science 233: 305–312
Oliff A, Agranovsky O, McKinney M D, Murty, V V V S, Bauchwitz R 1985 Proceedings of the National Academy of Sciences USA 82: 3306–3310
Padua R A, Carter G, Hughes D et al 1987 Blood 70 (Supplement 1) 284a (abstract No 990)
Pantaleo G, Olive D, Poggi A, Kozumbo W J, Moretta L, Moretta A 1987 European Journal of Immunology 17: 55–60
Park L S, Friend D, Gillis S, Urdal D L 1986 Journal of Biological Chemistry 261: 4177–4183
Patel M D, Samelson L E, Klausner R D 1987 Journal of Biological Chemistry 262: 5831–5838
Porfiri E Hoffbrand A V, Wickremasinghe R G 1988 Experimental Hematology (in press)
Rozengurt E, Rodriguez-Pena M, Smith K A 1983a Proceedings of the National Academy of Sciences USA 80: 7244–7248
Roussel M F, Dull T J, Rettenmeier C W, Ralph P, Ullrich A, Sherr C J 1987 Nature 325: 549–552
Samelson L E, Patel M D, Weissman A M, Harford J B, Klausner R D 1986 Cell 46: 1083–1090
Sasaki T, Hasegawa-Sasaki H 1987 FEBS Letters 218: 87–92
Sawyer S T, Krantz S B 1984 Journal of Biological Chemistry 259: 2769–2774
Schrader J W, Crapper R M 1983 Proceedings of the National Academy of Sciences USA 80: 6892–6896
Secker-Walker L M, Cooke H M G, Browett P J et al 1988 Blood (in press)
Sherr C J, Rettenmeier C W, Sacca R, Roussel M F, Look A T, Stanley E R 1985 Cell 41: 665–676
Sigal I S 1988 Nature 332: 485–486
Sorensen P, Mui A, Murthy S, Krystal G 1987 Blood 70 (Supplement 1) 186a (abstract No 598)

Studzinski G P, Brelvi Z S, Feldman S C, Watt R A 1986 Science 234: 467–470
Trahey M, McCormick F 1987 Science 238: 542–545
Treisman R 1986 Cell 46: 567–574
Truneh A, Albert F, Golstein P, Schmitt-Verhulst A-M 1985 Nature 313: 318–320
Tsien R Y, Pozzan T, Rink T J 1982 Nature 295: 68–71
Tsuda T, Hamamori Y, Yamashita T, Fukimoto Y, Takai Y 1986 FEBS Letters 208: 39–42
Wakelam M J O, Davies S A, Houslay M D, McKay I, Marshall C J, Hall A 1986 Nature 323: 173–176
Wedner H J, Bass G 1986 Journal of Immunology 136: 4226–4231
Wheeler E F, Rettenmeier C W, Look A T, Sherr C J 1986 Nature 342: 377–380
Whetton A D, Monk P N, Consalvey S D, Huang S J, Dexter T M, Downes C P 1988 Proceedings of the National Academy of Sciences USA 85: 3284–3288
Wickremasinghe R G, Mire-Sluis A R, Hoffbrand A V 1987 FEBS Letters 220: 52–56
Wiedemann L M, Karhi K K, Shivji M K K et al 1988 Blood 71: 349–355
Yamamoto M, Nishimura J, Ideguchi H, Ibayashi H 1988 Leukemia Research 12: 71–80

3. The thalassaemias

S. L. Thein   D. J. Weatherall

Since the last edition of Recent Advances in Haematology steady progress has been made in determining the molecular basis of the thalassaemias and in relating the underlying defects at the DNA level to the associated clinical phenotypes. This information has been applied successfully to the first trimester prenatal diagnosis of these conditions. And the advent of DNA technology has given a new lease of life to the study of the population genetics of the thalassaemias and how these conditions have reached their extraordinarily high gene frequencies in different populations. These topics will form the main part of this review. For more extensive coverage of the clinical and genetic aspects of thalassaemia, and its management, the reader is referred to several recent monographs and reviews (Collins & Weissman 1984, Bunn & Forget 1986, Weatherall et al 1988).

THE GENETIC CONTROL OF NORMAL HUMAN HAEMOGLOBIN

All the human haemoglobins have a tetrameric structure made up of two different pairs of globin chains. Adult and fetal haemoglobins have α chains combined with β chains (Hb A, $\alpha_2\beta_2$), δ chains (Hb A$_2$, $\alpha_2\delta_2$) or γ chains (Hb F, $\alpha_2\gamma_2$) (Fig. 3.1).

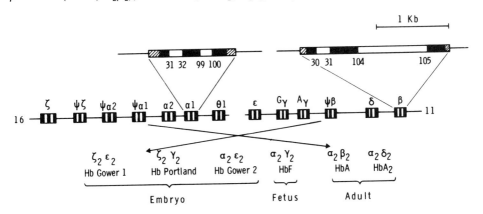

Fig. 3.1 The genetic control of human haemoglobin.

In embryos α-like chains called ζ chains combine with γ chains to produce Hb Portland ($\zeta_2\gamma_2$), or with ε chains to make Hb Gower 1 ($\zeta_2\varepsilon_2$), and α and ε chains combine to form Hb Gower 2 ($\alpha_2\varepsilon_2$). Fetal haemoglobin is heterogeneous; there are two types of γ chains which differ in their amino acid composition at position 136 where they have either glycine or alanine — those with glycine are called $^G\gamma$ chains and those with alanine are called $^A\gamma$ chains.

The α-like globin genes form a linked cluster on chromosome 16 (Fig. 3.1). Those genes denoted ψ are pseudogenes, that is they have sequences that resemble the functional ζ or α genes but which contain mutations which prevent them functioning as structural loci. They may be evolutionary remnants of once active genes. The α gene cluster contains no less than four pseudogenes, $\psi\zeta$, $\psi\alpha1$, $\psi\alpha2$, and θ. The latter has only been discovered recently (Marks et al 1986) and is remarkably conserved in different species. Although it appears to be expressed in early fetal life (Leung et al 1987) its function is unknown; it seems unlikely that it can produce a viable globin chain. Recent studies have shown that the α globin gene cluster is remarkably polymorphic (Higgs et al 1986). It contains a number of single base restriction fragment length polymorphisms (RFLPs), and several hypervariable regions, one downstream from the $\alpha1$ gene and the other between the ζ and $\psi\zeta$ genes. Both these regions have been sequenced (Goodbourne et al 1983, Jarman et al 1986) and they consist of a varying number of tandem repeats of nucleotide sequences. Taken together the single base RFLPs and hypervariable regions produce a level of heterozygosity of approximately 0.95, i.e. it is possible to identify individual α globin gene clusters in the majority of individuals.

The arrangement of the β globin gene cluster on the short arm of chromosome 11 is shown in Figure 3.1. Like the α globin genes this cluster contains a series of single point RFLPs although in this case no hypervariable regions have been identified. The arrangement of RFLPs, or haplotype, in the β globin gene cluster seems to fall into two domains (Antonarakis et al 1982). On the 5' side of the β gene, spanning about 32 kb from the ε gene to the 3' end of the $\psi\beta$ gene, there are three common patterns of RFLPs; those found in Mediterranean and Asian populations are similar. In the region containing about 18 kb to the 3' side of the β globin gene there are three common patterns in Mediterranean populations. Between these regions there is a DNA sequence of about 11 kb in which there is randomisation of the 5' and 3' domains and hence where a relatively higher rate of recombination may occur. Recent studies indicate that the β globin gene haplotypes are similar in most populations although differ markedly in individuals of African origin; these studies have been analysed in terms of the evolutionary development of different populations and are consistent with data obtained from mitochondrial DNA polymorphisms which point to the early emergence of a relatively small population from Africa with subsequent divergence into other racial groups (Wainscoat et al 1986).

Structural features of the globin genes

All globin genes contain two introns in identical positions relative to the coding sequence but of variable length, the shortest being the first of the α gene at 117 base pairs; the largest being 1264 base pairs in IVS1 of the ζ gene. Sequence analysis of the β-like genes shows very little homology among the larger IVS2 introns except in the case of the duplicated $^G\gamma$ and $^A\gamma$ genes, and only patchy homology among the smaller IVS1 introns. Comparison of the sequences of introns from many different genes shows only a few common features, most notably in the sequences immediately adjacent to and around the coding sequences they interrupt. At the 5' exon/intron junction the sequence GT is always present, while at the 3' junction the sequence AG is invariate.

The regions flanking the coding sequences of globin genes contain a number of conserved sequences that are essential for their expression. The first is the ATA box, which serves to accurately locate the site of transcription initiation at the CAP site, usually about 30 bases downstream, and which also appears to influence the level of transcription. In addition there are two so-called upstream promotor elements; 70 or 80 base pairs upstream is a second conserved sequence, the CCAAT box, and further 5', approximately 80–100 bp from the CAP site is a GC-rich region with a sequence that can be either inverted or duplicated. These sequences are also those required for optimal transcription, and as we shall see later mutations in this region of the β globin gene cause its defective expression.

Globin gene expression

The steps in globin gene synthesis are outlined in Figure 3.2. Transcription initiates

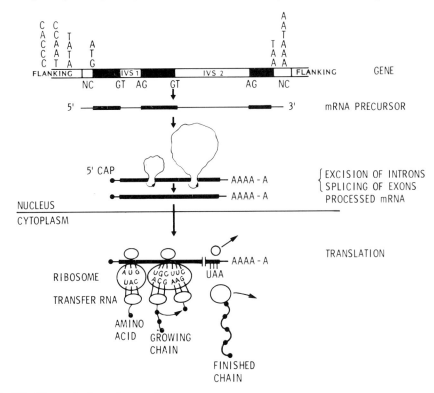

Fig. 3.2   The mechanisms of gene action.

at the CAP site which is approximately 50 base pairs upstream from the AUG initiation codon, and which forms the 5' end of the processed messenger RNA. Although processed mRNA terminates 10–20 base pairs downstream of the AATAAA polyadenylation signal sequence (see below) the initial transcript may run well beyond this site, and cleavage distal to the polyadenylation signal may take place subsequently.

The primary transcript is a large precursor mRNA containing both intron and exon sequences. During its stay in the nucleus it undergoes a good deal of processing. This entails 'capping' the 5' end and polyadenylation of the 3' end, both of which probably serve to stabilise the transcript. Capping involves a GTP mediated modification of the 5' residue while polyadenylation results in the addition of a long string of A residues to the 3' end of the transcript formed by cleavage of the initial precursor about 10–20 bp downstream of the AATAAA signal site (Fig. 3.2). Next the intervening sequences are removed from the mRNA precursor in a complex two-stage process. First, the mRNA precursor is cut at the 5' splice site to generate two intermediates, a linear first exon and a branched lariat-type molecule containing the intron and second exon. Then the 3' splice site is cleaved, the lariat intron released, and the two exons joined together. It seems likely that introns are removed in a sequential manner in this way until the mature messenger RNA is produced. The latter is then transported from the nucleus to the cytoplasm where ribosomal translation of mRNA to globin can take place. Details of the translational phase of globin chain synthesis are outlined in Figure 3.2 and have been extensively reviewed (Collins & Weissman 1984, Choi et al 1986).

Regulation of globin gene expression
There is very little known about the mechanisms involved in the regulation of globin gene expression. It appears that it is mediated mainly at the level of transcription, with some fine tuning during translation and the association of the globin subunits. Any scheme for the regulation of globin gene expression must take into account the fact that globin genes are expressed only in haemopoietic cells, and that different genes are expressed at particular stages of erythroid maturation and at different times during fetal development. While little is known about how these control mechanisms are mediated some recent progress has been made in determining the structure of expressed and unexpressed globin genes.

It is now clear that the methylation state of a gene has important influence on its ability to be expressed; actively transcribed genes are almost always hypomethylated and vice verse (Weisbrod 1982, Busslinger et al 1983). In human and other animal tissues globin genes are extensively methylated in nonerythroid organs and are relatively undermethylated while they are being expressed. For example in the 5' flanking region of the human γ genes, CG sites within the CCAAT-ATA region are hypomethylated in fetal liver erythroid cells but become methylated in adult bone marrow where haemoglobin F expression is turned off. However, hypomethylation of 5' flanking DNA is not the primary signal for gene expression, since situations are known where globin genes are hypomethylated but not expressed. Rather, it appears that the state of methylation is more of a permissive controller of gene expression than a positive expression signal.

Genes in mammalian cells contain DNA complexed with histones and other proteins to form chromatin. One of the results of this packaging of DNA is that the transcriptional activity of the genome is limited. This is reflected by changes in chromatin structure which can be identified experimentally by variability in sensitivity to digestion by nucleases such as DNAse I. This has been studied in detail in erythroid cells of chickens and several different DNAse I sensitivity states have been defined. First, there is increased sensitivity affecting a considerable region of DNA surrounding the active gene, indicating that the whole region is capable of being expressed. Secondly, there is a more specific region of greater sensitivity that correlates with active transcription, and, finally, DNAse I hypersensitive sites that occur are usually found in 5' flanking sequences of actively transcribed genes. Increased sensitivity to DNAse I seems to be related to the binding of a group of non-histone proteins

(HMG or high mobility groups) to the active gene. Experiments in normal human erythroid cells support the view that DNAse I sensitivity is associated with globin gene expression. Thus it appears that the activity of globin genes is associated with a change in chromatin configuration which appears to precede gene expression rather than to initiate it. And these observations parallel the changes in methylation status described earlier.

There is increasing evidence that the globin genes also come under the influence of so-called *trans*-acting factors. Thus a variety of gene transfer experiments using neoplastic cell lines that appear to be 'frozen' at different stages of development suggest that these cells may contain developmental-stage-specific *trans*-acting factors which are capable of activating globin genes that normally are expressed at particular stages of maturation. To date, none of these factors has been isolated, so that their mode of action, which may well involve specific DNA binding, remains to be determined.

Thus although a start has been made in defining the anatomy of globin gene activation very little is known about how this is controlled. It is clear that the promotor sites are involved in efficient transcription of the globin genes and that the latter may be regulated by stage specific *trans*-acting factors. In addition however there is evidence that other sequences are involved, particularly in the tissue-specific expression of the globin genes. There is evidence for the existence of so-called enhancer sequences which are thought to act by coming into spatial apposition with the promotor sequences to increase the efficiency of transcription of the particular genes. A number of putative enhancer sequences for the human globin genes have been defined although their precise role in the regulation and specificity of expression of the genes remains to be determined (Bodine & Ley 1987).

It is against this incomplete understanding of how the globin genes are regulated that the results of the different mutations which constitute the underlying pathology of the thalassaemia syndromes must be interpreted. Fortunately however, most of the thalassaemias that have been analysed to date seem to involve simple mutations of the exons or critical regions of the introns; the only lesions that involve regulatory sequences are those which lie within or near to the promotor elements at the 5' end of the β or γ globin genes.

THE DIFFERENT FORMS OF THALASSAEMIA

The genetic disorders of haemoglobin are divided into the structural haemoglobin variants and thalassaemias. The thalassaemias are characterised by a reduced rate of synthesis of one or more of the globin chains, and are classified into α, β, $\delta\beta$ and $\gamma\delta\beta$ types. The α and β thalassaemias are further subdivided into α° and β° forms in which no α or β chains are produced, and α^+ and β^+ forms in which some α or β chains are synthesised but at a reduced rate. The defective synthesis of one pair of globin subunits leads to imbalanced globin chain production; the characteristic abnormalities of red cell maturation and survival are caused by precipitation of the chains that are produced in excess (see Weatherall & Clegg 1981). In addition there is a group of mutations that interfere with the switching of fetal to adult haemoglobin production, known collectively as 'hereditary persistence of fetal haemoglobin' (HPFH). Although of no clinical significance, these conditions are interesting models for studying the regulation of gene switching.

Like all biological classifications this approach to dividing up the haemoglobin disorders is not entirely satisfactory. For example, some structural haemoglobin variants are synthesised at a reduced rate and hence produce the clinical phenotype of thalassaemia; the most important of these is haemoglobin E, probably the commonest abnormal haemoglobin in the world population.

THE α THALASSAEMIAS

The molecular defects underlying α thalassaemia are extremely heterogeneous but ultimately the severity of the clinical phenotype depends on the total output of α globin. Many of the α thalassaemia defects have been characterised making it possible to establish a more comprehensive system for classifying the mutant alleles and to relate the clinical phenotype to the molecular defects (Higgs & Weatherall 1983).

Classification of α thalassaemia

Alpha thalassaemias in which no α globin is produced from the α-gene complex are called α° thalassaemia and those in which the output is reduced, α^+ thalassaemia. The α° and α^+ thalassaemias are further subdivided according to the nature of the molecular defect, into deletion and non-deletion types. The homozygous state for α° thalassaemia produces the haemoglobin Bart's hydrops syndrome; the compound heterozygous state for α° and α^+ thalassaemia causes haemoglobin H disease. But, as we shall see later, the genotype/phenotype relationships are not quite as simple as this.

Molecular basis of α thalassaemia

Gene deletions

In contrast to β thalassaemia, the majority of α thalassemias result from gross deletions of DNA within the α gene complex. This is clearly related to the extensive homology surrounding the structural α genes which is not seen in the β globin complex (Lauer et al 1980). The deletion of one or other of the duplicated α globin genes ($-\alpha^{3.7}$ and $-\alpha^{4.2}$) gives rise to the most common molecular defects underlying α thalassaemia (Embury et al 1980). Triplicated α gene arrangements, $\alpha\alpha\alpha^{\text{anti-3.7}}$ and $\alpha\alpha\alpha^{\text{anti-4.2}}$, corresponding to the $-\alpha^{3.7}$ and $-\alpha^{4.2}$ gene deletions produced during misalignment and crossover have been observed in many populations (Higgs et al 1980, Trent et al 1981, Lie-Injo et al 1981). Furthermore, chromosomes with four α genes ($\alpha\alpha\alpha\alpha^{\text{anti-3.7}}$ and $\alpha\alpha\alpha\alpha^{\text{anti-4.2}}$) which presumably result from similar crossovers involving the $\alpha\alpha\alpha^{\text{anti-3.7}}$ and $\alpha\alpha\alpha^{\text{anti-4.2}}$ arrangements have also been found (Gu et al 1987). Generally, the extra α genes are functional. The mechanism by which the recently described $-\alpha^{3.5}$ deletion (Kulozik et al 1988a) identified in an Asian Indian, has arisen is still not clear.

Deletions of the α gene complex which abolish α globin output from both α genes cause α° thalassaemia (Fig. 3.3). To date, nine such deletions have been described. These deletions are large and unlike the $-\alpha^{3.7}$ and $-\alpha^{4.2}$ deletions, are of limited geographical distribution; individual deletions are defined by a superscript describing the geographical or individual origin of the mutation. Among these deletions, the $\alpha\alpha^{\text{RA}}$ mutation is unusual in that it deletes 62 kb of the α gene complex upstream

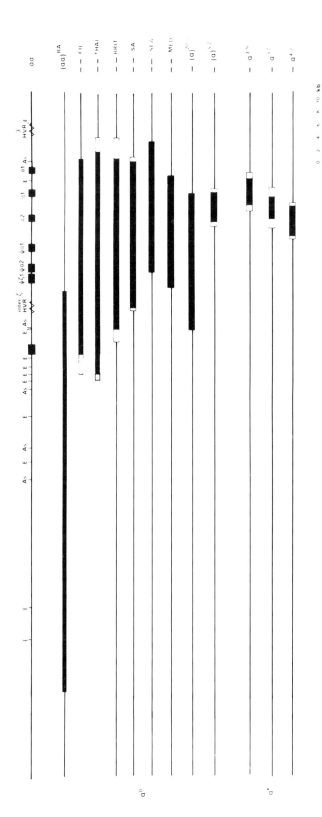

Fig. 3.3 Deletion map of the α globin locus. The upper line shows the restriction enzyme sites with genes as solid blocks and hypervariable regions (HVRs) as zigzag lines. As — Asp 718; E — EcoRI.

The first nine deletions result in an α° thalassaemia phenotype, and the other three deletions are associated with α⁺ thalassaemia. All deletions are listed according to standard nomenclature (Higgs & Weatherall 1983) with the deletion extent shown as solid black boxes or unfilled boxes where the end points have not been precisely determined.

Table 3.1   Non-deletion α thalassaemia

Mutant class	Site	Affected α gene	Nomenclature	Ethnic group
RNA processing mutations	IVS-1 donor site −5 bp	$\alpha2$	$\alpha^{Hph}\alpha$	Mediterranean
	*Polyadenylation signal AATAAA → AATAAG	$\alpha2$	$\alpha^{T\,Saudi}\alpha$	Saudi Arabia Mediterranean
RNA translation	Initiator codon			
	ATG → ACG	$\alpha2$	$\alpha^{Nco}\alpha$	Mediterranean
	?ATG → ACG	$\alpha1$	$\alpha\alpha^{Nco}$	Sardinian
	ATG → GTG	$-\alpha^{3.7}$	$-\alpha^{3.7Nco}$	Black
	−2 bp before ATG	$-\alpha^{3.7}$	$-\alpha^{3.7T}$	North African Mediterranean
	Nonsense mutation codon 116 (GAG → TAG)	$\alpha2$	$\alpha^{MS}\alpha$	Black
	Terminator codon 142			
	TAA → CAA	$\alpha2$	$\alpha^{CS}\alpha$	S.E. Asian
	TAA → AAA	$\alpha2$	$\alpha^{Ic}\alpha$	Mediterranean
	TAA → TCA	$\alpha2$	$\alpha^{KD}\alpha$	Asian Indian
	TAA → GAA	$\alpha2$	$\alpha^{SR}\alpha$	Black
Post translational instability	Exon 111 codon 125 (CTG → CCG)	$\alpha2$	$\alpha^{QS}\alpha$	S.E. Asian
	Exon 111 codon 101	?	Suan Dok	
	Exon 111 codon 110	?	Petah Tikva	

* This mutation has been found in both $\alpha2$-like genes in the $\alpha\alpha\alpha^{anti-3.7}$ chromosome from a Saudi Arabian individual.

of the α genes and appears to inactivate these genes although there is as yet no definite proof that the sequence of these α genes is entirely normal.

Analysis of some of the other deletions reveal a subset in which the 5′ breakpoints cluster and are staggered at approximately the same distance apart and in the same order as their respective 3′ breakpoints (Nicholls et al 1987). These findings are consistent with observations on a group of deletions in the β globin cluster (Vanin et al 1983). These staggered deletions are thought to result from illegitimate recombination events deleting an integral number of chromatin loops as they pass through their nuclear attachment points during replication.

Non-deletion forms of α thalassaemia

Most of the non-deletion α thalassaemias affect the $\alpha2$ gene (Liebhaber et al 1986a). This is probably because the $\alpha2$ gene is the dominant of the two α genes (Liebhaber et al 1986a, Shakin & Liebhaber 1986) and any mutations of the $\alpha2$ gene will have a greater effect on the phenotype and presumably a greater selective advantage. Unlike the deletion of the $\alpha2$ gene in the $-\alpha^{4.2}$ defect, in which there is a compensatory increase in the expression of the remaining $\alpha1$ gene (Liebhaber et al 1985), there appears to be no increase in the expression of the $\alpha1$ gene when the $\alpha2$ gene is inactivated by a point mutation. Hence, the non-deletion α thalassaemias produce a more severe phenotype than the $-\alpha$ mutants. As for the β thalassaemia mutations, they affect gene function by interfering with transcription, RNA processing or RNA translation. These molecular lesions are listed in Table 3.1 and briefly summarised below.

RNA PROCESSING MUTATIONS

Two mutations which affect processing of the primary mRNA transcript have been characterised. The first consists of a deletion of 5 bp in the 5' splice junction of IVS-1 of the $\alpha2$ globin gene ($\alpha^{Hph}\alpha$), including the invariant GT donor splicing sequence, thus abolishing normal RNA processing (Felber et al 1982, Orkin et al 1981a). The second mutation involves a base substitution in the polyadenylation signal (AATAAA $\rightarrow$ AATAAG) of the $\alpha2$ gene, originally identified in a Saudi Arabian individual (Higgs et al 1983a, Thein et al 1988). The mutation down regulates the $\alpha2$ gene by interfering with the 3' end processing and possibly with termination of transcription (Whitelaw & Proudfoot 1986), and appears to also affect the linked $\alpha1$ gene. In a Saudi Arabian individual with Hb H disease and the α genotype $\alpha\alpha\alpha/\alpha\alpha$, both the $\alpha2$-like genes in the $\alpha\alpha\alpha^{anti-3.7}$ complex and the $\alpha2$ gene on the other chromosome have been shown to contain this mutation, hence the revised genotype $(\alpha\alpha\alpha)^{T\ Saudi}/\alpha^{T-Saudi}\alpha$ (Thein et al 1988).

MUTATIONS THAT AFFECT RNA TRANSLATION

Several mutations prevent translation of mRNA by affecting the initiator codon. Two of these are single base substitutions; ATG $\rightarrow$ ACG, common in Mediterraneans (Pirastu et al 1984), and the recently identified ATG $\rightarrow$ GTG in a Black $-\alpha^{3.7}$ chromosome (Olivieri et al 1987). In a single Sardinian patient, an $\alpha1$ globin gene initiation codon mutation was inferred by Southern blotting (Paglietti et al 1986). These mutations are directly detectable by Southern blotting as they abolish a cleavage site for the restriction enzyme Nco 1. Another mutation deletes 2 bp of the sequence preceding the initiation signal (CCCACCATG $\rightarrow$ CCCCATG) (Morle et al 1985).

A recently described mutation identified in a Black individual from Mississippi ($\alpha^{MS}\alpha$) (Liebhaber et al 1986b) causes premature termination of RNA translation by a base substitution in codon 116 (GAG $\rightarrow$ TAG) changing an entire amino acid codon to an in-phase terminator. Four mutations affect termination of translation and give rise to elongated α globin variants; Hb Constant Spring ($\alpha^{CS}\alpha$), Hb Icaria ($\alpha^{Ic}\alpha$), Hb Koya Dora ($\alpha^{KD}\alpha$) and Hb Seal Rock ($\alpha^{SR}\alpha$). Each specifically changes the termination codon (TAA) (Weatherall & Clegg 1975) generating glutamine, lysine, serine and glutamic acid codons respectively, at position 142.

MUTATIONS CAUSING POST-TRANSLATIONAL INSTABILITY

A group of structural mutations give rise to highly unstable α globin variants that cannot form stable haemoglobin tetramers, resulting in α thalassaemia. The best characterised mutation of this class is Hb Quong Sze ($\alpha^{QS}\alpha$) (Liebhaber & Kan 1983) in which a single base substitution in codon 125 of the $\alpha2$ gene causes leucine to be replaced by proline. This class of α thalassaemia is analogous to β thalassaemia due to the unstable β chain variant, Hb Indianapolis.

Clinical phenotypes of α thalassaemia

The interactions of the different α genotypes result in four broad categories of clinical phenotypes; normal, α thalassaemia minor, Hb H disease and Hb Bart's hydrops fetalis syndrome.

The majority of normal individuals have four α globin genes ($\alpha\alpha/\alpha\alpha$) and about 2% of most populations have five α genes ($\alpha\alpha\alpha/\alpha\alpha$). Rarely, individuals with $\alpha\alpha\alpha\alpha/\alpha\alpha$ or $\alpha\alpha\alpha/\alpha\alpha\alpha$ genotypes have been identified. Although the extra α globin genes are functional, individuals with these α genotypes are phenotypically indistinguishable from normal.

The α thalassaemia minor phenotype includes a broad category in which individuals have mild haematological changes but no major clinical symptoms, spanning from the normal phenotype to Hb H disease. This phenotype often results from the interaction of a normal genotype $(\alpha\alpha)$ with one of the α^+ or α° determinants; the degree of α globin deficit, anaemia, hypochromia and microcytosis depending on the number of functional α genes. In general, chromosomes with a single α gene deletion $(-\alpha)$ produce the mildest phenotype, followed by the non-deletion mutants $(\alpha\alpha^T)$ that affect the dominant $\alpha2$ gene, with deletion mutants involving both α genes (e.g. $--^{MED}$ and $--^{SEA}$) producing the most severe phenotype. In view of the potential number of interactions, it is not possible to predict acccurately the α genotype from any given phenotype.

Hb H disease is characterised by a chronic haemolytic anaemia of variable severity and a clinical picture of thalassaemia intermedia. Although the genetic basis for Hb H disease is diverse, generally the disease results when the total output is equivalent to one functional α globin gene. Hb H disease is most frequent in SE Asia and the Mediterranean region, where it results from the interaction of α^+ and α° thalassaemia $(--/-\alpha)$. It may also result from homozygosity for non-deletion mutants affecting the dominant $\alpha2$ globin gene $(\alpha^{Nco}\alpha/\alpha^{Nco}\alpha,\ \alpha^{T\,Saudi}\alpha/\alpha^{T\,Saudi}\alpha,\ (\alpha\alpha\alpha)^{T\,Saudi}/\alpha^{T\,Saudi}\alpha)$ (Paglietti et al 1986, Higgs et al 1983a, Thein et al 1988). In Algeria, homozygotes for the $-\alpha^{3.7T}\ (-\alpha^{3.7T}/-\alpha^{3.7T})$ have typical Hb H disease (Morle et al 1985). Homozygotes for Hb Constant Spring $(\alpha^{CS}\alpha/\alpha^{CS}\alpha)$ have a phenotype more severe than that of α thalassaemia minor but milder than typical Hb H disease (Lie-Injo et al 1974). By comparing the phenotypes resulting from the different molecular interactions, it would appear that there is a critical threshold of α chain output below which the syndrome of Hb H disease results.

Haemoglobin Bart's hydrops fetalis is almost exclusively seen in the Southeast Asian and Mediterranean community where it is caused by the interaction of two α° determinants $(--^{SEA}/--^{SEA}$ and $--^{MED}/--^{MED})$ resulting in the complete absence of α globin synthesis. Recently however, there have been reports of hydrops fetalis in three Greek (Loukopoulos, D., personal communication; Trent et al 1986, Sharma et al 1979) and one Southeast Asian infant (Chan et al 1985) associated with very low levels of α chain synthesis. Gene mapping shows that they result from the interaction of the common α° determinants and non-deletion mutations $(\alpha\alpha^T)$ although the latter have not been characterised. The Greek mutation has been called $\alpha\alpha^T$ Karditsa. Hydrops fetalis has also been reported in some Chinese infants with a non-deletion mutation in which there is no α globin production, thus identifying an entirely different type of $\alpha\alpha^T$ determinant (Todd, D., personal communication).

Acquired α thalassaemia in myeloproliferative disorders and mental retardation

Although Hb H disease is almost always inherited, it has been described in several individuals as an acquired defect associated with the development of a myeloproliferative disorder (Higgs et al 1983b). It appears to be more frequent in males than females. The structure of the α globin complex is normal but virtually no α globin mRNA is detectable in the neoplastic marrow population. The molecular basis thus appears to be an acquired defect in α gene transcription but the precise mechanism is not known.

A second unusual type of α thalassaemia is associated with mental retardation and a variety of other developmental abnormalities including microcephaly, hypogonadism, hypotonia, and recurrent seizures (Weatherall et al 1981). Family studies show that in each case neither parent is a carrier for a severe α thalassaemia determinant, and that at least one chromosome 16 has been affected by a de novo mutation in the germ cell causing α thalassaemia. In several cases, this de novo mutation involves a deletion of the entire α globin complex; in others the molecular defect is not yet apparent. Cytogenetic analysis has not revealed any gross abnormality of chromosome 16 in any of these cases. It seems possible that in those cases where the α gene complex is intact, expression of the α genes is affected by a deletion of other parts of chromosome 16 that does not extend into the α complex but which is associated causally with mental retardation.

THE β THALASSAEMIAS

The β thalassaemias are a heterogeneous group of disorders characterised by deficiency or complete absence of β globin production. To a large extent, the diversity in clinical severity can now be related to the nature of the underlying mutations.

Molecular basis of β thalassaemia

The deficiency or absence of β chains that characterises β thalassaemia could potentially arise from defects affecting transcription, RNA processing or RNA translation (see Fig. 3.2). Beta thalassaemia mutations which cause a complete absence of production of normal β globin are called β° thalassaemia and those which cause a reduced output, β^+ thalassaemia. Since the last edition of 'Recent Advances in Haematology' several more β thalassaemia genes have been characterised bringing the total to a mere 48! The identification of new defects has been greatly facilitated by the observation that within any population, each mutation is in strong linkage disequilibrium with specific patterns of restriction fragment length polymorphisms in the β globin gene cluster (RFLP haplotypes) (Orkin et al 1982a). The defects characterised to date are summarised in Table 3.2, classified according to the mechanism by which they inactivate β gene expression.

Gene deletions

Five different deletions affecting only the β globin gene have now been described (Fig. 3.4, Table 3.2) (Spritz & Orkin 1982, Gilman et al 1984, Gilman 1987, Padanilam et al 1984, Popovich et al 1986, Diaz-Chico et al 1987). With one exception these are rare and appear to be isolated single events; the 619 bp deletion at the 3' end of the β gene is more common but even that is restricted to the Sind and Gujarati populations of Pakistan and India where it accounts for about 50% of the β thalassaemia alleles (Thein et al 1984b).

The Indian 619 bp deletion removes the 3' end of the β gene but leaves the 5' end intact, while the other four deletions remove the 5' end of the β gene but leave the δ gene intact. Heterozygotes for the Indian 619 bp deletion have raised Hb A_2 and F levels indistinguishable from the levels seen in individuals heterozygous for the other common forms of β thalassaemia (Fig. 3.4) (S. L. Thein, unpublished

Table 3.2 β thalassaemia mutations

Mutant class	Site	Type	Ethnic group
I Non-deletion			
A. Transcriptional	1. −88 C-T	+	Am Black, As Ind
	2. −87 C-G	+	Med
	3. −31 A-G	+	Jap
	4. −29 A-G	+	Am Black, Ch, SEA
	5. −28 A-C	+	Kurdish
	6. −28 A-G	+	Ch, SEA
	7. +1 A-C	+	As Ind
B. RNA processing			
Splice junction	1. IVS1-1 GT-AT	0	Med
	2. IVS1-1 GT-TT	0	As Ind
	3. IVS2-1 GT-AT	0	Med, Am Black
	4. IVS1 3′ end −17 bp		Kuwait
	5. IVS1 3′ end −25 bp	0	As Ind
	6. IVS2 3′ end AG-CG	0	Am Black
	7. IVS2 3′ end AG-GG	0	Am Black
Consensus region	8. IVS1-5 G-C	+	As Ind, Ch, SEA, Leb
	9. IVS1-5 G-T	+	Greek, N European
	10. IVS1-5 G-A	+	Corfu, Algerian
	11. IVS1-6 T-C	+	Med, M East
Internal IVS	12. IVS1-110 G-A	+	Med, Leb
	13. IVS1-116 T-G	0	Med
	14. IVS2-654 C-T	0	Ch, SEA
	15. IVS2-705 T-G	+	Med
	16. IVS2-745 C-G	+	Med, Leb
Coding region	17. cod 24 (T-A)	+	Am Black
	18. cod 26 (G-A)	+, βE	SEA
	19. cod 27 (G-T)	+, β Knossos	Med
	20. cod 29 (C-T)	+, β	Lebanese
Polyadenylation signal	21. AATAAA-AACAAA	+	Am Black
C. RNA translation			
Nonsense	1. cod 15 (G-A)	0	As Ind
	2. cod 17 (A-T)	0	Ch, SEA
	3. cod 37 (G-A)	0	S Arabian
	4. cod 39 (C-T)	0	Med, N Europe, Leb
	5. cod 43 (G-T)	0	Ch
	6. cod 121 (G-T)	0	Polish
Frameshift	7. −1 cod 6	0	Med
	8. −2 cod 8	0	Turk, Ital, Leb
	9. +1 cod 8/9	0	As Ind, Iranian
	10. −1 cod 16	0	As Ind
	11. −4 cod 41/42	0	As Ind, Ch, SEA
	12. −1 cod 44	0	Kurdish
	13. +1 cod 71/72	0	Ch
	14. +1 cod 106/107	0	Am Black
II. Deletions	1. 3′ β (−619 bp)	0	As Ind
	2. 5′ β (−1.35 kb)	0, ↑ HbA$_2$	Am Black
	3. 5′ β (−4.2 kb)	0, ↑ HbA$_2$	Czech
	4. β (−10 kb)	0, ↑ HbA$_2$	Dutch
	5. 5′ β (−300 bp)	0, ↑ HbA$_2$	Turkish
III. Unknown 'silent' carrier		+	Albanian

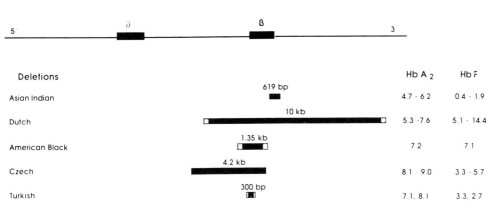

Fig. 3.4 β thalassaemia deletions. Summary of the deletions affecting only the β globin gene and their effect on the Hb A₂ and F levels. Deleted regions are indicated by the solid black boxes or hatched boxes where the end-points have not been precisely determined. Sizes of the deletions are shown above the boxes in kilobases (kb) or base-pairs (bp).

observations). However, heterozygotes for the other four deletions all have unusually high Hb A₂ levels. It is not clear whether the increased δ chain production results from increased δ gene transcription and, if so, whether it is only the gene in *cis* that is unusually active, possibly as a result of reduced competition from the deleted 5′ β gene for transcriptional factors.

Non-deletion forms of β thalassaemia

These defects result from single base substitutions or small deletions or insertions within or immediately upstream of the β globin gene and are so classified because analysis of DNA from patients with these defects reveal no gross abnormality by Southern blotting. These mutations ultimately affect gene function by interfering with transcription of the β gene into RNA, RNA processing, and translation into β globin.

TRANSCRIPTIONAL MUTATIONS

Six mutations resulting in β⁺ thalassaemia have been described; these mutations consist of single base substitutions within conserved DNA sequences that are known to be important in transcriptional efficiency (Table 3.2). Two of them, at position −88 and −87 (Orkin et al 1984a, Orkin et al 1982a) relative to the mRNA CAP site, are close to the CCAAT box and the others lie within the ATA box homology (Poncz et al 1982, Orkin et al 1983a, Antonarakis et al 1984, Surrey et al 1985, Takihara et al 1986). These mutant genes show decreased β mRNA production in transient expression systems, ranging from 10–25% of the output from a normal gene, confirming that these substitutions are responsible for their defective function. In general, the level of expression in vitro correlates well with the clinical severity of the condition, where this is known. These mutations have been found in diverse ethnic groups (Mediterraneans, Lebanese, Kurds, Chinese, Blacks and Asian Indians); the A → G substitution at position −29 is responsible for the mild β⁺ form of thalassaemia commonly found in Blacks (Antonarakis et al 1984) (see later section).

Recently an A→C substitution at the CAP site (+1) was described in an Asian Indian (Wong et al 1987) who, despite being homozygous for the mutation, appeared to have a phenotype typical of a β thalassaemia trait. The mechanism by which this novel mutation produces β thalassaemia is still uncertain.

RNA processing mutations
Precise processing of precursor RNA is critical to the synthesis of functional mRNA. This involves removal of the intervening sequences (or introns) from the primary transcript and the splicing together of exons. The boundaries of exons and introns are marked by the invariant dinucleotides, GT at the 5' (donor) and AG at the 3' (acceptor) sites. Mutations which affect either of these splice junctions (Treisman et al 1983, Kazazian et al 1984, Treisman et al 1982, Bunn & Forget 1986, Orkin et al 1983b, Padanilam & Huisman 1986, Atweh et al 1985) totally abolish normal RNA splicing and result in β° thalassaemia (see Table 3.2).

Surrounding the invariant dinucleotides at the splice junctions are fairly well conserved sequences. Four types of β thalassaemia involve single base substitutions within the consensus sequence of the IVS-1 donor site (Treisman et al 1983, Kazazian et al 1984, Atweh et al 1987a, Kulozik et al 1988a) and illustrate the importance of the consensus region in RNA splicing. Substitution of the G in position 5 of IVS-1 by C or T results in severe β^{+} thalassaemia whereas the G to A mutation at position 5, recently described in a Corfu family (Kulozik et al 1988a) and in Algeria (Lapoumeroulie et al 1986), and the T to C change at position 6 common in the Mediterranean region (Tamagnini et al 1983) result in a mild β^{+} thalassaemia. The G to C mutation at position 5 has also been found in Melanesia and appears to be the commonest cause of β thalassaemia in New Guinea (Hill et al 1988). The evidence that there have been at least two and probably three independent origins for the G→C mutation as well as two independent origins for the G→T mutation and the G→A mutation at position 5 of IVS-1 suggests that there is a mutational 'hotspot' at this position in the β gene.

RNA processing can also be affected by mutations which create new splice sites, either within introns or exons. The first β thalassaemia mutation characterised was of this type, a single base substitution at position 110 in IVS-1 (Spritz et al 1981, Busslinger et al 1981). During RNA processing the newly created splice site is preferentially used and the type of β thalassaemia that results depends on the amount of normal β mRNA produced. The G→A mutation at position 110 of IVS-1 leads to only about 10% splicing at the normal site resulting in a phenotype of severe β^{+} thalassaemia. More recently, another β thalassaemia mutation has been identified; a new acceptor site at position 116 in IVS-1 (Metherall et al 1986) results in little or no normal β mRNA and a phenotype of β° thalassaemia. Within exon 1 there is a cryptic donor site which covers codons 24–27 (Orkin & Kazazian 1984). Three mutations within this region can activate this cryptic site such that it is utilised during RNA processing (Orkin et al 1982b, Goldsmith et al 1983, Orkin et al 1984b). Two of them, GAG→AAG in codon 26 (Orkin et al 1982b) and GCC→TCC in codon 27 (Orkin et al 1984a), result in both reduced production of β mRNA and an amino acid substitution, so that the mRNA that is spliced normally is translated into protein. The abnormal haemoglobins produced are Hbs E and Knossos respectively. Recently, another β^{+} thalassaemia mutation due to a single base substitution, C→A at codon

29, was described in two Lebanese (Chehab et al 1987a); this creates a GT dinucleotide two bp 5′ to the normal GT donor site of IVS-1. It is not clear if this new GT dinucleotide acts as an alternative donor splice site or, as in the case of the mutations in codons 24–27, it activates the cryptic donor site present in this region of the β globin gene.

The sequence AAUAAA found near the 3′ end of most RNAs is the signal fore cleavage and polyadenylation of the gene transcript. A β globin gene isolated from an Afro-American has been shown to contain a single base substitution (AATAAA → AACAAA) within this conserved sequence (Orkin et al 1985); this resulted in the production of only one tenth of the normal amount of β mRNA, and hence β^+ thalassaemia. A small amount of β mRNA cleaved and polyadenylated 90 nucleotides downstream from the normal cleavage site was observed both in vitro and in the expression assay.

MUTATIONS THAT AFFECT RNA TRANSLATION

Several β thalassaemia genes contain nonsense or frameshift mutations that lead to premature chain termination during translation of β mRNA, with no β globin being produced, and hence result in β^0 thalassaemia. The nonsense mutations arise from base substitutions that change an amino acid codon to a chain termination codon, directly interfering with translation. Six mutations of this class have now been described (Table 3.2) (Chang & Kan 1979, Trecartin et al 1981, Kazazian et al 1984, Boehm et al 1986, Kazazian et al 1986a), the codon 17 mutation being common in SE Asia (Kazazian et al 1986b) and the codon 39 mutation in the Mediterranean region (Rosatelli et al 1987). Frameshift mutations arise from the insertion or deletion of one or a few nucleotides in the coding region which disrupts the normal reading frame and mRNA translation, and causes termination further downstream. The abnormal mRNA is found in very low levels in erythroid cells. Several mutations of this type have been described and two, the insertion of one nucleotide between codons 8 and 9 and the deletion of four nucleotides in codons 41 and 42 are common in Asian Indians (Kazazian et al 1984), the latter also being common in SE Asia (Kazazian et al 1986b).

Silent β thalassaemia

The β thalassaemias that are described in the preceding sections are due to *cis* acting mutations. However, in one reporterd Albanian family with two children with thalassaemia intermedia the thalassaemia lesion inherited from the father appeared not to be present in the β globin gene and was also shown to be unlinked to the β globin gene cluster (Semenza et al 1984). Although the precise nature of this defect is still unresolved, the existence of this entity illustrates the influence of other genes on globin chain balance. The reduction of β globin production in this condition, sometimes referred to as type 1 normal Hb A_2 thalassaemia, is minimal.

THALASSAEMIA INTERMEDIA

Thalassaemia intermedia is an ill-defined clinical term used to describe patients with phenotypes which are more severe than the usually asymptomatic thalassaemia trait but milder than transfusion-dependent thalassaemia major. The syndrome

Table 3.3   Molecular basis of thalassaemia intermedia

  I. Homozygosity for β thalassaemia mutations of usual severity with:
   a. Co-inheritance of α thalassaemia
   b. Co-inheritance of HPFH determinant, linked or unlinked to β gene cluster
   c. ? Co-inheritance of determinant for increased proteolysis of excess α chains

 II. $\delta\beta$ thalassaemia and Hb Lepore
   a. Homozygous $\delta\beta$ thalassaemia
   b. Compound heterozygotes for $\delta\beta$ thalassaemia and β thalassaemia
   c. Homozygous Hb Lepore (not all cases)

III. Inheritance of mild β thalassaemia genes

IV. Severe heterozygous β thalassaemia
   a. Co-inheritance of extra α globin genes ($\alpha\alpha/\alpha\alpha\alpha$ or $\alpha\alpha\alpha/\alpha\alpha\alpha$)
   b. Hb Indianapolis, a highly unstable β globin chain variant
   c. Syndrome of inclusion body formation and dyserythropoiesis in Northern Europeans

encompasses disorders with a wide spectrum of disability. At the severe end, patients present soon after the age of 2 years and are just able to maintain a haemoglobin level of about 6 g/dl without transfusion. At the other end, patients remain asymptomatic until adult life and are transfusion-independent with haemoglobin levels of 10–12 g/dl except at times of infection. There is no standard regime of management for thalassaemia intermedia but it is important to recognise that these patients can develop iron overload with its accompanying complications despite minimal blood transfusions. Patients with a more severe disease need blood transfusion although the requirements are not as great as those with thalassaemia major.

Molecular basis of thalassaemia intermedia
Table 3.3 lists the various molecular interactions that have been associated with thalassaemia intermedia. The majority of patients are homozygotes or compound heterozygotes for β thalassaemia and have usually co-inherited genes for α thalassaemia or hereditary persistence of fetal haemoglobin (HPFH), or have one or two mild β thalassaemia genes.

In homozygous β thalassaemia there is a large excess of α globin chains which precipitate in the red cell precursors causing ineffective erythropoiesis. It might be expected, therefore, that the co-inheritance of α thalassaemia leading to a reduction of α globin production would be an ameliorating factor. Two large surveys (Wainscoat et al 1983a, Wainscoat et al 1983b) have now established that α thalassaemia is an important factor in reducing the severity of homozygous β thalassaemia, the shift in clinical spectrum being more obvious in β^+ thalassaemia (Table 3.4).

Chain imbalance in homozygous β thalassaemia can also be reduced by the co-inheritance of one or more genetic determinants for enhanced production of γ chains. The interaction of the Swiss type of HPFH (characterised by slightly elevated levels of Hb F in normal individuals) in the amelioration of homozygous β thalassaemia has been clearly demonstrated in two large families, one from Sardinia (Cappellini et al 1981) and one of Asian Indian origin (S. L. Thein, unpublished data). The genetic basis for such types of HPFH is probably heterogeneous; it is clear that in some cases the HPFH determinant is not linked to the β globin gene cluster (Gianni et al 1983, Jeffreys et al 1986).

Table 3.4 Alpha genotypes of thalassaemia intermedia and thalassaemia major patients. The majority of the Cypriots (80%) have the severe form of β^+ thalassaemia (IVS 1 position 110), all the Sardinians are homozygous for $\beta°$ thalassaemia (codon 39 nonsense mutation), the Asian Indian TI patients have homozygous $\beta°$ thalassaemia while the TM patients have both $\beta°$ and β^+ thalassaemia. *Key*: TI, thalassaemia intermedia; TM thalassaemia major.

	Cypriot		Sardinian		Asian Indian	
α genotype	TI	TM	TI	TM	TI	TM
$\alpha\alpha/\alpha\alpha$	13	26	2	11	11	37
$-\alpha/\alpha\alpha$	9	4	4	4	3	5
$-\alpha/-\alpha$ or $--/\alpha\alpha$	3	0	2	2	0	0
$-\alpha/--$	2	0	0	0	0	0
Total	27	30	8	17	14	42

Table 3.5 Frequency of 5′ β haplotypes in homozygous β thalassaemia patients. *Key*: TI, thalassaemia intermedia; TM, thalassaemia major.

		Asian Indian		Italian	
5′ β halotypes		TI	TM	TI	TM
$-+-++/-+-++$		6	1	0	1
$-+-++/$others		2	8	12	3
Others/others		6	33	33	59
	Total	14	42	45	63

Recently, surveys have shown that there are other β thalassaemia homozygotes with a mild clinical course due to high levels of Hb F in whom family studies show no obvious increased Hb F levels in either parent (Labie et al 1985, Thein et al 1987). Many of these cases share a common RFLP haplotype in the region 5′ to the β gene, encompassing the ε, $^G\gamma$, $^A\gamma$ and $\psi\beta$ genes, $-+-++$. In one study of homozygous β thalassaemia (Thein et al 1987), 6 out of 7 Asian Indian patients who were homozygous for this haplotype had a mild disease, and of 15 Italian patients who were heterozygous for this haplotype, 12 had thalassaemia intermedia compared to 3 with thalassaemia major (Table 3.5). Unlike the other HPFH determinants, it appears that the increased $-$Hb F determinant associated with the $-+-++$ 5′ β haplotype confers the ability to increase Hb F only under conditions of erythropoietic stress. The $-+-++$ haplotype is also associated with increased Hb F production in patients with sickle cell disease (Gilman & Huisman 1985, Nagel et al 1985) and is clearly related to the $++-++$ haplotype, which is associated with high Hb F levels ($>20\%$) in sickle cell disease patients from Eastern Saudi Arabia and India (Kulozik et al 1986, 1987a). Both these haplotypes, but none of the other common haplotypes, share a sequence change $(C\rightarrow T)$ at position -158 relative to the $^G\gamma$ globin gene which creates a cleavage site for the restriction enzyme XmnI. It is not clear whether the Xmn I-γ polymorphism is simply a marker within the haplotype linked to the high Hb F determinant or whether the base substitution at -158 itself is the determinant since it lies within the region where other base substitutions responsible for the non-deletion HPFH conditions occur (see below).

Homozygous $\delta\beta$ thalassaemia tends to be relatively mild because the high level of Hb F associated with this disorder results in less chain imbalance between the α and non-α globin chains. Similarly, patients who are compound heterozygotes for $\delta\beta$ thalassaemia and β thalassaemia (Weatherall & Clegg 1981) tend to have a less severe disease. Individuals homozygous for Hb Lepore also have a milder disease than homozygous β thalassaemia whereas most compound heterozygotes for Hb Lepore and β thalassaemia have thalassaemia major (Weatherall & Clegg 1981).

Most β thalassaemia mutations cause a total absence or severe deficit of β globin synthesis and, in the homozygous state, produce thalassaemia major. However, several mutations associated with much less severe reduction in β chain synthesis have been described; one set is located in the promotor region of the β gene. Two, one at position -29 (Antonarakis et al 1984), which is very common, and the other at -88 (Orkin et al 1984a), have been found to be associated with mild β^+ thalassaemia in Blacks. Mild β thalassaemia mutations have also been characterised in the Mediterraneans; these include a base substitution at position 6 of IVS-1 (Tamagnini et al 1983) and at position -87 (Orkin et al 1982a) in the 5' flanking DNA of the β gene. The base substitution at position -31 described in a Japanese patient (Takihara et al 1986) is also associated with a mild disease. Another set of mild β thalassaemia mutations is associated with single base substitutions in the first exon of the β gene; the base substitution at codon 27 produces Hb Knossos and that at codon 26 Hb E. Heterozygotes for Hb Knossos have minimal red cell changes, normal Hb A_2 and F levels but globin chain imbalance, giving rise to a 'silent' carrier state for β thalassaemia. Co-inheritance of Hb Knossos with typical high Hb A_2 β thalassaemia results in thalassaemia intermedia. Hb E is associated with a more severe phenotype than Hb Knossos; compound heterozygotes for Hb E and β thalassaemia often have thalassaemia major. However, homozygotes for Hb E are clinically asymptomatic.

There are other well characterised forms of β thalassaemia which tend to produce a milder disease. These are associated with normal levels of Hb A_2 and F, and fall into two categories; type 1, the 'silent carrier' state for β thalassaemia, in which red cell indices are normal but globin chain synthesis shows a deficit of β chain production, and type 2 in which the usual haematological and morphological abnormalities are present but the Hb A_2 level is normal. The 'silent carrier' state for β thalassaemia was first described by Schwartz (1969) in an Albanian family in which two children had thalassaemia of intermediate severity. The mother had typical high Hb A_2 β thalassaemia trait, whereas the father had essentially normal haematology with an abnormal α/β chain synthesis ratio, characteristic of mild β thalassaemia. Subsequent studies have shown that this mild β thalassaemia determinant is not linked to the β globin gene (Semenza et al 1984). The phenotype of 'silent carrier' β thalassaemia has also been described in association with Hb Knossos. Type 2 normal Hb A_2 β thalassaemia also shows considerable heterogeneity. Many cases are likely to be due to the co-inheritance of a defective δ gene which may occur in cis or in trans to the β thalassaemia gene which may itself be of the β° or β^+ type. In contrast to the less severe disease associated with double heterozygosity for type 1 normal Hb A_2 β thalassaemia and typical high Hb A_2 thalassaemia, compound heterozygotes for type 2 normal Hb A_2 β thalassaemia and typical high Hb A_2 β thalassaemia have thalassaemia major. An unusual case of normal Hb A_2 β thalassaemia from Corfu is due to a small deletion of 7 kb which removes the δ globin gene but leaves the β gene intact (Wainscoat et al 1985a, Kulozik et al 1988a). Homozygotes for this deletion have a mild disease.

Occasionally β thalassaemia heterozygotes present with thalassaemia intermedia. In the majority of cases this is due to the co-inheritance of extra α globin genes directing an increased production of α globin. The co-inheritance of two extra α

globin genes as, in the homozygous state for the triplicated α globin gene complex ($\alpha\alpha\alpha/\alpha\alpha\alpha$) with heterozygous β thalassaemia, results in thalassaemia intermedia (Galanello et al 1983, Thein et al 1984a). Some β thalassaemia heterozygotes with a single extra α globin gene ($\alpha\alpha\alpha/\alpha\alpha$) are clinically and haematologically indistinguishable from simple heterozygotes for β thalassaemia while others clearly have the clinical picture of thalassaemia intermedia (Sampietro et al 1983, Kulozik et al 1987b). The reason for this difference remains unexplained; it does not seem to be due to the nature of the β thalassaemia allele. It appears that there is a critical threshold of α globin chain excess in each individual above which clinical symptoms develop.

Heterozygous β thalassaemia of unusual severity associated with inclusion body formation and haemolysis or with features of dyserythropoiesis has been described in northern Europeans (Weatherall et al 1973). In most cases, the molecular basis for the disorder is not known. In cases in which the defect has been identified it has been due to the inheritance of a β chain structural variant e.g. Hb Indianapolis (Adams et al 1979) and the recently described Hb Showa-Yakushiji (β^{110}Leu-Pro) (Kobayashi et al 1987). The severe phenotype in such cases is probably the result of the combination of the unstable β chain and the concomitant α chain excess overwhelming the cells' proteolytic capacity. Recently another unstable haemoglobin variant, Hb Shanghai (Zeng et al 1987), which leads to thalassaemia intermedia in a heterozygote has been described in a Chinese.

THE $\gamma\delta\beta$ THALASSAEMIAS AND HEREDITARY PERSISTENCE OF FETAL HAEMOGLOBIN (HPFH)

With the exception of the rare $\gamma\delta\beta$ thalassaemias, this group of disorders are milder than the β thalassaemias and hence are of less clinical interest. However, they provide models for studying the genetic control of the switch from fetal to adult haemoglobin.

Notation and classification
The notation and classification of this group of conditions is confusing and still needs revision. Hitherto, it has been customary to categorise them as $\delta\beta$ thalassaemia or HPFH depending on the haematological changes, globin chain synthesis ratios and intercellular distribution of Hb F, and to further divide them, according to the structure of the Hb F which is produced, into $^{G}\gamma$, $^{A}\gamma$ or $^{G}\gamma^{A}\gamma$ varieties. Using gene mapping techniques, it has been possible to further subdivide them into deletion and non-deletion types.

It is now apparent that division of conditions which result from long deletions of the $\gamma\delta\beta$ globin gene cluster into $\delta\beta$ thalassaemia and HPFH is artificial; in effect they form a spectrum of disorders in which there is a variable (but never complete) compensation for absent δ and β chain production by $^{G}\gamma$, or $^{G}\gamma$ and $^{A}\gamma$ chain production. Hence, if we define thalassaemia as a disorder characterised by imbalanced globin chain synthesis, they are all forms of $\delta\beta$ thalassaemia. Furthermore, it is illogical to designate them by the type of Hb F that is produced. $^{G}\gamma$ $\delta\beta$ thalassaemia should be called $(^{A}\gamma\delta\beta)^{\circ}$ thalassaemia; it is the $^{A}\gamma$, δ and β genes which are inactive (i.e. thalassaemic) and the $^{G}\gamma$ genes which remain active! Similarly $^{G}\gamma^{A}\gamma$ $\delta\beta$ thalassaemia should be called $(\delta\beta)^{\circ}$ thalassaemia. Perhaps the term HPFH should be restricted to those conditions in which there is no globin chain imbalance in homozygotes.

Hopefully, as the molecular basis for more of these disorders is worked out it will become possible to classify them more logically.

Deletion forms of δβ thalassaemia and pancellular HPFH

The δβ thalassaemias are milder than the β thalassaemias because there is efficient compensation for the absence of β chain synthesis by γ chain production. Homozygotes have the clinical phenotype of thalassaemia intermedia with 100% Hb F; heterozygoes have hypochromic microcytic red cells and between 5 and 15% Hb F. The condition is currently subdivided into $^G\gamma$ and $^G\gamma^A\gamma$ $(\delta\beta)°$ forms according to the structure of the Hb F. They all result from deletions which remove the β and δ globin genes. In the case of $^G\gamma$ δβ thalassaemia the deletions also involve the $^A\gamma$ genes. In one form of $^G\gamma$ δβ thalassaemia most of the region between the $^G\gamma$ and δ globin genes is inverted and there are small deletions involving the $^A\gamma$ and δ genes (Jones et al 1981). $^G\gamma^A\gamma$ HPFH is very similar to $^G\gamma^A\gamma$ δβ thalassaemia except that heterozygotes have higher levels of Hb F and homozygotes have a haematological picture and a degree of globin chain production similar to heterozygous β thalassaemia; like δβ thalassaemia homozygotes they have 100% Hb F. $^G\gamma^A\gamma$ HPFH is also heterogeneous. Each type results from a different-length deletion of the γδβ gene cluster (for references see Bunn & Forget 1986, Weatherall et al 1988).

The particular interest of these conditions is that they are all associated with relatively effective γ chain synthesis in adults. Several explanations have been proposed, none entirely satisfactory.

Based on the observation that, as a group, the HPFH deletions (i.e. those with a relatively higher output of γ chains) tend to extend further upstream than those which produce δβ thalassaemia, attempts have been made to define putative regulatory regions in the β globin gene cluster which may or may not be involved in the deletion. One approach has been to compare the 5′ ends of the HPFH and δβ thalassaemia deletions that are closest together. It has been found that the two deletions end in a pair of Alu 1 repeats 5′ to the δ gene (Jagadeeswaren et al 1982, Ottolenghi et al 1982). The HPFH deletion ends in the 5′ Alu 1 repeat of the bipolar pair and the δβ thalassaemia in the 3′ Alu 1 repeat. Thus the two deletions have endpoints which are within 500 nucleotides of each other; the larger deletion causes a significantly higher output of γ chains than the smaller one. Hence, unless the different phenotypes are due entirely to differences in the DNA sequences at the 3′ end of the deletions, the 5′ Alu 1 repeat and the non-repetitive DNA connecting it to the 3′ Alu 1 repeat must be considered to have an important regulatory role. Alternatively, Tuan et al (1983) have pointed out that the deletions which cause HPFH are situated at least 52–57 kb from the 3′ extremity of the β globin genes, while those which cause δβ thalassaemia are shorter and located no more than 5–10 kb from the β gene. They suggest that the nature of the DNA brought into the vicinity of the γ genes by these deletions (?enhancer sequences) may be an important factor in determining the phenotype. On the other hand, three $^G\gamma$ δβ thalassaemias have been shown to have different 3′ sequences yet their phenotypes are essentially the same (Trent et al 1984).

Another form of δβ thalassaemia (Wainscoat et al 1984) breaks the rule that the putative 'regulatory region' is absent from all deletion types of HPFH but is present in the δβ thalassaemias. Heterozygotes show characteristics intermediate between δβ and HPFH (20% Hb F, almost normal red cell indices, and α/non-α globin chain synthesis ratios of 1.3), but compound heterozygotes with β^+ thalassaemia have the clinical picture of thalassaemia intermedia, much more typical of a patient with the $\delta\beta/\beta^+$ thalassaemia genotype. A tentative explanation for these findings is that there has been a deletion of the same regulatory region that is responsible for the HPFH phenotype (i.e. relatively high γ chain production), but that the proximity of the deletion 3' to the $^A\gamma$ gene has down-regulated this locus; this idea is supported by the $^G\gamma/^A\gamma$ ratio of the Hb F of 3:1. Using a similar argument it has been suggested that an individual with $^G\gamma$ $\delta\beta$ thalassaemia would have had the HPFH phenotype (due to loss of the presumptive regulatory region) if it were not for the loss of the $^A\gamma$ gene; the $^G\gamma$ gene, even if fully active, may not be able to compensate fully for the lack of β chain production (Jones et al 1981).

Finally, as originally suggested by Bernards & Flavell (1980) it is possible that the phenotypic expression of these deletions simply reflects the degree of involvement of functional 'fetal' or 'adult' domains within the cluster. But so far deletion mapping has not resulted in clear definition of these regions.

$\gamma\delta\beta$ Thalassaemia

The $\gamma\delta\beta$ thalassaemias have only been observed in heterozygotes. They are characterised by neonatal haemolysis and haematological changes of β thalassaemia with a normal haemoglobin A_2 level in adults (Weatherall & Clegg 1981). Four deletions have now been described in this condition, all originating 5' to the $\gamma\delta\beta$ gene complex. Two of these (Pirastu et al 1983a, Fearon et al 1983) remove the entire complex; the other two end within the complex, in one case including the 5' end of the β gene and hence inactivating it (Orkin et al 1981b), in the other case ending 2 kb upstream from the β gene (Van der Ploeg et al 1980). Interestingly, in the latter case the β gene does not function in vivo, although when cloned and expressed in vitro it appears to function normally (Kioussis et al 1983). This may mean that a normally inactive locus has been brought into contact with the intact β locus on the affected chromosome, thus altering its expression, possibly by a local change in chromatin configuration.

Non-deletion form of HPFH

So far, this section has dealt with conditions that result from major deletions of the $\gamma\delta\beta$ globin gene cluster. Because of the major pertubations in the structure of this region which must follow from deletions of this magnitude it seems likely that the value of these conditions as models for analysing the regulation of globin gene switching may be limited. However, there is recent evidence that there are forms of HPFH in which there appear to be no major gene deletions but which may, in the long term, tell us much more about the developmental regulation of the globin gene cluster.

It is already apparent that non-deletion HPFH is heterogeneous. Formal genetic studies have shown that some of these conditions result from lesions within the β gene cluster, while the genetic determinants for others seem to be at some distance away or even on another chromosome (Gianni et al 1983). Very little is known about the latter group as yet. However, the non-deletion forms of HPFH which are determined by lesions within the $\gamma\delta\beta$ gene cluster are proving to be of particular interest. Initially these were designated as the Greek or British forms of HPFH and $^G\gamma\beta^+$

HPFH. In fact they are all forms of either $^G\gamma\beta^+$ or $^A\gamma\beta^+$ HPFH. That is they are characterised by the persistence of fetal haemoglobin production beyond the neonatal period; the γ chains are predominantly $^G\gamma$ or $^A\gamma$ varieties, but not both. Furthermore, from the study of interactions between these conditions and various β globin structural variants it is quite clear that the linked β globin genes are active, although with a lower output than normal. There is recent evidence that these conditions result from point mutations upstream from either the $^G\gamma$ or $^A\gamma$ globin genes which cluster in a region of DNA stretching from -150 to -202 i.e. 50–200 bases upstream from the initiation site (Fig. 3.5) (Collins et al 1984, Giglioni et al 1984,

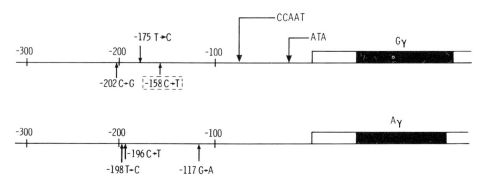

Fig. 3.5 The point mutations upstream from the γ globin genes that are associated with hereditary persistence of fetal haemoglobin (for reference see text).

Gelinas et al 1985, Tate et al 1986). Studies on the British family with the $^A\gamma\beta^+$ variety of non-deletion HPFH are particularly instructive. At birth affected heterozygotes or homozygotes have normal $^G\gamma^A\gamma$ globin chain ratios but during subsequent development, while the level of $^G\gamma$ chain production declines as normal, $^A\gamma$ chain synthesis remains active. These findings suggest that these upstream point mutations somehow interfere with the interaction of proteins which normally are responsible for the neonatal suppression of γ chain activity and that somehow this process is ineffective when mutations occur at these critical regulatory sites. Thus the existence of these mutations offers a direct approach to defining these critical regulatory regions and, hopefully, to isolating the putative regulatory proteins with which they interact.

In a type of non-deletion $\delta\beta$-thalassaemia characterised by decreased expression of the β globin gene and increased expression of the γ globin genes, a mutation has been identified that leads to decreased expression of the β gene e.g. a nonsense mutation at codon 39 in the β gene in the Sardinian $\delta\beta^\circ$ thalassaemia (Ottolenghi et al 1987) and an A to G mutation in the 'ATA' sequence of the promotor region of the β gene in the Chinese $\delta\beta$ thalassaemia (Atweh et al 1987b). Increased expression of the $^A\gamma$ gene in the Sardinian $\delta\beta^\circ$ thalassaemia is ascribed to the point mutation at position -196 upstream of the $^A\gamma$ gene previously described (Giglioni et al 1984).

POPULATION GENETICS

Recent estimates suggest that approximately 4% of the world population are carriers for an important haemoglobin disorder and that by the end of this century this figure may rise to 7%. The world distribution of the thalassaemias has been summarised in several reviews (Weatherall & Clegg 1981, Bunn & Forget 1986, Weatherall et al 1988) and progress has been made in understanding some of the factors which have maintained the thalassaemia polymorphisms at such remarkable high levels in some populations.

In 1949 J. B. S. Haldane suggested that individuals with red cell disorders such as thalassaemia might be protected against malaria. Recent studies have tended to validate Haldane's prediction. It is now apparent that in each of the high frequency areas for the β thalassaemias there are a few common mutations together with varying numbers of rare ones. Furthermore, in each of these regions the pattern of mutations is different. And even where the same mutation occurs in different populations it is usually found together with a different β globin gene RFLP haplotype. These studies make it very likely that the β thalassaemias have arisen independently in different populations and then achieved their high frequency by selection. Although there may have been some movement of the β thalassaemia genes between populations by drift and so on, there is little doubt that independent mutation and selection provides the overall basis for the world distribution of β thalassaemia. Recent molecular studies of the α thalassaemias lead to similar conclusions.

Early studies in Sardinia, which show that β thalassaemia is less common in the mountainous regions where malarial transmission was low, suggested that β thalassaemia might have reached its high frequency due to protection against malarial infection. For many years these data remained the only evidence for this protective effect. However, recent studies utilising malaria endemicity data together with globin gene mapping have shown a very clear altitude related effect on the frequency of α thalassaemia in Papua New Guinea. In addition, a sharp decline in the frequency of α thalassaemia has been found in a region stretching south from Papua New Guinea through the island populations of Melanesia to New Caledonia; this is mirrored by a similar gradient in the distribution of malaria as based on parasite data together with spleen rate studies collected in this region over many years. The effect of drift and founder effect in these island populations has been excluded by analysing other DNA polymorphisms which show a random distribution and no evidence of a decline similar to that which characterises the distribution of α thalassaemia in this region (Flint et al 1986). These studies provide strong evidence, albeit circumstantial, that the α thalassaemias have reached their high frequencies by protection against *P. falciparum* malaria. The cellular mechanism for this protection remains unknown.

PREVENTION AND TREATMENT

Prenatal diagnosis

Many successful programmes for the prenatal diagnosis of β thalassaemia have been set up utilising fetal blood sampling followed by globin chain synthesis studies. This approach has been used widely throughout the Mediterranean region, the Middle East and in Britain and North America and data are available on over 4000 cases (Alter 1984, 1985). The application of this technique has reduced the incidence of homozygous β thalassaemia very considerably in many Mediterranean populations, a remarkable example of the application of basic science to the control of a common genetic disease.

However, because of the inherent disadvantages of a second trimester prenatal

Table 3.6 β thalassaemia mutations directly detectable by restriction analysis

Mutation	Restriction enzyme
β^o thalassaemia	
1. Indian deletion	Various enzymes, -619 bp
2. American Black deletion	Various enzymes, -1.35 kb
3. Dutch deletion	Various enzymes, -10 kb
4. Czech deletion	Various enzymes, -4.2 kb
5. Turkish deletion	Various enzymes, -300 bp
6. -1 codon 6	Mst II
7. IVS 2 splice junction	Hph I
8. IVS 1 $(-25$ bp$)$	Fnu 4H, Mst II
9. IVS 1 $(-17$ bp$)$	Fnu 4H, Mst II
10. IVS 1-position 116	Mae I
11. IVS 1 position 6	Sfa N1
12. IVS 2 3' end AG $\rightarrow$ GG	Alu I
13. β^o39	Mae I
14. β^o17	Mae I
15. β^o37	Ava II
16. β^o121	Eco RI
β^+ thalassaemia	
17. IVS 2 position 745	Rsa I
18. -87 C $\rightarrow$ G	Avr II
19. Hb E	Mnl I

diagnosis there has been much interest in the application of fetal DNA analysis following chorion villus sampling (CVS) for the prenatal diagnosis of thalassaemia, and in the last few years this technique has become widely used for the prenatal identification of all the important haemoglobin disorders (Old et al 1986). It is currently estimated that fetal loss following CVS is in the region of 1–2%, but to date there are no good follow-up studies on infants who have been born following this procedure. Its safety is therefore subjudice.

It is possible to obtain 20–100 μg of fetal DNA following CVS and, if the procedure is carried out correctly, it is uncontaminated by maternal tissue. There is a variety of diagnostic procedures available for identifying the thalassaemias by DNA analysis. In the deletion forms of α and β thalassaemia the lesion can be identified directly by Southern blotting. This is also the case if the underlying mutations alter restriction enzyme sites or result in major gene rearrangements; about a third of the β thalassaemia mutations can be identified directly in this way (Table 3.6). If this is not possible prenatal diagnosis can be achieved by RFLP linkage analysis. This entails carrying out a family study to attempt to track the parental chromosomes that carry the particular mutations. Extensive studies in Europe have shown that this approach is feasible in about 40–80% of families of Mediterranean background (Old et al 1986). The success rate is higher, in the region of 80%, if an RFLP can be found that is in strong linkage disequilibrium with a common β thalassaemia mutation (Wainscoat et al 1985b).

More recently it has become possible to construct short DNA probes, oligonucleotide probes, that will detect directly single base mutations (Pirastu et al 1983b, Thein et al 1985). Feasibility studies suggest that, since most populations have only one or two common mutations, it is possible to set up a prenatal diagnosis programme with a few oligonucleotide probes. However, because some β thalassaemics in every population studied to date are compound heterozygotes for a common and a rare mutation this method will only cover about 80% of 'at risk' pregnancies (Thein et al 1985).

The approaches to developing a comprehensive prenatal diagnosis programme for β thalassaemia have been reviewed recently (Weatherall 1985, Thein & Weatherall 1987). The first priority, after public education and setting up a screening programme, is to determine the common mutations in the population. This should tell us if forms of thalassaemia exist that can be identified directly by Southern blotting and the proportion of cases that can be identified with oligonucleotide probes. In most cases in which the mutation is not known RFLP linkage analysis can be carried out. If none of these approaches is feasible it is necessary to have the backup of fetal blood sampling. Potential difficulties of RFLP linkage analysis include plasmid contamination, crossing over within the β globin gene cluster, and non-paternity.

Recent developments promise to simplify first trimester prenatal diagnosis (Chehab et al 1987b, Kogan et al 1987, Wong et al 1987). It is possible by the use of the polymerase chain reaction to amplify small amounts of DNA very rapidly. Using this approach together with oligonucleotide probes it should be possible to obtain a diagnosis within 24 hours. Current research is directed towards the development of non-radioactive methods for labelling the oligonucleotide probes; it may well be possible to use a simple dot blot technique without the necessity of separation of DNA fragments. If this can be combined with non-radioactive labelling of probes the whole process of first trimester prenatal diagnosis will be greatly simplified and become widely applicable in the developing world. Even in those cases in which the mutation is not known these new amplification techniques promise to simplify RFLP linkage analysis and obviate the need for radioactive labelling of probes; sufficient DNA can be generated to be visible by direct staining of gels (Kogan et al 1987).

Symptomatic treatment

There have been few major advances in the symptomatic treatment of thalassaemia; the main standbys remain regular transfusion, the judicious use of splenectomy, and regular chelation with subcutaneous desferrioxamine delivered by an infusion pump. There are still insufficient data to determine whether this approach will prolong the life of β thalassaemics, although this seems likely. At the time of going to press there are some promising reports of the development of oral chelating drugs which, if confirmed, may facilitate the symptomatic treatment of these disorders (Hershko & Weatherall 1987, Kontoghiorghes et al 1988, Kontoghiorghes & Hoffbrand, Ch. 4).

Bone marrow transplantation

Since the first report of successful bone marrow transplantation in β thalassaemia (Thomas et al 1982) large numbers of cases have been reported (Lucarelli et al 1985). There is still an unacceptable rate of graft versus host reaction and this procedure should be limited to patients who, for some reason or other, cannot receive adequate symptomatic treatment.

Specific gene therapy

One of the main difficulties in developing specific gene therapy for the haemoglobin disorders is that so little is known about how mammalian genes are regulated.

Mechanisms must exist that ensure that genes are switched on in the right tissues at the correct stage of development and that, once activated, are transcribed at an appropriate rate. Some genes, like the globin genes, only function at specific developmental stages and require very precise regulation of their rates of transcription. Others, so-called housekeeping genes, are transcribed at a fairly constant rate in most cells and at all phases of development. For this reason, current interest is directed mainly towards attempts at correction of genetic disorders due to defective production of genes like those for adenosine deaminase which probably do not require very tight regulation. The problems of correcting the haemoglobinopathies, in which gene regulation must be particularly tight, are even more formidable.

In considering gene transfer a clear distinction must be made between somatic gene therapy, in which only non-germline cells are involved, and transgenic approaches in which the transferred genes will be expressed in subsequent generations.

METHODS OF SOMATIC GENE TRANSFER

Genes can be inserted directly into cells, or attached to carriers, or vectors (Anderson 1984).

Direct insertion of genes into cells is still inefficient. One of the earlier methods was based on the principle of the uptake of calcium microprecipitates of DNA. Although very selective it is relatively inefficient and the rate of stable transfection is probably about 1 cell in 10^5. Attempts have also been made to microinject DNA directly into the nucleus of cells. This requires considerable technical expertise and because it involves treating one cell at a time it is unlikely to have any practical application. Most recently a method has been developed called electroporation which involves the exposure of cells to a pulsed electric field which opens up pores in the plasma membranes. Some very recent modifications of this technique (Chu et al 1987) have resulted in more than 1% of viable cells showing stable expression of a selectable marker gene.

Retroviruses are adapted by evolution for the efficient delivery of their genome into cells, with integration into the host genome and a high level of expression of their internal sequences. Currently this approach seems to be the most promising method for gene therapy (Anderson 1984, Williams & Orkin 1986, Anderson et al 1986, Miller et al 1986, Yee et al 1986, Dzierzak et al 1988).

Retroviruses contain a dimer of viral RNA within a protein coat surrounded by a lipid bilayer that contains viral-specific glycoproteins that attach themselves to cells during infection. The virion contains the virus-coded enzyme, reverse transcriptase. After entering cells the coat is shed and the RNA genome is copied into DNA by reverse transcriptase. A double-stranded DNA circle is formed and specific retroviral sequences direct the integration of viral DNA into the host genome. After integration, viral sequences transcribe full-length and spliced RNAs. The spliced RNAs are translated to generate glycoproteins while the full length RNA is either translated into internal structural proteins of the virion core and reverse transcriptase or packaged into viron particles as new genomic RNA. The subsequent assembly and budding of virion particles from infected cells is non-lytic.

By some ingenious genetic engineering a variety of recombinant retrovirus vectors have been constructed; the viral genome needed for the infection, integration and transcriptional control of the genome, which is all contained in the long terminal repeat sequences (LTRs) are preserved but viral sequences, the function of which can be supplied in *trans*, are deleted. Thus the *gag* sequences which encode internal structural proteins of the virion core, *pol* genes which encode reverse transcriptase, and *env* genes which encode the envelope glycoproteins are all deleted and are replaced by a dominant selectable marker and a restriction enzyme site into which the gene that is to be transferred can be cloned.

The recombinant DNA and now defective retroviral genome in the form of plasmid DNA is then introduced by transfection into murine fibroblasts to generate cell lines that produce the recombinant retrovirus. Simultaneous infection with wild-type helper viruses can provide the required packaging proteins although it is now possible to achieve the same result by the use of specialised packaging cell lines. Virus particles are shed into the surrounding medium which can then be harvested and used to infect the recipient cells, or the latter can be incubated directly with the cells budding off the viral particles.

Experiments using recombinant retroviruses of this type have demonstrated that gene transfer can be achieved. For example, murine bone marrow has been cultivated with packaging cell lines that produce recombinant retroviruses, harvested, and injected into lethally irradiated recipient mice (Williams & Orkin 1986). Since injected stem cells colonise the spleen it is possible to follow the fate of the transfected genes by analysis of the DNA of colonies formed in the spleen of the irradiated mice. Studies of this kind have shown that genes have been transferred into pluripotential haemopoietic stem cells and that the transfected cells appear to be long-lived, at least up to four months after transplantation. Furthermore, they are totipotential i.e. they give rise to both lymphoid and myeloid progeny.

A variety of genes have been transferred into intact mice using retroviral vectors including G418 (a neomycin resistant gene), hypoxanthine phosphoribosyl transferase (HPRT), dihydrofolate reductase (DHFR) and human adenosine deaminase (ADA). In addition to murine stem cells, retrovirus-mediated transfer and expression of drug resistance genes has also been carried out using human haemopoietic progenitors in culture (Miller et al 1986). And the human ADA gene has been transferred into and expressed in diploid skin fibroblasts obtained from an ADA-deficient human (Willis et al 1984). While these results are encouraging the level of expression of many of these transferred genes has been extremely variable, and often low.

It is clear that many problems remain, in particular the efficiency of transfection and level of expression using retroviral vectors for gene transfer. A number of ingenious attempts have been made to improve the level of expression (reviewed by Anderson 1984).

Finally, it should be emphasised that very little is known about the safety of retrovirus delivery systems. There is no doubt that they can rearrange their own structure as well as exchange sequences with other viruses. There is still a distinct possibility that a retroviral vector might recombine with an endogenous viral sequence to produce an infectious recombinant virus. Although the properties of a virus of this type are difficult to anticipate the possibility remains that they might be oncogenic.

Targeted modification of genes by exogenous DNA has been possible in yeast for many years. However, it is only recently that preliminary studies of this approach to the alteration of the human genome have been attempted (Gregg & Smithies 1986).

In principle, this approach to the replacement of defective genes has many attractions. In particular, it is site-directed and hence should not cause the problems of random integration. The idea is that the exogenous DNA should contain a region with the same nucleotide sequence as the target gene so that homologous recombination can occur between the regions of sequence identity. In other words the method uses nature's way of gene mixing. Depending on the arrangement of the incoming sequences relative to the target the recombination could either introduce new sequences into the recipient chromosome by a single crossover or substitute sequences by gene conversion or double crossover events.

Several ingenious attempts at targeted gene modification have been made recently. Plasmids have been linearised with restriction enzymes to produce a double strand break within the region homologous to the gene target. These have tended to be much more efficient than closed circular molecules which are also capable of generating recombination. It is presumed that the ends of the DNA molecules are more active in recombination. Although there have been some spectacular successes many problems remain. In particular the efficiency is low and there is a worrying tendency to introduce new mutations after recombination with the 'foreign' DNA. However, because of its specificity it is very important to continue work to develop this method.

Several forms of thalassaemia result from so-called nonsense mutations. These are single base changes that produce premature stop codons in the middle of exons and hence which make it impossible for the affected genes to produce full length protein products. It is possible to correct these defects by the use of so-called *suppressor transfer RNAs* i.e. transfer RNAs which will insert amino acids into the altered codons (see Ho et al 1986).

Recent work has suggested that functional suppressor genes of this type can be constructed by site-specific mutagenesis. Unfortunately however, these molecules mediate only low levels of suppression. Thus a major problem is whether it would be possible to achieve a level of suppression at which the appropriate genes could function in such a way as to produce adequate amounts of gene product. Current work in this field is directed towards constructing retrovirus vectors that contain the suppressor transfer RNA genes so that they can be inserted with high efficiency into bone marrow cells.

Again, there is a long way to go before this equally ingenious approach to gene therapy could have practical application. However, this method should be developed further because it also has the advantage of being a precise site-directed approach to gene therapy.

TRANSGENIC APPROACHES

The experimental introduction of DNA into fertilised eggs and subsequent integration into both somatic cells and germ cells has been achieved successfully in a variety of species. These experiments have been carried out with the object of developing the transgenic animal system as a model for studying gene regulation. DNA has been injected directly into fertilised eggs and have also been transferred using retroviral vectors.

There is no doubt that foreign DNA introduced either by microinjection or retroviral transfection integrates into chromosomal DNA and is carried in germ cells and is then transmitted to subsequent generations (see Palmiter & Brinster 1985). Some remarkable results have been obtained. For example, the introduction of metallothionein/growth hormone fusion genes into mice stimulates the production of growth hormone in tissues that normally synthesise metallothionein. Induction of the metallothionein genes with metals has caused treated mice to grow to about twice their normal size. Tissue specific expression of a variety of genes has been obtained and a number of genetic diseases of mice, including thalassaemia, have been corrected. This model is also extremely useful for studying the effects of oncogene expression and for the analysis of defective embryonic development by insertional mutagenesis.

At the present time the transgenic approach is restricted to the experimental study of gene regulation. Its application to human gene therapy is not contemplated; the modification of the genomes of human populations in this way would raise serious ethical problems.

ACKNOWLEDGEMENTS

We thank Dr D. R. Higgs for providing Figure 3.3 and Mrs Janet Watt for her help in the preparation of the manuscript.

REFERENCES

Adams, J G, Boxer L A, Baehner R L, Forget B G, Tsistrakis G A, Steinberg M A 1979 Journal of Clinical Investigation 69: 931–938
Alter B P 1984 Blood 64: 329–340
Alter B P 1985 Annals of the New York Academy of Sciences 445: 393–407
Anderson W F 1984 Science 226: 401–409
Anderson W F, Kantoff P, Eglitis M et al 1986 Cold Spring Harbor Symposium on Quantitative Biology 51: 1065–1072
Antonarakis S E, Boehm C D, Giardina P J V, Kazazian H H 1982 Proceedings of the National Academy of Sciences of the United States of America 79: 137–141
Antonarakis S E, Orkin S H, Cheng T-C et al 1984 Proceedings of the National Academy of Sciences of the United States of America 81: 1154–1158
Atweh G F, Agnanou N P, Shearin J, Forget B G, Kaufman R E 1985 Nucleic Acids Research 13: 777–790
Atweh G F, Wong C, Reed R et al 1987a Blood 70: 147–151
Atweh G F, Zhu X-X, Brickner H E, Dowling C H, Kazazian H H Jr, Forget B G 1987b Blood 70: 1470–1474
Bernards R, Flavell R A 1980 Nucleic Acids Research 8: 1521–1534
Bodine D M, Ley T J 1987 EMBO Journal 6: 2997–3004
Boehm C D, Dowling C E, Waber P G, Giardina P J V, Kazazian H H Jr 1986 Blood 67: 1185–1188
Bunn H F, Forget B G 1986 Hemoglobin: molecular, genetic and clinical aspects. Saunders, Philadelphia
Busslinger M, Moschonas N, Flavell R A 1981 Cell 27: 289–298
Busslinger M, Hurst J, Flavell R A 1983 Cell 34: 197–206
Cappellini M D, Fiorelli G, Bernini L F 1981 British Journal of Haematology 48: 561–572
Chan V, Chan T K, Liang S T, Ghosh A, Kan Y W, Todd D 1985 Blood 66: 224–228
Chang J C, Kan Y W 1979 Proceedings of the National Academy of Sciences of the United States of America 76: 2886–2889
Chehab F F, Der Kaloustian V, Khouri F P, Deeb S S, Kan Y W 1987a Blood 69: 1141–1145
Chehab F F, Doherty M, Cai S, Kan Y W, Cooper S, Rubin E M 1987b Nature 329: 293–294
Choi Y D, Grabowski P J, Sharp P A, Dreyfus G 1986 Science 231: 1534–1539
Chu G, Hayakawa, H, Berg P 1987 Nucleic Acids Research 15: 1311–1326
Collins F S, Weissman S M 1984 In: Cohn W E, Moldave K (eds) Progress in nucleic acids research and molecular biology. Academic Press, New York p 315–437
Collins F S, Stoeckert C J, Serjeant G R, Forget B G, Weissman S M 1984 Proceedings of the National Academy of Sciences of the United States of America 81: 4894–4898
Diaz-Chico J C, Yang K G, Kutlar A, Reese A L, Aksoy M, Huisman T H J 1987 Blood 70: 583–586
Dzierzak E A, Papayannopoulou T, Mulligan R C 1988 Nature 331: 35–41

Embury S H, Miller J A, Dozy A M, Kan Y W, Chan V, Todd D 1980 Journal of Clinical Investigation 66: 1319–1325
Fearon, E F, Kazazian H H, Waber P G et al 1983 Blood 61: 1269–1274
Felber B K, Orkin S H, Hamer D H 1982 Cell 29: 895–902
Flint J, Hill A V S, Bowden D K et al 1986 Nature 321: 744–749
Galanello R, Ruggeri R, Paglietti E, Addis M, Melis M A, Cao A 1983 Blood 62: 1035–1040
Gelinas R, Endlich B, Pfeiffer C, Yagi M, Stamatoyannopoulos G 1985 nature 313: 323–325
Gianni A M, Bregni M, Cappellini M D et al 1983 EMBO Journal 2: 921–925
Giglioni B, Casini C, Mantovani R et al 1984 EMBO Journal 3: 2641–2645
Gilman J G 1987 British Journal of Haematology 67: 369–372
Gilman J G, Huisman T H J 1985 Blood 66: 783–787
Gilman J G, Huisman T H J, Abels J 1984 British Journal of Haematology 56: 339–348
Goldsmith M E, Humphries R K, Ley T, Cline A, Kantor J A, Nienhuis A 1983 Proceedings of the National Academy of Sciences of the United States of America 88: 2318–2322
Goodbourn S E Y, Higgs D R, Clegg J B, Weatherall D J 1983 Proceedings of the National Academy of Sciences of the United States of America 80: 5022–5026
Gregg R G, Smithies O 1986 Cold Spring Harbor Symposium on Quantitative Biology 51: 1093–1100
Gu Y C, Landman H, Huisman T H J 1987 British Journal of Haematology 66: 245–250
Hershko C, Weatherall D J 1988 Iron chelating therapy. Submitted for publication
Higgs D R, Weatherall D J 1983 In: Piomelli S, Yachnin S (eds) Current topics in hematology 4th edn Liss, New York, p 37–97
Higgs D R, Old J M, Pressley L, Clegg J B, Weatherall D J 1980 Nature 284: 632–635
Higgs D R, Goodbourn S E Y, Lamb J, Clegg J B, Weatherall D J, Proudfoot N J 1983a Nature 306: 398–400
Higgs D R, Wood W G, Barton C, Weatherall D J 1983b American Journal of Medicine 75: 181–191
Higgs D R, Hill A V S, Bowden D K, Weatherall D J, Clegg J B 1984 Nucleic Acids Research 12: 6965–6967
Higgs D R, Wainscoat J S, Flint J et al 1986 Proceedings of the National Academy of Sciences of the United States of America 83: 5165–5169
Hill A V S, Bowden D K, O'Shaughnesy D F, Weatherall D J, Clegg J B 1988 Blood 72: 9–14
Ho T-S, Norton G P, Palese P, Dozy A M, Kan Y W 1986 Cold Spring Harbor Symposium on Quantitative Biology 51: 1033–1040
Jagadeeswaran P, Tuan D, Forget B G, Weissman S M 1982 Nature 296: 469–470
Jarman A P, Nicholls R D, Weatherall D J, Clegg J B, Higgs D R 1986 EMBO Journal 5: 1857–1863
Jeffreys A J, Wilson V, Thein S L, Weatherall D J, Ponder B A J 1986 American Journal of Human Genetics 39: 11–24
Jones R W, Old J M, Trent, R J, Clegg J B, Weatherall D J 1981 Nature 291: 39–44
Kazazian H H Jr, Orkin S H, Antonarakis S E et al 1984 EMBO Journal 3: 593–596
Kazazian H H Jr, Orkin S H, Boehm, C D et al 1986a American Journal of Human Genetics 38: 860–867
Kazazian H H Jr, Dowling C E, Waber P G, Huang S, Lo W H Y 1986b Blood 68: 964–966
Kioussis D, Vanin E, de Lange T, Flavell R A, Grosveld F G 1983 Nature 306: 662–666
Kobayashi Y, Fukumaki Y, Komatsu N, Ohba Y, Miyaji T, Miura Y 1987 Blood 70: 1688–1691
Kogan S C, Doherty M, Gitschier J 1987 New England Journal of Medicine 317: 985–990
Kontoghiorghes G J, Aldouri M A, Hoffbrand A V et al 1987 British Medical Journal 295: 1509–1512
Kulozik A E, Wainscoat J S, Serjeant G R 1986 American Journal of Human Genetics 39: 239–244
Kulozik A E, Kar B C, Satapathy R K, Serjeant B E, Serjeant G R, Weatherall D J 1987a Blood 69: 1742–1746
Kulozik A E, Thein S L, Wainscoat J S et al 1987a British Journal of Haematology 66: 109–112
Kulozik A E, Yarwood N, Jones R W 1988a Blood 71: 457–462
Kulozik A, Kar B C, Serjeant B E, Serjeant G R, Weatherall D J 1988b Blood 71: 467–472
Labie D, Pagnier J, Lapoumeroulie C et al 1985 Proceedings of the National Academy of Sciences of the United States of America 82: 2111–2114
Lapoumeroulie C, Pagnier J, Bank A, Labie D, Krishnamoorthy R 1986 Biochemical and Biophysical Research Communications 139: 709–713
Lauer J, Shen C-K J, Maniatis T 1980 Cell 20: 119–130
Leung S, Whitelaw E, Proudfoot N J 1987 Nature 329: 551–554
Liebhaber S A, Kan Y W 1983 Journal of Clinical Investigation 71: 461–466
Liebhaber S A, Cash F E, Main D M 1985 Journal of Clinical Investigation 76: 1057–1064
Liebhaber S A, Cash F E, Ballas S K 1986a Journal of Biological Chemistry 261: 15327–15333
Liebhaber S A, Coleman M B, Adams J G III, Cash F E, Steinberg M H 1986b ASH Abstract. Blood 68: 75

Lie-Injo L E, Ganesan J, Clegg J B, Weatherall J B 1974 Blood 43: 251–259
Lie-Injo L E, Herrera A R, Kan Y W 1981 Nucleic Acids Research 9: 3707–3717
Loukopoulos D Personal communication
Lucarelli G, Polchi P, Galimberti M et al 1985 Lancet i: 1355–1357
Luzzatto L, Testa U 1978 Current Topics in Hematology 1: 1–70
Marks J, Shaw J-P, Shen C-K J 1986 Nature 321: 785–788
Metherall J E, Collins F S, Pan J, Weissman S M, Forget B G 1986 EMBO Journal 5: 2551–2557
Miller A D, Palmer T D, Hock R A 1986 Cold Spring Harbor Symposium on Quantitative Biology 51: 1013–1020
Morle F, Lopez B, Henni T, Godet J 1985 EMBO Journal 4: 1245–1250
Nagel R L, Fabry M E, Pagnier J et al 1985 New England Journal of Medicine 312: 880–884
Nicholls R D, Fischel-Ghodsian N, Higgs D R 1987 Cell 49: 369–378
Old J M, Fitches A, Heath C et al 1986 Lancet 2: 763–767
Olivieri N F, Chang L S, Poon A O, Michelson A M, Orkin S H 1987 Blood 70: 729–732
Orkin S H, Goff S C 1981 Cell 24: 345–351
Orkin S H, Kazazian H H 1984 Annual Review of Genetics 18: 131–171
Orkin S H, Goff S C, Hechtman R L 1981a Proceedings of the National Academy of Sciences of the United States of America 78: 5041–5045
Orkin S H, Goff S C, Nathan D G 1981b Journal of Clinical Investigation 67: 878–884
Orkin S H, Kazazian H H Jr, Antonarakis S E et al 1982a Nature 296: 627–631
Orkin S H, Kazazian H H Jr, Antonarakis S E, Ostrer H, Goff S C, Sexton J P 1982b Nature 300: 768–769
Orkin S H, Sexton J P, Cheng T C et al 1983a Nucleic Acids Research 11: 4727–4734
Orkin S H, Sexton J P, Goff S C, Kazazian H H Jr 1983b Journal of Biological Chemistry 258: 7249–7251
Orkin S H, Antonarakis S E, Kazazian H H Jr 1984a Journal of Biological Chemistry 259: 8679–8681
Orkin S H, Antonarakis S E, Loukopoulos D 1984b Blood 64: 311–313
Orkin S H, Cheng T-C, Antonarakis S E, Kazazian H H Jr 1985 EMBO Journal 4: 453–456
Ottolenghi S, Giglioni B, Taramelli R et al 1982 Proceedings of the National Academy of Sciences of the United States of America 79: 2347–2351
Ottolenghi S, Giglioni B, Paluzzini A et al 1987 Blood 69: 1058–1061
Padanilam B J, Huisman T H J 1986 American Journal of Hematology 22: 259–263
Padanilam B J, Felice A E, Huisman T H J 1984 Blood 64: 941–944
Paglietti E, Galanello R, Moi P, Pirastu M, Cao A 1986 British Journal of Haematology 63: 485–496
Palmiter R D, Brinster R L 1985 Cell 41: 343–345
Pirastu M, Kan Y W, Lin C C, Baine R, Holbrook C T 1983a Journal of Clinical Investigation 72: 602–609
Pirastu M, Kan Y W, Lao A, Conner B J, Teplitz R K, Wallace R B 1983b New England Journal of Medicine 309: 284–287
Pirastu M, Saglio G, Chang J C, Cao A, Kan Y W 1984 Journal of Biological Chemistry 259: 12315–12317
Poncz M, Ballantine M, Soliwiejczyk D, Barak I, Schwartz E, Surrey S 1982 Journal of Biological Chemistry 257: 5994–5996
Popovich B W, Rosenblatt D S, Kendall A G, Nishioka Y 1986 American Journal of Human Genetics 39: 797–810
Rosatelli C, Leoni G B, Tuveri T, Scalas M T, DiTucci A, Cao A 1987 Journal of Medical Geneteics 24: 97–100
Sampietro M, Cazzola M, Cappellini M D, Fiorelli G 1983 British Journal of Haematology 55: 709–717
Schmickel R D 1986 Journal of Pediatrics 109: 231–241
Schwartz E 1969 New England Journal of Medicine 281: 1327–1333
Semenza G L, Delgrosso K, Poncz M, Malladi P, Schwartz E, Surrey S 1984 Cell 39: 123–128
Shakin S H, Liebhaber S A 1986 Journal of Clinical Investigation 78: 1125–1129
Sharma R S, Yu V, Walters W A W 1979 Medical Journal of Australia 2: 433–434
Spritz R A, Orkin S H 1982 Nucleic Acids Research 10: 8025–8029
Spritz R A, Jagadeeswaran P, Choudary P V et al 1981 Proceedings of the National Academy of Sciences of the United States of America 78: 2455–2459
Surrey S, Delgrosso K, Malladi P, Schwartz E 1985 Journal of Biological Chemistry 260: 6507–6510
Takihara Y, Nakamura T, Yamada H, Takagi Y, Fukumaki Y 1986 Blood 67: 547–550
Tamagnini G P, Lopes M C, Castanheira M E, Wainscoat J S, Wood W G 1983 British Journal of Haematology 54: 189–200
Tate V E, Wood W G, Weatherall D J 1986 Blood 68: 1389–1393
Thein S L, Weatherall D J 1987 Acta Haematologica (Basel) 78: 159–167
Thein S L, Al-Hakim I, Hoffbrand A V 1984a British Journal of Haematology 56: 333–337
Thein S L, Old J M, Wainscoat, J S, Weatherall D J 1984b British Journal of Haematology 57: 271–278

Thein S L, Wainscoat J S, Old J M et al 1985 Lancet ii: 345–347
Thein S L, Wainscoat J S, Sampietro M et al 1987 British Journal of Haematology 65: 367–373
Thein S L, Wallace R B, Pressley L, Clegg J B, Weatherall D J, Higgs D R 1988 Blood 71: 313–319
Thomas E D, Buckner C D, Saunders J E 1982 Lancet ii: 227
Todd D Personal communication
Trecartin R F, Liebhaber S A, Chang J C et al 1981 Journal of Clinical Investigation 68: 1012–1017
Treisman R, Proudfoot N J, Shander M, Maniatis T 1982 Cell 29: 903–911
Treisman R, Orkin S H, Maniatis T 1983 Nature 302: 591–596
Trent R J, Higgs D R, Clegg J B, Weatherall D J 1981 British Journal of Haematology 49: 149–152
Trent R J, Jones R W, Clegg J B, Weatherall D J, Davidson R, Wood W G 1984 British Journal of
    Haematology 57: 279–289
Trent R J, Wilkinson T, Yakas J, Carter J, Lammi A, Kronenberg H 1986 Scandinavian Journal of
    Haematology 36: 272–279
Tuan D, Feingold E, Newman M, Weissman S M, Forget B G 1983 Proceedings of the National Academy
    of Sciences of the United States of America 80: 6937–6941
Van der Ploeg L H T, Konings A, Oort M, Roos D, Bernini L, Flavell R A 1980 Nature 283: 637–642
Vanin E F, Henthorn P S, Kioussis D, Grosveld F, Smithies O 1983 Cell 35: 701–709
Wainscoat J S, Bell J I, Old J M et al 1983a Molecular Biology and Medicine 1: 1–10
Wainscoat J S, Kanavakis E, Wood W G et al 1983b British Journal of Haematology 53: 411–416
Wainscoat J S, Old J M, Wood W G, Trent R J, Weatherall D J 1984 British Journal of Haematology
    58: 353–360
Wainscoat J S, Thein S L, Wood W G, et al 1985a Annals of the New York Academy of Sciences 445:
    20–27
Wainscoat J S, Hill A V S, Boyce A et al 1986 Nature 319: 491–493
Wainscoat J S, Old J M, Thein S L, Weatherall D J 1985b Lancet 2: 1299–1301
Weatherall D J 1985 Clinics in Haematology 14: 747–774
Weatherall, D J, Clegg J B 1975 Philosophical Transactions of the Royal Society of London. Series B:
    Biological Sciences 271: 411–455
Weatherall D J, Clegg J B 1981 The thalassaemia syndromes 3rd edn. Blackwell Scientific, Oxford
Weatherall D J, Clegg J B, Knox-Macaulay, H H M, Bunch C, Hopkins C R, Temperley I J 1973
    British Journal of Haematology 24: 681–687
Weatherall, D J Higgs D R, Bunch C et al 1981 New England Journal of Medicine 305: 607–612
Weatherall D J, Clegg J B, Higgs D R, Wood W G 1988 In: Scriver C R, Beaudet A L, Sly W S,
    Valle D (eds) The metabolic basis of inherited disease 6th edn McGraw-Hill, New York (in press)
Weisbrod S 1982 Nature 297: 289–295
Whitelaw E, Proudfoot N 1986 EMBO Journal 5: 2915–2922
Williams D A, Orkin S H 1986 Journal of Clinical Investigation 77: 1053–1056
Willis R C, Jolly D J, Miller A D et al 1984 Journal of Biological Chemistry 259: 7842–7849
Wong C, Dowliong C E, Saiki R K, Higuchi R G, Erlich H A, Kazazian H H 1987 Nature 330: 384–386
Yee J-K, Jolly D J, Moores J C, Respess J D, Friedman T 1986 Cold Spring Harbor Symposium on
    Quantitative Biology 51: 1021–1026
Zeng Y T, Ren Z R, Chen M J, Zhao J Q, Qui X K, Huang S Z 1987 British Journal of Haematology
    67: 221–223

4. Prospects for effective and oral chelation in transfusional iron overload

G. J. Kontoghiorghes   A. V. Hoffbrand

In this chapter the prospects for treating transfusional iron overload with an orally active iron chelating drug are discussed. In the last few years, the possibility for this major therapeutic advance have improved dramatically. The development of different groups of chelators intended for clinical use and their interaction with iron at the molecular, cellular and tissue level and also in vivo is examined; major emphasis is given to the α-ketohydroxypyridines and in particular to the 1,2-dimethyl-3-hydroxypyrid-4-one which has been shown to be orally effective at iron removal in man. The results of a decade of chelation therapy with parenterally administered desferrioxamine (DF) are also briefly reviewed. The potential value of new oral iron chelators at removing other metals from the body and for treating disturbed iron metabolism other than tissue overload are also dealt with in a final section. Other recent reviews of iron chelation therapy include those by Modell & Berdoukas (1984), Marcus & Huehns (1986), Jacobs (1985), Kontoghiorghes (1987b), Cohen (1987), Brittenham (1988) and Hershko & Weatherall (in press).

CHELATORS

In aqueous solution positively charged metal ions such as Fe^{3+}, Cu^{2+} and Zn^{2+} form complexes with electronegative molecules called ligands, such as —COOH, —OH, —SH, —NH$_2$ etc. Chelator (Greek *chele*—claw of a crab) is a molecule capable of forming a heterocyclic ring with a metal atom as the closing member. It must possess at least two functional groups, with donor atoms (e.g. O, S, N) which can donate a pair of electrons for the formation of a bond with the metal. Depending on the number of the functional groups the chelators are classified as bidentates (e.g. 1,2-dimethyl-3-hydroxypyrid-4-one, L1), tridentates (e.g. pyridoxal isonicotinoyl hydrazone, PIH), hexadentates (e.g. desferrioxamine, DF), etc. (Fig. 4.1). Many structural factors influence the affinity of a chelator for metal ions, such as the molecular composition of the binding site, the chemical composition of the remaining molecule, steric, electronic and other physicochemical properties. Furthermore, the binding of a chelator to a certain metal ion in vivo is affected by the presence of other metal ions and chelating molecules (Kontoghiorghes 1987a). The specificity of a chelator for a particular metal, however, is not absolute so that no chelator has exclusive specificity for one metal ion (Ringborn 1963, Nicholls 1974).

Several other factors limit the effectiveness of a chelator in vivo, such as bioavailability, rate of excretion, rate of biotransformation and toxicity of the chelator and its metal complex (Kontoghiorghes 1982, 1987a,b).

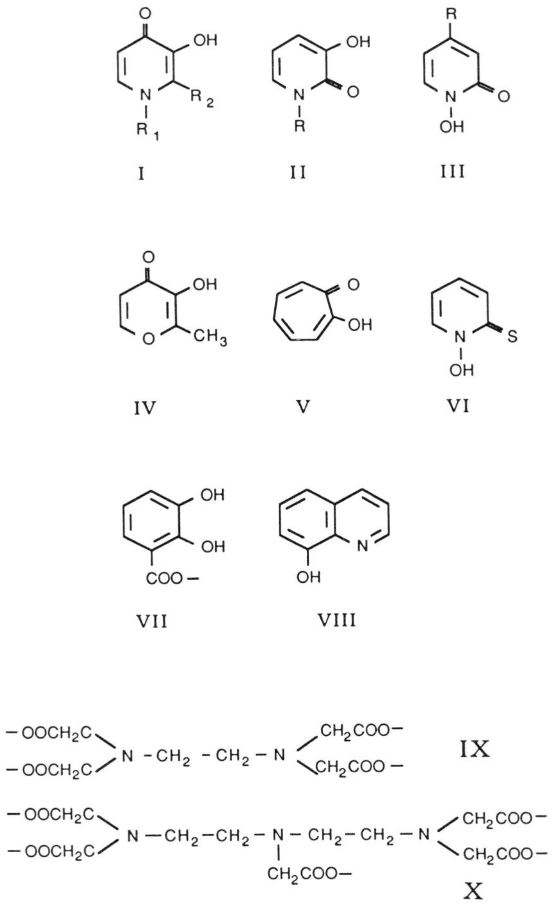

Fig. 4.1 Iron chelators.

I: 1,2-Disubstituted-3-hydroxypyrid-4-ones. 1,2-Dimethyl-3-hydroxypyrid-4-one, L1, $(R_1 = R_2 = -CH_3)$; 1-ethyl-3-hydroxy-2-methylpyrid-4-one, L1NEt, $(R_1 = -CH_2CH_3, R_2 = -CH_3)$; 3-hydroxy-2-methyl-1-propylpyrid-4-one, L1NPr, $(R_1 = CH_2CH_2CH_3, R_2 = -CH_3)$; 3-hydroxy-1-(2-methoxyethyl)-2-methylpyrid-4-one, L1-methoxyethyl, $(R_1 = -CH_2CH_2 - OH_3, R_2 = -CH_2CH_3)$; 2-ethyl-3-hydroxypyrid-4-one, EL1, $(R_1 = -CH_3, R_2 = -CH_2CH_3)$; 1,2-diethyl-3-hydroxypyrid-4-one, EL1NEt, $(R_1 = R_2 = -CH_2CH_3)$; 2-ethyl-3-hydroxy-1-propylpyrid-4-one, EL1NPr, $(R_1 = -CH_2CH_2CH_3, R_2 = -CH_2CH_3)$; 2-ethyl-3-hydroxy-1-(2-methoxyethyl)-pyrid-4-one, EL1-methoxyethyl, $(R_1 = -CH_2 - CH_2 - OCH_3, R_2 = -CH_2 - CH_2)$; mimosine, $(R_1 = -CH_2CHNH_2COOH, R_2 = -H)$.

II: 1-substituted-3-hydroxypyrid-2-ones. 3-hydroxy-1-methylpyrid-2-one, L2, $(R = -CH_3)$.

III: 4-substituted-1-hydroxypyrid-2-ones. 1-hydroxypyrid-2-one, L4, $(R = -H)$; 1,4-dihydroxypyrid-2-one, L3, $(R = -OH)$; 1-hydroxy-4-methoxypyrid-2-one, L6, $(R = -OCH_3)$.

IV: Maltol.

V: Tropolone.

VI: Omadine.

VII: 2,3-Dihydroxybenzoic acid, 2,3-DHB.

VIII: 8-Hydroxyquinoline.

IX: Ethylenediaminetetraacetic acid, EDTA.

X: Diethylenetriaminepentaacetic acid, DTPA.

XI: Desferrithiocin.

XII: Pyridoxal isonicotinoyl hydrazone, PIH.

XIII: Cholylhydroxamic acid.

XIV: Rhodotorulic acid.

XV: Desferrioxamine, DF.

XVI: Ethylenediamine-N,N'-bis-(2-hydroxyphenylacetic acid), EDHPA, or N,N'-ethylenebis-(2-hydroxyphenylglycine), EHPG.

XVII: Enterobactin (enterochelin).

XVIII: N,N',N''-tris-(2,3-dihydroxy-benzoyl)-1,3,5-triaminoethyl benzene, MECAM.

XI

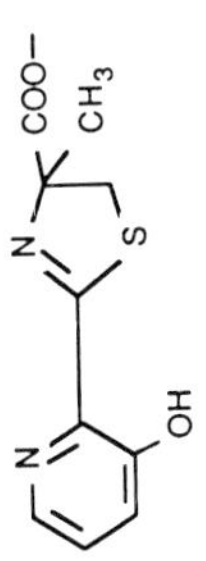

XII

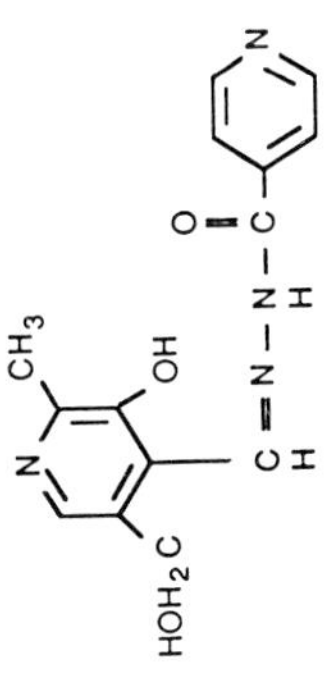

XIII

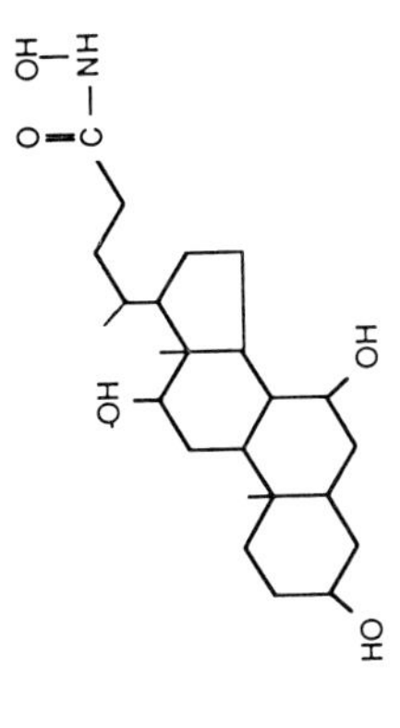

XIV

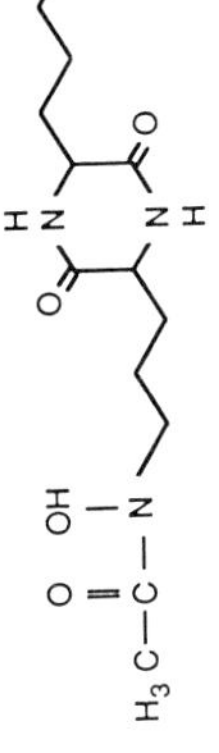

XV

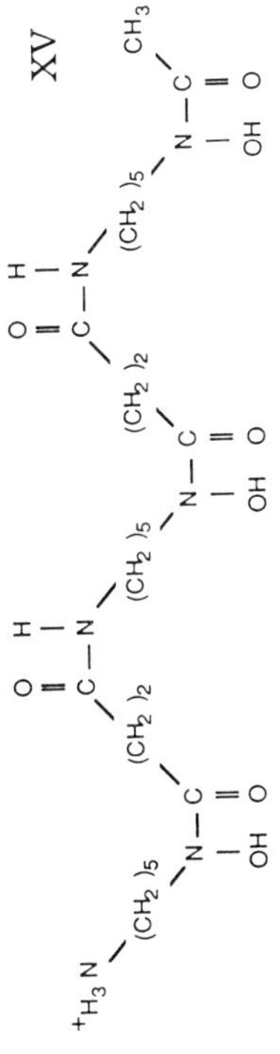

XVI

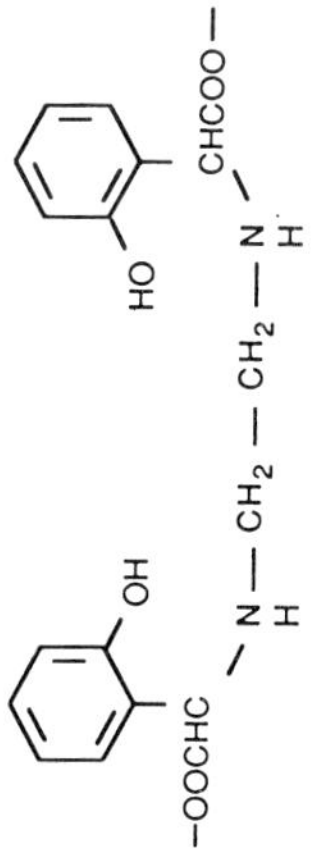

XVII

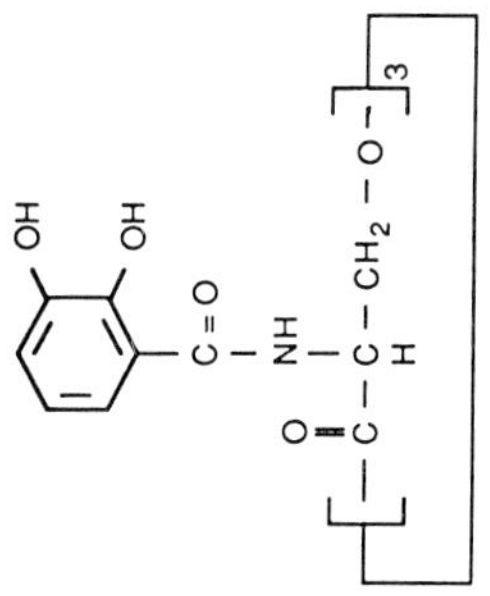

XVIII

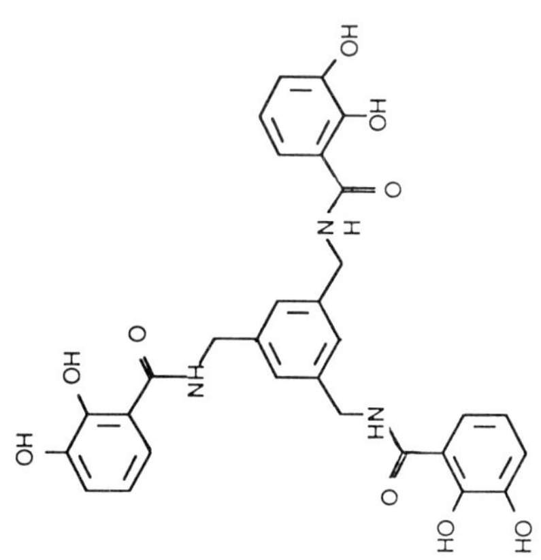

Iron chelators

Naturally occurring iron chelators, called siderophores (Greek: *sideros*—iron, *phero*—carry) were synthesised early in evolution by bacteria and fungi in order to mobilise iron needed in many biological reactions from insoluble iron deposits in the earth's crust (Neilands 1980). Three major iron binding sites occur widely in siderophores: the hydroxamates which are mainly found in fungi, the catechols which are mainly found in bacteria and the carboxylates which are found in both types of organisms. Iron binding substances in plants have been less well characterised but catechols and carboxylates dominate (Sugiura & Nomoto 1984, Kontoghiorghes 1987b).

In addition, the powerful α-ketohydroxy iron binding site found in the orally active chelator L1, is widely distributed in compounds of some plant species e.g. mimosine, maltol and tropolone and is also found in bacteria (Akers et al 1980). In animals and in man, specific proteins with high affinity for iron have evolved for transporting iron e.g. transferrin and lactoferrin and for storing iron e.g. ferritin. Several other low molecular weight chelators such as citrate, phosphate and ATP, have also been implicated in iron metabolism in man and are thought to participate in intracellular iron transport (Jacobs 1977, Kontoghiorghes 1987b).

Synthetic iron chelators

Many synthetic iron chelators, most of which resemble the naturally occurring compounds have been designed and tested for clinical use with limited success (Anderson & Hiller 1975, Martell et al 1981). The most promising synthetic chelators which show some activity in vivo are listed in Table 4.1. DF, its derivatives and other

Table 4.1   Effective iron chelators in vivo

	Log β*
1. Desferrioxamine derivatives and polymeric hydroxamates	31
2. Phenolic ethylene diamines	34–40
3. Pyridoxal isonicotinoyl hydrazones	25–28
4. Desferrithiocins	30
5. DTPA, EDTA	25–29
6. 2,3-DHB and other oligomeric catechols	40–52
7. α-ketohydroxypyridines	30–37

* Log β: is the iron stability constant obtained at ideal conditions. It is a general indicator but not directly related to iron binding at physiological pH or in vivo (Kontoghiorghes 1982).

polymeric hydroxamates (Winston et al 1982) are all effective chelators, specific in removing iron but suffer from the high cost of preparation and oral inactivity. The phenolic ethylene diamine derivatives are in general cheaper to prepare and effective by the parenteral route and also to a lesser extent active orally. It is expected from their structure that these chelators will have an affinity for other metals such as Ca^{2+}, Mg^{2+} and Zn^{2+}. PIH and related derivatives are orally active and more specific iron chelators which are easy to synthesise. Desferrithiocin is a naturally occurring iron chelator derived from streptomyces which is orally active but toxic. Derivatives of this chelator may eliminate the toxicity (Peter 1983, Longueville & Crichton 1986). The polycarboxylic polyamine derivatives diethylenetriaminepentaacetic acid (DTPA) and ethylenediaminetetra-acetic acid (EDTA) are chelators which are non specific for iron and are not orally active. They are cheap to produce and DTPA is effective clinically but supplementation with zinc is required to avoid serious side effects (Pippard et al 1986). 2,3-Dihydroxybenzoic acid (2,3-DHB) and other catecholic chelators have high specificity for iron but suffer from autoxidation and the possibility of supporting the growth of microbes in vivo. The α-ketohydroxypyridines (α-KHPs) are divided into three classes: the 1-hydroxypyrid-2-ones, 1-substituted 3-hydroxypyrid-2-ones and 1-substituted 2-alkyl-3-hydroxypyrid-4-ones. The last group was designed to mimic tropolone and mimosine which were shown to be orally active in iron removal in vivo previously (Kontoghiorghes 1988a). The 1-substituted 2-alkyl-3-hydroxypyrid-4-ones are the most promising chelators for clinical use and several of its members are cheap to synthesise and orally active.

Several attempts to substantially improve chelation with the most widely used drug DF by incorporating it into red blood cell ghosts (Green et al 1977) or liposomes or by structural modifications of the DF molecule have also been unsuccessful. Limited success has been repeatedly found following the administration of oral DF and also with the drug as a suppository (Kontoghiorghes et al 1983).

IRON METABOLISM

Body iron levels are regulated by the gut through absorption and the erythropoietic activity of the bone marrow. Transfusion and increased iron absorption result in iron overload because there is no regulatory process of iron excretion in man. There are many iron containing proteins which are involved in metabolic pathways essential for normal growth, development and detoxification of toxic substances in man (Table 4.2). Transferrin, which transports iron from the sites of absorption and storage to the sites of utilisation is thought to be in equilibrium with all the other intracellular

Table 4.2 Examples of iron proteins and their function

Function	Proteins	Iron form
Oxygen transport	Haemoglobin	Haem
Oxygen storage	Myoglobin	Haem
Electron transfer	Cytochromes	Haem
	Adrenoxin	Fe, S
	Xanthine oxidase	Fe, S
Drug detoxification	Cyt P_{450} and b_5	Haem
DNA synthesis	Ribonucleotide reductase	Non-haem
Collagen synthesis	Proline hydroxylase	Non-haem
Tricarboxylic acid cycle	Aconitase	Non-haem
Other enzymatic functions	Peroxidases	Haem
	Catalase	Haem
	Cytochrome b_2	Haem
	Tyrosine hydroxylase	Haem
	Cyclooxygenase	Haem
	Nitrite reductase	Fe, S
	Lipoxygenase	Non-haem
Iron transport	Transferrin	Non-haem
	Lactoferrin	Non-haem
Iron storage	Ferritin	Inorganic FeOOH
	Haemosiderin	(Polynuclear)

iron pools. This equilibrium may be affected in several ways such as disease e.g. anaemia of chronic disease, haemodialysis, in atransferrinaemia, by chelation etc. In iron overload, non-haem iron as ferritin and mainly haemosiderin increases substantially in tissues especially in the liver and the spleen. Under these conditions transferrin is saturated with iron and a non-transferrin iron pool of serum ferritin iron (Pootrakul et al 1988) and possibly also of a low molecular weight (MW) (Hershko et al 1978) may be present in the serum. In transfusional iron overload the major pools of chelatable iron are those found in the serum, liver parenchymal cells, the cells of the endocrine organs and in the reticuloendothelial system as macrophages following the catabolism of effete red cells. During chelation one or more of the chelatable iron pools could be primarily affected depending on the physicochemical properties of the chelators (see later).

The effect of chelators on the molecular iron pools

Low MW pool

The interaction of a chelator with the various iron containing proteins and other molecules in vitro gives an indication of the site of action of the chelators in vivo. Iron removal or incorporation in iron-containing proteins including haemoglobin, transferrin, haemosiderin and ferritin is mononuclear, that is a low MW complex with one molecule of iron bound to the ligand. Iron excreted in the urine of iron loaded patients following DF or L1 treatment is also of a low MW complex form, of one to one (DF) or one to three (L1) iron to chelator molar ratio (Kontoghiorghes et al 1987a,b, Kontoghiorghes et al 1988b). Low MW iron is mainly found intracellularly, and in serum of iron loaded patients in whom transferrin is saturated. All effective chelators, including those in Table 4.1 bind such low MW iron within minutes, whether this is found intracellularly (Jacobs 1977), secreted by macrophages (Saito et al 1986) or in the serum of iron overloaded patients. The ability of the chelator and its complex to diffuse across the cell membrane and to compete for iron with transferrin and other biomolecules with iron binding capacity are important considerations in the removal of iron from low MW iron pools (Kontoghiorghes 1987b).

Ferritin

Iron removal by chelators from polynuclear iron forms such as ferritin (which has a storage capacity of up to 4500 molecules of iron per protein molecule) and haemosiderin (which is the main storage protein in iron overload) both of which contain a highly concentrated iron precipitate form ($FeOOH$ polymer, Gray 1975) is very slow, taking days to reach completion (Kontoghiorghes 1986a, 1987c). Ferritin is a water soluble spherical-shaped protein (MW 450 000) with 6 hydrophobic and 8 hydrophilic channels through which iron is deposited or removed (Rice et al 1983). Large chelators such as the trimeric catechols 3,4-LICAMS and MECAM and to some extent DF are not effective in mobilising substantial amounts of iron from ferritin (Tufano et al 1981), possibly due to their inability to pass through the protein channels (Kontoghiorghes 1986a). PIH and its analogues also mobilise iron from ferritin but less than DF (Vitolo et al 1984). The most successful chelators so far in iron removal from ferritin are the bidentate 1-hydroxypyrid-2-one derivatives L3 and L6 (Kontoghiorghes 1986a, Kontoghiorghes 1987d) and the 1,2-dialkyl-3-

hydroxypyrid-4-ones including L1 (Kontoghiorghes et al 1987c,d, 1988 in press). Two other α-ketohydroxy chelators namely 1-methyl-3-hydroxypyrid-2-one (L2) and the natural product maltol are less effective.

The mechanism of iron release from ferritin by chelators appears to be: (1) diffusion of the chelator through the channels; (2) the displacement of the hydroxyl ligands and the breaking of the oxo bridges of the iron core; (3) formation of a ternary complex of the chelator with the iron core; (4) formation of iron chelator complexes of different stoichiometry; (5) diffusion of the iron complex through the channels out of ferritin and (6) the formation of the normal chelator-iron complex stoichiometry e.g. 1:1 for DF and 3:1 for L1. Iron mobilisation from ferritin by chelators is also limited by other factors such as the relative concentrations and iron solubility constant of the chelator, the concentration of protein and iron in ferritin, and the presence of mediators such as ascorbic acid which further augments iron mobilisation. Iron mobilisation by chelators is also higher at acid pH (Kontoghiorghes unpublished) and under reducing conditions (Sirivech et al 1974).

Iron incorporated more recently into ferritin was shown to be mobilised faster than iron previously incorporated into ferritin (Hoy et al 1974). Decreased solubility of ferritin iron and of a freshly prepared iron precipitate was observed following repeated in vitro exposure to chelators such as DF and L1 (Kontoghiorghes 1987c). These results are consistent with the observations that as the iron content of ferritin, or for that matter of stored iron in iron overload decreases, the proportion of iron chelated using the same amount of chelator also decreases.

Haemosiderin

Haemosiderin is an armorphous non water soluble, variable mixture of non haem iron precipitates, other metals, protein and lipid fractions (Weir et al 1984). It may be formed from the proteolysis and polymerisation of ferritin (Hoy & Jacobs 1981). Iron mobilisation in vitro by chelators from haemosiderin is slow taking days to reach completion but is faster than from ferritin probably due to restrictions imposed by channels in the latter (Kontoghiorghes et al 1987c). DF was found to be more effective than the α-KHP chelators in the mobilisation of iron from haemosiderin (Kontoghiorghes et al 1987c). Intensive treatment of thalassaemia patients with DF particularly reduces the amount of iron found as haemosiderin in the liver (Hoffbrand 1980, Cohen et al 1984).

Transferrin

The central role of transferrin in iron transport between the sites of absorption, storage, utilisation and iron recycling following the breakdown of haemoglobin is of major importance in the chelation strategy. One molecule of transferrin binds two molecules of iron at two different domains, via a two tyrosine, one histidine, one aspartate and possibly one water and one carbonate or bicarbonate ligand complex. The transferrin iron pool is thought to be in equilibrium with the low MW intracellular iron pool, and in turn with ferritin, haemosiderin and other proteins containing iron. Since transferrin is normally 25–35% saturated with iron and is turning over several times during the day to provide 20–25 mg of iron needed daily for the production of haemoglobin, its contribution to the chelatable iron is potentially substantial. It is estimated that at least 75 mg of transferrin bound iron may be available for chelation each day in transfusional iron overload patients whose transferrin is 100% saturated.

Furthermore chelation of transferrin bound iron will minimise accumulation of iron in the tissues, which may be less toxic because it will take place extracellularly or on the surface of cells and it will be faster than mobilisation of intracellular polynuclear iron (Kontoghiorghes 1982).

Iron removal from transferrin by DF in vitro at physiological pH is very slow although the presence of mediators such as citrate, ADP and ATP may accelerate this process (Pollack et al 1977). The trimeric catechols 3,4-LICAMS and MECAM (Carrano & Raymond 1979) and the aminoalkyl phosphonic acid derivatives (Harris 1984), all remove iron from transferrin at pH 7.4. The most effective chelators of transferrin iron mobilisation at physiological pH are the α-KHPs (Kontoghiorghes 1982). Of these, the 1,2-dialkyl-3-hydroxypyrid-4-ones including L1 (Kontoghiorghes 1986b, Kontoghiorghes et al 1987d) and the 2-hydroxypyridine-1-oxides (Kontoghiorghes 1987a) are the most effective causing the release of more than 80% of transferrin iron within a few hours. The rate of iron mobilisation from the two sites of transferrin using the α-KHP is different and with L1 is much faster from the C-terminal than from the N-terminal (Kontoghiorghes & Evans 1985). The mechanism of iron removal from transferrin by chelators involves: (1) the transfer of the chelator to the iron binding site; (2) displacement of bicarbonate and other transferrin ligands; (3) formation of ternary chelator-iron-tranferrin complex; (4) displacement of all transferrin ligands by the chelator and the formation of a chelator iron complex (Kontoghiorghes 1986b).

Other sources
The mobilisation of iron from the other iron containing proteins contributes only a small proportion to the total iron chelatable pool. For example iron could be mobilised from lactoferrin when effective chelators like L1 are used (Kontoghiorghes 1986c) in contrast to haem iron in proteins such as the major pool, haemoglobin (Kontoghiorghes 1987f).

CELLULAR IRON METABOLISM

The major iron storage cellular pools are parenchymal cells mainly of the liver and macrophages of the RE system. Iron mobilisation from isolated ^{59}Fe labelled hepatocytes has been studied using a variety of chelators such as DF, PIH and its analogues (Baker et al 1985), L1 and mimosine (Mostert et al 1987). Several chelators including PIH and L1 were found to be more effective than DF in releasing iron from hepatocytes. The mechanism of iron release from these and probably of other cells seems to be stepwise: (1) diffusion of the chelator into the cell; (2) binding of a small low MW iron pool; (3) mobilisation of ferritin/haemosiderin iron; (4) formation of a large intracellular chelator-iron low MW complex and (5) gradual diffusion of the chelator-iron complex out of the cell. Iron release from macrophages prelabelled with ^{59}Fe is enhanced in vitro in the presence of DF (Esparza & Brock 1981, Kleber et al 1981, Saito et al 1986). In other studies several 1,2-dialkyl-3-hydroxypyrid-4-ones including L1 were shown to be as effective as DF at increasing iron release from mouse peritoneal macrophages (Brock et al, unpublished).

Of 40 chelators derivatives of 2,3-DHB and hydroxamic acid which were tested on Chang cells, 2,3-DHB the ethyl ester of 3,4-dimethoxybenzoic acid and cholyl-hydroxamic acid were identified as the most effective (White et al 1976). The study of 10 chelators, mostly of microbial siderophore origin, in cultured rat myocytes has identified agrobactin as more effective than DF at reducing cellular iron uptake (Sciortino et al 1980). Screening of PIH using ^{59}Fe-labelled reticulocytes indicated increased ^{59}Fe removal mainly from mitochondia by this chelator (Ponka et al 1979).

Eight chelators including L1 and PIH have been studied for their effects on iron donation, transferrin iron donation, transferrin membrane binding and DNA synthesis in the leukaemic cells lines K562 and U937. Increased transferrin receptor synthesis due to the removal of an intracellular iron pool was shown with hydrophilic chelators e.g. L1 which were non cytotoxic. In contrast, lipophilic chelators such as PIH were found to be toxic in these cell systems (Forsbeck et al 1987).

Study of 36 chelators mainly of hydroxamate and benzoate origin on DNA synthesis in phytohaemagglutin (PHA) stimulated lymphocytes, has also shown inhibitory effects on ribonucleotide reductase by some chelators such as DF, but also cytotoxic effects unrelated to this enzyme by chelators such as tropolone (Ganeshaguru et al 1980). A chelator structure/cytotoxic activity correlation of several iron chelators with different physicochemical properties have been studied in the human leukaemia cell lines U937, K562, ML2 and HL60. While lipophilic chelators such as 8-hydroxyquinoline, tropolone and omadine were found to have similar cytotoxic effects to those of the anti-cancer drugs doxorubicin and mitoxantrone, hydrophilic ones such as L1 and DF did not inhibit cell growth or cause any toxic effects at 4 h incubations. Addition of iron potentiated the cytotoxic activity of the lipophilic chelators, indicating that with these compounds iron removal is not the only mechanism of toxicity by chelators (Kontoghiorghes et al 1986a,b). In a more detailed examination of the effect of 20 chelators on transmembrane cellular uptake of iron in mature erythrocytes it was shown that chelators forming neutral lipophilic iron complexes such as L6, 8-hydroxyquinoline and tropolone, cause the incorporation of iron into the cells at different rates, which are proportional to the lipid/water partition coefficient of the chelator iron complexes. In contrast charged or neutral/hydrophilic chelators, such as L1 and DF did not cause iron to be incorporated into the cells. Thus, chelators forming lipophilic iron complexes may enhance iron uptake into cells, resulting in toxicity, while hydrophilic chelators may be less toxic because of their more rapid excretion and a minimal accumulation in cells (Kontoghiorghes 1988). Similar results have been obtained using human erythroid cells. Iron from lipophilic chelator iron complexes was incorporated mainly into ferritin and partly into haem. Hydrophilic chelator iron complexes on the other hand did not make iron available to these cells (May & Kontoghiorghes, unpublished).

EVALUATION OF CHELATORS IN ANIMALS

Several animal models have been used in the past for evaluating hundreds of chelators intended for clinical use. From those studies only a few chelators have been shown to be promising e.g. 2,3-DHB, rhodotorulic acid and ethylene diamine-N,N'-bis-2-hydroxyphenylacetic acid (EDHPA) (Pitt et al 1979, Graziano et al 1974, Grady et al 1979). In recent studies normal rats, and rats loaded with iron from a fortified iron diet and radiolabelled with ^{59}Fe ferritin, were used to identify the efficacy and site of action of DF, DHB, DTPA, EDHPA and PIH (Pippard et al 1981). Of the chelators tested, EDHPA and PIH were shown to be orally active and comparable to DF in iron release, which was almost completely biliary. This, and the previous model, were used to screen several analogues of pyridoxal, some of which were highly effective e.g. pyridoxal benzoyl hydrazone or PIH (Avramovici-Grisaru et al 1983).

Identification of potentially effective α-KHP chelators for clinical use was carried out using normal and iron dextran loaded animals, ^{59}Fe labels and ^{59}Fe/^{56}Fe estimations (Kontoghiorghes 1982, 1985). Mice were loaded by intraperitoneally administered iron dextran and labelled with ^{59}Fe lactoferrin, which directs the ^{59}Fe initially into the liver but then equilibrates with the other iron pools in the body (Kontoghiorghes 1986d).

A study of 12 analogues of L1 and L2, at doses of 200 mg/kg, identified at least 4 alkyl derivatives of such chelators, which were orally and intra-peritoneally effective at increasing iron excretion. Three, L1, L1NEt and L1NPr (Fig. 4.1), had an equivalent effect to intraperitoneal DF (Kontoghiorghes 1986d). In the same model, using dose response studies, the range of effective doses for iron removal was identified to be >30 mg/kg for the above three chelators (Kontoghiorghes 1986e). Repeated administration of L3 (2 × 200 mg/kg), a slightly less effective chelator than DF, caused an increase in iron excretion to levels equivalent to those achieved by single doses of DF and L1 (300 mg/kg) (Kontoghiorghes 1987e). Such chelators therefore may be effective in achieving negative iron balance following repeated administrations, despite the relatively low iron output from a single dose. Studies in iron loaded/radioactively labelled rabbits confirmed that oral L1 and L1NEt are effective iron chelators and suggested that they chelated iron from different pools than DF (Kontoghiorghes & Hoffbrand 1986). There was no increase in the urinary excretion of Cu, Zn, Mg and Ca in these studies (Kontoghiorghes 1987f). Iron dextran loaded or normal ^{59}Fe-lactoferrin labelled mice showed equivalent amounts of ^{59}Fe excretion following intraperitoneal DF and intraperitoneal or oral L1, or L1NEt (Kontoghiorghes 1987f). Furthermore in three different rat models, parenteral or oral L1 was shown to be as effective as parenteral DF (Kontoghiorghes et al 1987e). From the above animal studies it appears that: (1) only a few % of the ^{59}Fe is removed during chelator treatment; (2) in animals ^{59}Fe from all three radiolabels ^{59}Fe transferrin, lactoferrin and citrate is predominantly excreted in the faeces, but in different proportions (>70), (>90) and (>97) in rabbits, rats and mice respectively; (3) different chelators have different affinities for different iron pools (Kontoghiorghes et al 1986d).

STUDIES IN MAN

Results of desferrioxamine therapy

Patients with refractory anaemias requiring regular red blood cell transfusions usually receive about 30 units of blood each year, equivalent to 7 g of iron. Approximately 20 mg iron must be excreted daily in order to maintain iron balance. Following earlier observation of prevention of progression of hepatic fibrosis in thalassaemia major with daily intramuscular injections of DF, daily subcutaneous (SC) DF infusions were introduced for the management of transfusional iron overload in 1976–7. In previously unchelated teenage patients with thalassaemia major, up to 200 mg of iron was excreted daily at doses of 40–60 mg/kg SC DF. More recent studies have assessed the value of long-term intensive DF chelation therapy on survival, cardiac, liver and endocrine damage in patients with refractory anaemias requiring regular transfusion therapy. These include those with congenital disorders such as Diamond Blackfan syndrome, Fanconi anaemia, sickle cell anaemia and sideroblastic anaemia and also acquired anaemias including myelodysplasia, red cell aplasia, aplastic anaemia and myelofibrosis. By far the largest group are, however, patients with thalassaemia major and most of the studies on the effect of SC DF are based on this disease. These have also revealed a number of side-effects of DF therapy. The major problems with DF therapy, however, remain its cost and its mode of administration which make the introduction of a cheap effective oral chelator of prime importance.

Thalassaemia major

Although serious organ damage was thought to occur only after about 100 units (or 20 g iron) have been transfused, it is clear from sensitive tests of organ function that damage e.g. to the liver, heart or endocrine organs may occur with lesser amounts of iron. It is now usual, therefore, to commence SC DF soon after blood transfusions have started, and well before irreversible organ damage can occur. The dose recommended is 40–60 mg/kg given over 12 hours on 5–7 nights each week. DF can also be given intravenously at the time of blood transfusion e.g. 2 g with each unit of blood. A plateau of urine iron excretion occurs in most iron loaded patients at doses of 50–60 mg/kg/day although with severely iron loaded patients more iron is excreted at higher doses. Pippard et al (1982) have shown that there is no plateau to faecal iron excretion induced by DF and at high doses of DF, particularly when the haemoglobin level is also high, faecal excretion may account for 40% or more of the total iron excreted.

It is usual to give oral vitamin C, 100–200 mg daily at the beginning of SC DF therapy since this enhances urine iron excretion in vitamin C deficient iron loaded patients. Iron overload is itself a potent cause of vitamin C deficiency due to increased catabolism. Vitamin C appears to expand the chelatable iron pool, increase serum iron and serum ferritin and there is some anecdotal experience that vitamin C at larger doses (500 mg or more daily) may lead to cardiac decompensation.

The benefits of iron chelation include the immediate removal of a toxic intracellular iron pool as well as free non-protein bound iron from serum but the major effect is to reduce or prevent iron loading.

Survival and cardiac disease

It is too early to assess the life expectancy of children with thalassaemia major and other genetically determined anaemias who begin regular transfusions and SC DF therapy in the first few years of life. Before the introduction of DF and transfusions to maintain adequate haemoglobin levels, survival in thalassaemia major over the age of 20 was unusual. In one series studied between 1964 and 1977, the mean age at death was 18 (range 9–33, Ehlers et al 1980). Over 50% of patients now survive to this age, no doubt partly due to DF chelation therapy, although better general management (e.g. of transfusion, infections and splenectomy) may also contribute. Modell et al (1982) reported that patients in Britain who had received more than 4 g DF weekly over the previous few years were less likely to die in the near future than those who had received less or no DF. Giardina et al (1987) have compared the survival of 70 thalassaemia-major patients maintained at pretransfusion haemoglobin levels of 8 g/dl and not chelated (median survival 17.1 years, 51 of 70 dead) and 89 patients given SC DF 3 or more days per week with pretransfusion haemoglobin levels 11 g/dl (median survival 30 years, 27 of 89 dead). Although these findings confirm the value of DF therapy the results in the chelated group are rather disappointing perhaps due to the rather low doses of DF (20 mg/kg/day) given to at least some of the patients.

Hyman et al (1985) noted that all 6 non-chelated patients who had received 40–100 g iron in transfused blood died whereas none of their 7 DF treated patients with the same iron load died. More detailed studies of cardiac function provide more direct evidence of the value of chelation. Wolfe et al (1985) found that 12 of 19 non-compliant (with SC DF) patients developed clinical or laboratory evidence of cardiac disease, and 7 died, whereas only 1 of 12 compliant patients developed cardiac abnormalities and died. All 31, however, had commenced DF therapy over the age of 10. Freeman et al (1983) had earlier shown cardiac abnormalities in 18 of 23 thalassaemia major patients, the mean serum ferritin being 1043 μg/l in the 5 with normal left ventricular (LV) function and 3732 μg/l in those of comparable age with abnormal LV function. In 4 of 7 with an abnormal LV function on exercise, this became normal after a year of intensive DF therapy although 1 deteriorated and died.

Reversal of clinical apparent cardiac disease has also been described in a number of thalassaemic patients given intensive DF therapy. Marcus et al (1984), treated 5 such patients; 3 improved and were alive 18 months later. Hyman et al (1985) reversed congestive heart failure in 3 patients who were alive 2, 7 and 8 years later and 1 of our patients, now aged 28 is alive and clinically well having been in congestive heart failure 11 years ago (Hussain, Hoffbrand & Politis, unpublished). All these patients whose heart disease improved, received high doses of DF ranging from 40–235 mg/kg/day and generally continuous, 24 hour infusions either by insertion of an indwelling intravenous catheter (e.g. Port-A-Cath or Hickman) or by admission to hospital and intravenous line.

Liver disease

Within a year of commencement of SC DF it was apparent that liver iron content (and serum ferritin levels) could be reduced despite the need for continuing transfusions (Hoffbrand et al 1979). More recent studies have shown that liver iron stores are maintained about 5–10 times normal in thalassaemia major with doses of SC DF of 40–60 mg/kg 5 times weekly (Al-Douri et al 1987). Progression of liver failure in these well chelated patients was found to be related more to viral hepatitis than to iron overload. More intensive SC and intravenous DF may even bring liver iron stores and serum ferritin levels down to normal (Cohen et al 1984) but in view of the side-effects of such intensive DF therapy, particularly if used for prolonged periods, it may not be justified except in an attempt to reverse cardiac dysfunction.

Endocrine function

Although it is clear that SC DF may prevent endocrine damage in a proportion of patients leading to increased growth and sexual development, there is little evidence for reversal of damage already present. Moreover, diabetes mellitus, hypothyroidism, hypoparathyroidism, failure of puberty and of growth and secondary amenorrhoea continue to occur frequently in teenage and young adult patients even though they commenced SC DF 10 years ago and have complied with the therapy. For example, De Sanctis et al (1987) found that of 29 patients with normal glucose tolerance at the start of chelation therapy, in 17 this became abnormal, 6 patients developing overt diabetes mellitus over a period of 6.2–8.8 years.

Adult transfusional iron overload
Subcutaneous DF therapy (40–60 mg/kg 5 nights weekly) has proved effective at preventing organ damage due to iron and indeed reversing this in adults with acquired transfusion dependent anaemias. In a typical study, Schafer et al (1985) found that liver iron content decreased, liver function normalised and plasma cortisol response to insulin induced hypoglycaemia improved but there was no improvement in glucose tolerance in a substantial proportion of their patients and there was no cardiac deterioration over a 13–66 month period. Compliance with SC DF therapy is good in patients commencing SC DF as adults.

Side-effects of desferrioxamine therapy
DF has proved a remarkably safe drug. However, a number of unwanted side-effects have now been documented. The best described are neurological, ophthalmic and auditory complications which become apparent when high doses of DF have been used. Earlier reports included occasional anaphylactic reactions or skin sensitivity and one of cataracts.

Ophthalmic toxicity
Davies et al (1983) described visual failure, particularly night and colour blindness and annular field loss in patients given 75–235 mg/kg/day DF intravenously for advanced iron induced cardiac disease. Borgna-Pignatti et al (1984) described a further case while Olivieri et al (1986) in an extensive study described 4 of 89 patients receiving 34–150 mg/kg/day to have symptomatic visual loss with optic neuropathy and delayed visual evoked potential and loss of colour vision while a further 5 showed changes in retinal epithelial pigment but were asymptomatic. Arden et al (1984) detected retinal abnormalities in 29 of 43 patients, more closely related to diabetes or an abnormal glucose tolerance than to dose of DF received. They suggested that diabetes, by altering the retinal vascular permeability may cause increased susceptibility in some patients to DF toxicity. De Virgilliis et al (1988a) suggest acute zinc, copper or 'iron' deficiency as possible causes of eye toxicity after high IV closes on the basis of excretion studies and tests of leucocyte alkaline phosphatase.

Auditory toxicity
Olivieri et al (1986) found significant loss of high tone hearing in 22 of 89 patients receiving SC DF, with clinical deafness in 6. The affected patients tended to be of a younger age, with lower serum ferritin levels and receiving higher doses of DF than patients with normal hearing. Wonke et al (1988) have confirmed these observations, finding 5 patients with clinical deafness of 50 patients (not unselected) studied. A further 6 (12%) showed high tone hearing loss. Interestingly, in all 5 patients, hearing loss improved to normal over periods up to 18 months when DF treatment was discontinued and regular SC DTPA with oral zinc supplements used instead. More serious cerebral toxicity has been described in non-iron loaded patients with rheumatoid arthritis given SC DF. Coma for 48–72 h developed in 2 given 3 g DF/day with prochlorperazine and nausea and vomiting occurred in 5 of 6 given 2 g SC DF daily (Blake et al 1985).

Other side-effects

Gabutti et al (1987) have described failure of growth in children receiving SC DF 60 mg/kg/day or more, reversed by stopping DF therapy. De Virgilliis et al (1988b) showed growth failure and bone abnormalities in children who had commenced high dose SC DF at age 8 ± 6 months. Wonke (1988, unpublished) noted bone changes in 3 of 128 patients, ascribed to DF, with decreased spinal growth, flattening and increased density of the vertebral bodies.

The mechanism for these side-effects of DF are unclear. They are all most marked in patients receiving the highest doses of DF and with the lowest iron stores. Access of DF is restricted by the blood-brain and blood-retinal barrier, but diabetes, or drugs such as prochlorperazine may reduce this barrier. Chelation of iron from key enzymes, chelation of other metals e.g. copper or zinc, and oxidation of proteins (Kontoghiorghes 1987f) have all been suggested as possible mechanisms.

CHELATORS TESTED IN CLINICAL TRIALS

Of the many hundreds of chelators other than DF, tested in vitro and in animals, only a handful have reached the stage of clinical trials. One of these, 2,3-DHB was studied in 8 β-thalassaemia patients receiving a low iron diet, at oral doses of 25 mg/kg/d for a maximum of 21 days. Iron excretion during the metabolic iron balance studies varied, with an estimated mean of 6.5 mg/d. The drug was generally well tolerated, with the exception of some gastrointestinal complaints which stopped when food was taken with the drug (Peterson et al 1976).

Rhodotorulic acid, administered intravenously to 5 thalassaemia patients at a dose of 25 mg/kg caused a mean iron excretion of 46 mg, 98% of which appeared in the urine. The amount of iron excretion was comparable to that caused by DF. Although the intramuscular (im) and subcutaneous (sc) administration of rhodotorulic acid was less effective than the intravenous (iv) route e.g. 35 mg iron following 25 mg/kg in 1 patient, major drawbacks to its use in therapy are the generation of pain on the site of injection which persists over several days probably due to its low water solubility and also increased excretion of Zn (Grady et al 1979).

Cholyhydroxamic acid was another orally promising chelator which when it was administered at 25 mg/kg in 4 thalassaemia patients 4 times a day for 7 days caused sufficient iron excretion to maintain iron balance. During the trials there were no major side-effects other than transient diarrhoea (Cerami et al 1980). Disappointing results were obtained when the chelator ethylenediamine-N,N'bis (2-hydroxyphenyl-glycine) EHPG or EDHPA was given orally to 4 thalassaemia patients at 25 mg/kg each day for 7 days. Urine and stool analysis revealed net iron excretion increases of only 1 mg/kg/day (Cerami et al 1980).

EDTA and DTPA are some of the few chelators which have been tested in man since the early 1950s mainly for the detoxification of radioactive elements but also of heavy metals such as lead and mercury. When the disodium calcium salt of EDTA was administered orally using doses of up to 9 g/day there was no increase in urinary iron excretion. In contrast the intravenous administration of this drug at 4 g/day to normal and iron loaded subjects caused an increase in urinary iron excretion of up to 3 mg and 8 mg of iron respectively. No major side-effects were reported. In more encouraging studies with trisodium calcium DTPA it was shown that its parenteral administration resulted in much higher urinary iron excretion than EDTA. Intravenous doses of 2.5–4.0 g of DTPA in 5 iron loaded patients resulted in urinary iron excretion of up to 109 mg in a day. Despite the effectiveness of DTPA at increasing iron excretion, its general use was curtailed by reports that it increased the excretion of other bivalent metals including Ca, Mg, Mn, Cu and particularly Zn. Administration of Zn-DTPA did not increase iron excretion but Ca-DTPA with oral Zn supplements in combination with DF was suggested to be more effective than DF and also less toxic than DTPA (Pippard et al 1986). Studies with DTPA in 5 patients who had damage from DF showed it to be possible to give DTPA for up to 18 months without side-effects provided adequate Zn supplementation is given (Wonke et al 1988). Initial clinical studies with PIH have also been carried out with some successes (Brittenham, personal communication). It seems that PIH causes a net increase in faecal iron excretion in iron loaded patients. It is not sufficiently effective at increasing urinary iron excretion, however, for the total effect to be a sufficiently net negative iron balance for it to replace DF in thalassaemia major patients.

ORAL CHELATION THERAPY IN MAN WITH 1,2-DIMETHYL-3-HYDROXYPYRID-4-ONE AND OTHER α-KHPS

The equivalence in iron excretion following oral or parenteral administration of α-KHPs with parenteral DF in three different animal species, as well as the lack of toxicity during long term (3 months) animal studies, and of many in vitro studies (see previous section) prompted the clinical investigation with these drugs.

A small dose (0.5 g in gelatin capsules) of L1 was initially administered in a few patients to determine acceptibility. The dose was then increased gradually to levels that were sufficiently high to cause an increase in iron excretion but not greater than 100 mg/kg/day. Repeated daily administration at 4–6 h intervals of effective doses was then used to increase daily iron excretion to levels equivalent to or higher than the amount of iron taken in from blood transfusions (20–25 mg/day) (Kontoghiorghes et al 1987a,b).

These studies were initially carried out on four multiply transfused patients with myelodysplasia (MDS). In each case the amount of iron excreted was found to depend on the dose of the drug taken and the initial iron load of the patient. In subsequent studies more iron (up to 99 mg in 24 h) was excreted from β-thalassaemia major patients with greater iron loads. In preliminary studies the co-administration of ascorbic acid at 200 mg/day caused a further increase in urinary iron excretion in most, but not all the patients. This discrepancy is not related solely to initial vitamin C stores. Iron metabolic balance studies in four patients receiving low iron diet and doses of L1 of up to 4 g revealed that increased iron excretion is predominantly found in the urine and not in the faeces (Kontoghiorghes et al 1988). This indicates that the major site of clearance of chelator iron complexes such as that of L1 and presumably closely related chelators is probably through the kidneys and not the liver.

The red iron chelator complex is maximally excreted to over a 2–4 h period after oral dose and returns to almost background levels within 8–12 h. If the 2–3 g doses are taken every 4–6 h for 18 h, iron excretion continues to increase indicating that over the period of administration L1 has not exhausted the chelatable pools.

Urinary iron excretion caused by L1 ranged from 2–11 mg with 2 g L1, 4–28 mg with 3 g L1, 7–29 mg with 2×2 g L1 (at 6 h intervals) in patients who had received 50–80 units of red blood cells and serum ferritin levels of 960–2400 μg/l. Urinary iron excretion ranging from 17–59 mg with 2 g L1, 22–99 mg with 3 g L1 and 31–67 mg with 2×2 g L1 were observed in thalassaemia patients who received more than 100 units of red blood cells and serum ferritin of 3000–8000 μg/l. Further work is needed to explore the role of repeated doses, of ascorbic acid, and other factors influencing the daily iron excretion output.

Other precautions taken included no intake of food or other drugs within 1 hour before and after taking L1 as these could affect the solubility as well as the absorption of the chelator. In particular metal ions such as iron and aluminium found in the diet or drugs will inhibit both the absorption of the metal and of the chelating agent (Kontoghiorghes, unpublished).

Toxicity studies
Long term and toxicological studies have not yet been carried out with L1 or other α-KHPs. However, based on studies of animals and preliminary studies of patients the prospects of the oral treatment of transfusional iron overload with L1 or a related drug are encouraging.

In preliminary studies the median lethal dose of a single intraperitoneal injection of L1 was estimated to be between 600–700 mg/kg in rats and daily intraperitoneal or intragastric administration for 1 month of 200 mg/kg and for 2 further weeks of 200 mg/kg twice daily in mice was found to be without apparent toxicity (Kontoghiorghes 1986e, Kontoghiorghes & Sheppard 1987).

The need for long term and repeated daily administration of the oral chelators for the effective treatment of iron overload requires the use of a hydrophilic substance like L1, which is rapidly cleared and does not accumulate in the tissues. Similar conditions apply for the metabolites and the iron complex of the chelator. No apparent toxicity has been observed so far in over 20 volunteers and patients who received L1 either as single doses or as daily therapy for up to 4 months and up to 4×2 g dose in a day. Ten patients treated daily for 2 weeks with over a total of 30 g of L1 have no symptoms ascribed to the drug up to $1\frac{1}{2}$ years after the treatment. Similar studies on 4 patients who have received 3–4 g of L1 daily for up to 4 months have not revealed any toxic side-effects. Clinical (including ophthalmic and auditory), biochemical and haematological monitoring of the treated patients have also not revealed toxic side-effects. Cardiac studies including ECG and MUGA scanning have also not shown any side-effects or deterioration of the heart. The identification in animals of several other orally active α-KHPs and particularly 1-substitute-2-alkyl-3-hydroxypyrid-4-ones which have equivalent effects to that of L1 and DF e.g. L1NEt, EL1, EL1NEt, L1N-Methoxyethyl and EL1-Methoxyethyl (Fig. 4.1) increases the prospects of future oral chelation therapy with one of this group of drugs should toxic side effects occur with one or other of them. Several other α-KHP chelators are in the process of being developed for oral use and it is hoped that they will be as non-toxic as L1.

Pharmacological, toxicological and metabolic aspects of the oral chelators
DF's bioavailability is limited by its rapid clearance from the blood ($T\frac{1}{2}$ 5–10 min), enzymatic breakdown in the plasma and other tissues, rapid excretion by filtration

and tubular secretion. Blood clearance of the iron complex of DF is slower, of about T_2^1 90 min (Kruck et al 1985) and it may be associated with partial tubular reabsorption in the kidney. The slow subcutaneous infusion of DF overcomes most of the rapid clearance problems and increases its efficacy in iron removal. The rapid clearance of DF is associated with its hydrophilicity and low lipid/water partition (Kpar = 0.02). L1 is also hydrophilic (Kpar = 0.2) and its rapid clearance requires the use of repeated daily administration for maximum iron removal efficacy. Although the site and mechanisms of absorption and excretion of L1 and the other α-KHPs have not yet been identified, some clues on their pharmacology/metabolism could be obtained from studies of chelators with similar structure.

Maltol, ethyl maltol, mimosine, tropolone and omadine
When the α-ketohydroxypyrones maltol and ethyl maltol were administered orally or intravenously to beagle dogs, both were rapidly and extensively absorbed, metabolised and excreted in the urine as the glucuronide and ethereal sulphate conjugates, which are common to phenolic compounds (Rennhard 1971). Metabolic radioassay (^{35}S) studies with oral omadine (Fig. 4.1) and its sodium and zinc salts in rats, rabbits and monkeys also revealed substantial absorption (60–80%), rapid urinary excretion and a small biliary excretion. About 50% of the ^{35}S label was absorbed from the stomach of fasted rats within 2 h and rapidly excreted in the urine without the compound or its metabolites accumulating in the tissues (Ziller 1977). S-glucuronides, disulphide and sulphonic acid conjugates were the major metabolites of intravenous and dermal omadine salts (Wedig et al 1978). Because of the close structural relation (Fig. 4.1) similar sites and rates of absorption, biotransformation and excretion are likely to hold for L1 and the other α-KHPs.

The natural plant amino acid product mimosine, which is an α-KHP chelator, is known to effect several metal containing enzymes and also enzymes which utilise substances which are structurally similar to mimosine such as tyrosine and dopa. Mimosine inhibits competitively and reversibly tyrosinase and uncompetitively dopamine 8-hydroxylase, DNA synthesis in wool follicles and mitosis in H.Ep-2 cells. It also causes shedding in sheep and its metabolic product in the rumen namely 3-hydroxypyrid-4-one and its 3-0-glucuronide derivative caused goitre in mice (Hegarty et al 1979). In almost all the above cases the addition of iron or other metals such as copper or aluminium reversed the toxicity of mimosine. L1 and other α-KHP derivatives which have 2-alkyl substituents are unlikely to have the same toxic effects as mimosine.

Catecholamines
The structural similarity of the catechol ring in catecholamines and the α-ketohydroxy site in a heteroaromatic ring envisages the possibility of interference in the hormonal action and metabolism of catecholamines. Indeed it was shown that tropolone and other α-ketohydroxy heteroaromatic chelators cause inhibition of catechol-O-methyl transferase, which is one of the major enzymes of catecholamines metabolism (Guldberg & Marsden 1975, Borchardt 1973). There is no evidence that L1 and other 1-substituted 2-alkyl 3-hydroxypyrid 4-ones will have the same effect on catechol-O-methyl-transferase as the above chelators.

Salivation

A side-effect of L1, its analogue L1NEt and their iron complexes is their ability to increase salivation after parenteral or oral administration in rats for 2–3 h (Kontoghiorghes et al 1987). However, when these chelators were administered when the rats were under anaesthetic, no salivation occurred. The precise cause of the salivation is not known but this could be due to their bitter taste. No increased salivation has occurred in patients nor in mice or rabbits given L1 or L1NEt.

The effects of the α-KHPs on the excretion of other metals

L1 and its analogues have been shown to be highly specific in iron removal and ineffective in the mobilisation of Zn, Mg and Ca in the urine and serum of animals and man (Kontoghiorghes 1985, 1987f, et al 1987a,b).

Protein and enzyme inhibition

Formation of iron complexes or the oxidation of metal ions might lead to inhibition or inactivation of metal containing proteins. For example maltol and 1-methyl-3-hydroxypyrid-2-one form ternary complexes with transferrin iron (Kontoghiorghes 1986b), the anti-cancer agent hydroxyurea inhibit DNA synthesis by bonding to iron in ribonucleotide reductase and DF may oxidise haemoglobin to methaemoglobin. This oxidation of other biomolecules by DF could theoretically be the cause of some of the side-effects observed with high doses of this drug (Kontoghiorghes 1987f). Despite the above effects, chelators do not usually inhibit the many essential iron containing proteins present in cells unless severe iron depletion occurs or a chelator is designed specifically to attack such proteins.

Stimulation of microbial growth

Synthetic chelators are usually designed to mimic microbial siderophores which have a high affinity for iron. One of the drawbacks of some of such chelators is their ability to supply iron to and support the growth of microbes. DF has been shown to increase the susceptibility of patients to infection with *Yersinia enterocolitica* and other pathogenic bacteria (Melby et al 1982). The growth of *Y. enterocolitica, E. coli, P. aeruginosa* and *S. epidermidis* in human serum was examined using DF, L1 and other α-ketohydroxy heteroaromatic chelators. DF enhanced the growth of all the bacteria species except for *E. coli* while L1, L1NEt and L1NPr inhibited the growth of all the organisms except for mild stimulation of growth in *S. epidermidis* (Brock et al 1988). Other metabolic/toxicological effects would be anticipated from the structure of the metal binding site and the remaining backbone structure of the different chelators. Such effects, however, and also allergic and anaphylactic reactions, caused by many drugs, require further investigation.

Iron toxicity

Although it has been suggested that iron may be involved in the pathogenesis of many diseases, transfusional iron overload still remains the main disease where iron toxicity is the cause of death.

Ingestion of large quantities of ferrous iron salts in children is usually fatal. In such cases iron causes damage to the gut leading to haemorrhage, serum iron is elevated, blood acidosis accompanied by lactic and citric acid acidosis follows. Liver mitochondrial, microsomal and lysosomal damage, heart mitochondrial and myofibril damage hepatic fibrosis perhaps through stimulation of collagen synthesis in hepato-cytes are further consequences of iron toxicity which may also play a role in the cause of death in chronic iron overload such as transfusional iron overload in thalassae-mia. Hydrogen peroxide, superoxide and hydroxyl radicals formed during iron cataly-sis could attack and damage all known biomolecules (Willson 1977). Lipids on the cell and mitochondrial membranes are particularly vulnerable to toxic oxygen stress forming lipid peroxides which then may cause cellular and tissue damage. This oxidative process of damage is similar to rancidification (Dormandy 1978) where a cascade of oxygen activated products occur. Under normal conditions the formation of such cas-cades of oxygen species is controlled by glutathione perioxidase, superoxide dismutase, catalase, vitamin E and other mechanisms. The possible role of iron in the catalytic formation of oxygen activated products in tissue damage in iron overload and other diseases has been reviewed (Slater 1984, Halliwell & Gutteridge 1984, Editorial 1985).

Most chelators, including DF, the α-KHPs, α-ketohydroxypyrones and the catechols are potent inhibitors of free radical formation induced by iron in vitro but few may exacerbate its toxicity e.g. EDTA and purpurogallin (Kontoghiorghes et al 1986c).

OTHER POTENTIAL USES OF ORAL IRON CHELATORS

Aluminium toxicity
Aluminium shares the same metabolic pathways as iron, e.g. being carried by transfer-rin. It accumulates in renal dialysis patients because of the use of aluminium hydroxide as a phosphate binder in the gut or the high aluminium content of water used during renal dialysis. Aluminium overload is associated with hypercalcaemic osteomalacia and encephalopathy and possibly anaemia. DF has been shown to be effective in increasing aluminium excretion in dialysis osteomalacia patients (Brown et al 1982) and it is routinely used for aluminium intoxication in such patients. Recent develop-ments in treatment of aluminium overload in dialysis patients have been reviewed overload (Seminars in Nephrology, Vol VI, No. 4, Suppl. 1, 1986). The α-KHPs are as effective as DF in aluminium binding and could therefore be used for treating this condition, providing they are not toxic to these patients.

Plutonium
DTPA is the main chelator used for the removal of actinides in vivo, but DF and the tetracatecholic chelator LICAM (C) (Volf 1986) were also shown to be effective in rats. The need for rapid application of chelating agents for decreasing the incorporation of [238]Pu in tissues during accidental contamination would be best achieved with an oral drug. Studies using [238]Pu labelled transferrin and ferritin with some orally active α-KHPs revealed that L1, L3 and mimosine are almost as effective as DTPA and LICAM(C) in the release of [238]Pu from these two proteins (Taylor & Kontoghiorghes 1986).

Radiopharmaceuticals
Two other radioactive metals namely [67]Ca and ^{111}In also share the metabolic pathways of iron. ^{111}In-8-hydroxyquinoline complexes are used for labelling cells and platelets for kinetic studies, e.g. Hodgkins disease (Lavender et al 1977) and for tissue imaging.

The use of strong ^{67}Ca complexes which do not exchange ^{67}Ca with transferrin could be used for imaging the renal or hepatobiliary system and for positron emission tomography (Hunt 1984). 8-Hydroxyquinoline and other lipophilic chelators were amongst the few successful chelators of a group of 19 chelators tested which were able to label red blood cells with ^{59}Fe and may also have a use as ^{67}Ca and ^{111}In chelators (Kontoghiorghes 1988b).

Inhibition of free radical formation

Chelators could inhibit the catalytic formation of oxygen activated products formed by iron and this may have application in the treatment of diseases related to this toxicity such as post-ischaemic injury following reperfusion after cardiac arrest, myocardial infarction or stroke (Nayini et al 1985). Similarly this method of treatment may also be applied during the reperfusion or storage of organs in transplantation.

In the adult respiratory distress syndrome (ARDS), rheumatoid arthritis and other inflammatory conditions the accumulation and clumping of neutrophils and their adhesion to the endothelial cells results among other events (Harlan 1985) in the release of oxygen activated products which may cause damage to the tissue (Ward et al 1983). The presence of DF and lactoferrin was shown to minimise and of iron to exacerbate such injury (Frigid et al 1984). In rheumatoid arthritis the presence of iron deposits in the joints which may stimulate further oxygen activated product toxicity is the one condition where DF has actually been administered in a clinical trial. The results were highly disappointing in that there was no improvement in the joints of the patients and DF caused serious side-effects (Polson et al 1985). Although until now the suspected site of toxicity in the above conditions was thought to be low MW iron which can be inactivated by chelators, recent studies have shown that DF and the α-KHPs, L1, L1NEt and L1NPr are all potent inhibitors of prostacyclin synthesis (Jeremy et al 1988). Inhibition of proinflammatory prostacyclins and related oxygen activated products by chelators may be through the inhibition of the iron containing enzyme cyclooxygenase and possibly lipoxygenase.

Porphyria Cutanea Tarda

Iron has also been implicated in the pathogenesis of porphyria cutanea tarda through inhibition of the enzyme uroporphyrinogen decarboxylase. SC DF (1.5 g/day, 5 days/week) was shown to be as effective as phlebotomy in the treatment of this condition (Rocchi et al 1986) but the expense and mode of administration of DF does not make it a viable alternative.

Malaria

In the search for alternative drugs for the treatment of drug-resistant malaria it has been found that iron chelators may have a use in this disease because P. falciparum and other malaria strains require iron for growth and acquire iron by synthesising a transferrin receptor on infected erythrocytes (Rodriguez & Jungery 1986). The lipophilic cytotoxic chelators 8-hydroxyquinoline and omadine ($7–8 \times 10^{-10}$ M) are potent inhibitors of P. falciparum in vitro (Scheibel & Alder 1980) and are thought to act through the intracellular toxicity of their iron complexes (Kontoghiorghes et al 1986b, Scheibel & Stanton 1986). DF (15×10^{-6} M) is inhibitory under similar conditions by acting through iron deprivation. L1, L1NEt, L1NPR, EL1, EL1NEt and EL1NPr are also highly inhibitory of the growth of *P. falciparum* in vitro at $1–10 \times 10^{-5}$ M but in particular L1 is 50% more effective than DF at the low concentration (10×10^{-6} M) (Heppner et al, 1988). Although the precise mechanism of the inhibition of the parasites is not known it appears that following the formation of iron complexes by the chelators described above iron is not available to the parasite for growth. Inhibition of parasite ribonucleotide reductase or other important iron containing enzyme is clearly a possibility.

Cytotoxic therapy

Chelators may have a use in cytotoxic therapy by interacting with ribonucleotide reductase and with intracellular iron linked to this enzyme which may inhibit DNA synthesis (Robbins & Peterson 1970, Hoffbrand et al 1976, Kontoghiorghes 1982). Such an effect was shown using 8-hydroxyquinoline in a cell free system (Thelander & Reinhard 1979), with DF in a variety of cell and culture systems (Brockman 1974, Hoffbrand et al 1976, Ganeshaguru et al 1980), and with 8-hydroxyquinoline and omadine in human myeloid cell lines (Kontoghiorghes et al 1986a,b, Forsbeck et al 1987). In preliminary studies DF in combination with cytosine arabinoside may have caused leukaemic cytoreduction in neonatal acute leukaemia (Estrov et al 1987).

In contrast the anticancer iron chelating drugs doxorubicin, bleomycin and mitoxantrone are thought to cause DNA damage through the oxidative toxicity of their iron complexes (Sansville et al 1976, Elliot et al 1984) which was also observed with the iron complexes of omadine and 8-hydroxyquinoline (Kontoghiorghes et al 1986a,b). Since the side-effects of these drugs such as lung toxicity with bleomycin and cardiotoxicity with doxorubicin may also be through the action of their iron complexes, the use of chelators may potentially eliminate these side-effects.

Iron deficiency anaemia

Although the main role of chelators is in iron detoxification and removal, their beneficial roles could include increased absorption of iron and other metals (e.g. of Zn) in nutritional metal deficiencies. Chelators intended for the prevention of iron deficiency are those which form neutral lipophilic iron complexes and are able to transfer iron across the gut wall and donate it to transferrin or ferritin. Such effects of increased iron donation have been previously shown with maltol, 8-hydroxyquinoline, L2 and L6 (Kontoghiorghes 1982). Maltol in particular, holds a promise for development because it is already being used as a food additive (flavouring agent) and is non-toxic (Kontoghiorghes 1987a).

CONCLUSION

The mode of action of chelators intended for clinical use is determined by their structural features. Effectiveness in iron binding is not the only criterion for assessing their efficacy. Toxicity, pharmacology, metabolism, biotransformation and the binding of other metals are some of the many properties which have to be considered and assessed during the designing of chelators for specific use. The observation of increased iron excretion to levels equivalent to those caused by the same doses of desferrioxamine in iron loaded patients given oral 1,2-dimethyl-3-hydroxypyrid-4-one (L1) increases the prospects for development of oral chelating drugs for the treatment of iron overload and of other diseases of iron and other metal imbalance and toxicity.

REFERENCES

Akers H A, Abrego V A, Garland E 1980 Journal of Bacteriology 141: 164–168
Al-Douri M, Wonke B, Hoffbrand A V et al 1987 Journal of Clinical Pathology 40: 1353–1359
Anderson W F, Hiller M C (eds) 1975 National Institute of Health, Bethesda, Maryland, USA: 1–277
Arden G B, Wonke B, Kennedy C, Huehns E R 1984 British Journal of Ophthalmology 68: 873–877
Avramovici-Grisaru S, Sarel S, Ling G, Hersko C 1983 Journal of Medicinal Chemistry 26: 298–302
Baker E, Vitolo Ml, Webb J 1985 Biochemical Pharmacology 34: 3011–3017
Blake D R, Winyard P, Lunec J et al 1985 Quarterly Journal of Medicine 56: 345–355
Borchardt R T 1973 Journal of Medicinal Chemistry 16: 581–583
Borgna-Pignatti C, De Stefano P, Broglia A M 1984 Lancet i: 681
Brittenham G M 1988 In: Brain M C, Carbone P P, Decker B C (eds) Current therapy in haematology-oncology 3. Toronto, p 149–153
Brock J H, Liceaga J, Kontoghiorghes G J 1988 FEMS 47: 55–60
Brockman R W 1974 Cancer Chemotherapy Reports 4: 115–129
Brown D S, Ham K N, Dawborn J K, Xipell J M 1982. Lancet i: 343–345
Carrano C J, Raymond K N 1979 Journal of the American Chemical Society 101: 5401–5404
Cerami A, Grady R W, Peterson C M, Bhargava K K 1980 Annals of the New York Academy of Sciences 344: 425–435
Cohen A 1987 Haematology/Oncology Clinics of North America 1: 521–524
Cohen A, Mizanin J, Schwartz E 1984 British Journal of Haematology 58: 369–373
Davies S C, Hungerford J L, Arden J B, Marcus R E, Miller M H, Huehns E R 1983 Lancet ii: 181–184
De Sanctis V, D'Ascola G, Wonke B 1986 Postgraduate Medical Journal 62: 831–836
De Virgilliis S, Congia M, Turco M P et al 1988a Archives of Disease in Childhood 63: 250–255
De Virgilliis S, Congia M, Frau F (1988b) Journal of Pediatrics (in press)
Dormandy T L 1978 Lancet i: 647–650
Editorial 1985 Lancet i: 143–145
Ehlers K H, Levin A R, Markenson A L, Klein A A, Hilgartner M W, Engle M A 1980 Annals of the New York Academy of Sciences 344: 397–404
Elliot H, Gianni L, Meyers C 1984 Biochemistry 23: 928–936
Esparza I, Brock J H 1981 British Journal of Haematology 49: 603–614
Estrov Z, Tawa A, Wang X H 1987 Blood 69: 757–761
Forsbeck K, Nilson K, Kontoghiorghes G J 1987 European Journal of Haematology 39: 318–326
Freeman A P, Giles R W, Berdoukas V A, Walsh W F, Choy D, Murray R E 1983 Annals Internal Medicine 99: 450–454
Frigid S E G, Ward P A, Johnson K J, Till G O 1984 American Journal of Pathology 115: 375–382
Gabutti V, Luzzatto L, Saudi A et al 1987 2nd International Conference on Thalassaemia and the Haemoglobinopathies, Heraklion, Crete. 27 (Abstract)
Ganeshaguru K, Hoffbrand A V, Grady R W, Cerami A 1980 Biochemical Pharmacology 29: 1275–1279
Giandina P J V, Ehlers K H, Engle M A, Grady R W, Hilgartner M W 1985 Annals of the New York Academy of Science 445: 282–292
Giardina P J, Ehlers K, Lesser M et al 1987 Paediatric Research 21: 299
Grady R W, Peterson C M, Jones R L, Graziano J H et al 1979 Journal of Pharmacology Experimental Therapeutics 209: 342–348
Gray H B 1975 In: Crichton R R (ed) Proteins of iron storage and transport in biochemistry and medicine. North Holland, Elsevier, p 3–13
Graziano J H, Grady R W, Cerami R W 1974 Journal of Pharmacology Experimental Therapeutics 190: 570–575
Green R, Lamon J L, Curran D 1977 Lancet ii: 327–330
Guldberg H C, Marsden C A 1975 Pharmacological Reviews 27: 135–206
Halliwell B, Gutteridge J M C 1984 Biochemical Journal 219: 1–14
Harlan J M 1985 Blood 65: 513–525
Harris W R 1984 Journal of Inorganic Biochemistry 21: 263–276
Hegarty M P, Lee C P, Christie G S, Court R D, Haydock K P 1979 Australian Journal of Biological Science 32: 27–40
Heppner D G, Holloway P E, Kontoghiorghes G J, Eaton J W 1988 Blood 72: 358–361
Hershko C, Graham G, Bates G N, Rachmilewitz E A 1978 British Journal of Haematology 40: 255–263
Hershko C, Weatherall D J 1988 Iron Chelation Therapy CRC Critical Reviews (in press)

Hoffbrand A V 1980 In: Jacobs A, Worwood M (eds) Iron in biochemistry and medicine (II). Academic Press, London, p 499–527

Hoffbrand A V, Ganeshaguru K, Hooton J W L, Tattersall M H N 1976 British Journal of Haematology 33: 517–526

Hoffbrand A V, Gorman A, Laulicht M et al 1979 Lancet i: 947–949

Hoy T G, Harrison P M, Shabir M 1974 Biochemical Journal 139: 603–607

Hoy T G, Jacobs A 1981 British Journal of Haematology 49: 595–602

Hunt F C 1984 Nuklearmedizin 23: 123–125

Hyman C B, Agress C L, Rodriguez-Funes R, Zednikova M 1985 New England Journal of Medicine 312: 1600–1603

Jacobs A 1977 Blood 50: 433–439

Jacobs A 1985 CRC Critical Review 3: 143–186

Jeremy J Y, Kontoghiorghes G J, Hoffbrand A V, Dandona P 1988 Biochemical Journal 254: 239–244

Kleber E E, Torrance J D, Bothwell T H, Simon M D, Charlton R W 1981 Scandinavian Journal of Haematology 27: 209–218

Kontoghiorghes G J 1982 The design of orally active iron chelators for the treatment of thalassaemia. PhD Thesis. Essex University. Colchester UK. British Library Microfilm D66194/86

Kontoghiorghes G J 1985 Lancet i: 817

Kontoghiorghes G J 1986a Biochemical Journal 233: 299–302

Kontoghiorghes G J 1986b Biochimica Biophysica Acta 869: 141–146

Kontoghiorghes G J 1986c Biochimica Biophysica Acta 882: 267–270

Kontoghiorghes G J 1986d Molecular Pharmacology 30: 670–673

Kontoghiorghes G J 1986e Scandinavian Journal of Haematology 37: 63–70

Kontoghiorghes G J 1987a Inorganica Chimica Acta 135: 145–150

Kontoghiorghes G J 1987b In: Rice-Evans C (ed) Free radicals, oxidant stress and drug action. Richelieu Press, London, p 277–303

Kontoghiorghes G J 1987c Inorganica Chimica Acta 138: 35–39

Kontoghiorghes G J 1987d Biochimica Biophysica Acta 924: 13–18

Kontoghiorghes G J 1987e Clinica Chimica Acta 163: 137–141

Kontoghiorghes G J 1987f Acta Haematologica 78: 212–216

Kontoghiorghes G J 1988a 1,2-Dimethyl-3-hydroxypyrid-4-one. Drugs of the future 13: 413–415

Kontoghiorghes G J 1988b Inorganica Chimica Acta 151: 101–106

Kontoghiorghes G J, Evans R W 1985 FEBS Letters 189: 141–144

Kontoghiorghes G J, Hoffbrand A V 1986 British Journal of Haematology 62: 607–613

Kontoghiorghes G J, Sheppard L 1987 Inorganica Chimica Acta 136: L11–L12

Kontoghiorghes G J, Marcus R E, Huehns E R 1983 Lancet ii: 454

Kontoghiorghes G J, Piga A, Hoffbrand A V 1986a FEBS Letters 204: 208–212

Kontoghiorghes G J, Piga A, Hoffbrand A V 1986b Haematological Oncology 4: 195–204

Kontoghiorghes G J, Jackson M J, Lunec J 1986c Free Radical Research Communications 2: 115–124

Kontoghiorghes G J, Chambers S, Dodd A, Thompson H 1986d British Journal of Haematology 64: 839–840

Kontoghiorghes G J, Aldouri M A, Sheppard L, Hoffbrand A V 1987a Lancet i: 1294–1295

Kontoghiorghes G J, Aldouri M A, Hoffbrand et al 1987b British Medical Journal 295: 1509–1512

Kontoghiorghes G J, Chambers S, Hoffbrand A V 1987c Biochemical Journal 241: 87–92

Kontoghiorghes G J, Sheppard L, Chambers S 1987d Arzneimittel Forsch/Drug Research 37: 1099–1102

Kontoghiorghes G J, Sheppard L, Hoffbrand A V, Charalambous J, Tikerpae J, Pippard M J 1987e Journal of Clinical Pathology 40: 404–408

Kontoghiorghes G J, Sheppard L, Barr J et al 1988a British Journal of Haematology 69: 129

Kontoghiorghes G J, Sheppard L, Barr J 1988b Inorganica Chimica Acta 152: 195–199

Kruck T P A, Kalow W, McLachlan D R C 1985 Journal of Chromatography 341: 123–130

Lavender J P, Goldman J M, Arnot R N, Thaakur M L 1977 British Medical Journal 2: 797–799

Longueville A, Crichton R R 1986 Biochemical Pharmacology 36: 3669–3678

Marcus R E, Davies S C, Bantock H M, Underwood S R, Walton S, Huehns E R 1984 Lancet i: 392–393

Marcus R E, Huehns E R 1986 Clinical and Laboratory Haematology 7: 195–212

Martell A E, Anderson W F, Badman D G (eds) 1981 Development of iron chelators for clinical use. Elsevier, North Holland, p 1–311

Melby K, Slordahl S, Gutteberg T J, Nordbo S A 1982 British Medical Journal 285: 467–468

Modell B, Berdoukas V 1984 The clinical approach to thalassaemia. Grune and Stratton, London

Modell C B, Letsky E, Flynn D M et al 1982 British Medical Journal 284: 1081–1084

Mostert L J, Van Dorst J A L M, Koster J F, Van Eijk H G, Kontoghiorghes G J 1987 Radical Research Communications 3: 379–388

Nayini N R, White B C, Aust S D et al 1985. Post resuscitation iron delocalisation and malonaldehyde production in the brain following prolonged cardiac arrest. Journal of Free Radicals in Biology and Medicine 1: 111–116

Neilands J B 1980 In: Jacobs A, Worwood M (eds) Iron in biochemistry and medicine (II). Academic Press, London, 529–572

Nicholls D 1974 Complexes and first-row transition elements. Macmillan Press, London, p 1–215

Olivieri N F, Buncic J R, Chew E et al 1986 New England Journal of Medicine 314: 869–873

Peter H H 1983 Schweiz Med. Wschr 113: 1428–1433

Peterson C M, Graziano J H, Grady R W et al 1976 British Journal of Haematology 33: 477–485

Pippard M J, Johnson D K, Finch L A 1981 Blood 58: 685–692

Pippard M J, Callendar S T, Finch C A 1982 Blood 60: 288–294

Pippard M J, Jackson M J, Hoffman K, Petrou M, Modell C B 1986 Scandinavian Journal of Haematology 36: 466–472

Pitt C G, Gupta G I, Estes W E et al 1979 Journal of Pharmacology Experimental Therapeutics 208: 12–18

Pollack S, Vanderhoff G, Lasky F 1977 Biochimica Biophysica Acta 497: 481–487

Polson R J, Jawd A, Bomford A, Berry H, Williams R 1985 British Medical Journal 291: 448

Pootrakul P, Josephson B, Huebers H A, Finch C A 1988 Blood 71: 1120–1123

Ponka P, Borova J, Neuwirt J, Fuchs O 1979 FEBS Letters 97: 317–321

Rennhard H H 1971 Journal of Agricultural and Food Chemistry 19: 152–154

Ringborn A 1963 In: Elving P J, Kolthoff I M (eds) Chemical analysis. Complexation in analytical chemistry. Volume XVI. Interscience, New York, p 1–374

Rise D W, Ford G C, White J L, Smith J M A, Harrison P M 1983 In: Aisen P, Listowsky I, Drysdale J W (eds) Structure and function of iron transport and storage proteins. Elsevier, Amsterdam, p 11–116

Robbins E, Peterson T 1970 Proceedings of the National Academy of Science, USA 60: 1244–1251

Rocchi E, Gibertini P, Cassanelli M et al 1986 British Journal of Dermatology 114: 621–629

Rodriguez M H, Jungery M 1986 Nature 324: 388–391

Saito K, Nishisato T, Grasso J A, Aisen P 1986 British Journal of Haematology 62: 275–286

Sansville E A, Pelsach J, Horwitz S B 1976 Biochemistry 17: 2740–2746

Schafer A I, Rabinowe S, Le Boff M S, Bridges K, Cheron R C, Dluhy R 1985 Archives of Internal Medicine 145: 1217–1221

Scheibel L W, Alder A 1980 Molecular Pharmacology 18: 320–325

Scheibel L W, Stanton G G 1986 Molecular Pharmacology 30: 364–369

Sciortino C V, Byers B R, Prentiss Cox 1980 Journal of Laboratory and Clinical Medicine 96: 1081–1085

Sirivech S, Frieden E, Osaki S 1974 Biochemical Journal 143: 311–315

Slater T F 1984 Biochemical Journal 222: 1–15

Sugiura Y, Nomoto K 1984 Structure and Bonding 58: 107–135

Taylor D M, Kontoghiorghes G J 1986 Inorganica Chimica Acta 125: L35–L38

Thelander L, Reinhard P 1979 Annual Review of Biochemistry 48: 133–158

Tufano T P, Pecoraro V L, Raymond K N 1981 Biochimica Biophysica Acta 668: 420–428

Vitolo M L, Webb J, Saltman P 1984 Journal of Inorganic Biochemistry 20: 255–262

Volf V 1986 Journal of Radiation Biology 49: 449–462

Ward P A, Till G O, Kinkel R, Beauchamp C 1983 Journal of Clinical Investigation 72: 789–801

Wedig J H, Mitoma C, Howd R A, Thomas D W 1978 Toxicology and Applied Pharmacology 43: 373–379

Weir M P, Gibson J F, Peters T J 1984 Biochemical Journal 223: 31–38

White G P, Jacobs A, Grady R W, Cerami A 1976 British Journal of Haematology 27: 209–218

Willson R L 1977 In: Iron metabolism. CIBA Symposium Elsevier, Excerpta Medica, North Holland 51: 331–349

Winston A, Rosthauser J, Fair D, Bapasola J, Lerdthusnel W 1982 American Chemical Society Series 176: 107–117

Wolfe L, Olivieri I, Sallan D et al 1985 New England Journal of Medicine 312: 1600–1603

Wonke B, Hoffbrand A V, Al-Douri M et al 1988 Archives Disease in Childhood (in press)

Ziller S A 1977 Food, Cosmetic Toxicology 15: 49–54

5. Gene rearrangements in leukemias and lymphomas

M. D. Reis   H. Griesser   T. W. Mak

The last 10 years have witnessed a remarkable progress in the development of techniques in molecular biology that have led to recombinant DNA technology. Two critical conquests in immunology were the cloning of genes coding for the B lymphocyte antigen receptors, the immunoglobulins, and for the T lymphocyte antigen receptor. As a consequence, the mechanisms responsible for the generation of antibody diversity have been unveiled, stages in the ontogeny of B and T cells have begun to be understood, the molecular aspects of the recognition of self- and foreign antigens and of events implicated in the pathogenesis of lymphoid neoplasias are being elucidated, and diagnostic tools for the detection of lymphoid clonal expansions and for determination of their lineage have become available. Furthermore, the links between histocompatibility antigens and disease associations can be probed, and a potential exists for exploiting the knowledge now available on these receptor structures for therapeutic purposes. In this review, we will analyse some of these issues. An up-to-date knowledge of the use of these receptor genes in the definition of clonality and possible lineage of lymphoproliferative disorders as well as the role of these genes in chromosomal translocations in T cell malignancies will be discussed.

B CELL ANTIGEN RECEPTOR

B cells form the effector arm of the humoral immune response, as precursors of antibody-producing cells. The immunoglobulin (Ig) molecules serve as cell membrane antigen receptors and exhibit the property of reacting with soluble antigens. Functional and structural characteristics of the B cell antigen receptor were elucidated before those of the T cell antigen receptors because large amounts of Ig were available from Ig-producing myelomas. The basic units of these polypeptides were found to form a heterodimer, consisting of a pair of light (L) and heavy (H) chains. Amino acid sequences of these chains revealed a remarkable pattern, with marked variation in the sequences of the N terminal portion of the molecules when compared to each other. The sequences of the C terminal half of the molecules of a given class were, however, practically identical. Antigen recognition has been ascribed to the variable regions of the light and heavy chains, and contain hypervariable segments that have been implicated in antigen contact. These studies have also shown that the heavy and light chains consist of a series of homology units or domains.

The fundamental issue of how a limited number of genes can generate a vast number of antibodies with unique specificities was elucidated by Tonegawa. The genes specifying the structure of each Ig molecule are organized as discontinuous DNA segments in their germline configuration, the form present in essentially all non-B lymphoid cells. As a mandatory event in B cell differentiation, an uncommitted pre-B cell undergoes an orderly sequence of events that activate Ig genes with ensuing somatic recombination, that is, these genes become rearranged. The genes for kappa (κ) and lambda (λ) light chains contain variable (V) and joining (J) gene segments, and constant (C) region genes. The heavy chain genes contain diversity (D) segments, in addition to V, J and C region genes. The rearrangement and joining of one of each V-(D)-J segments leads to the assembly of a V region gene whose product is an Ig variable region polypeptide.

There are several genetic mechanisms thought to contribute to the generation of antibody specificities, including the multiple germline variable region gene segments and the random combinatorial joining of the numerous V, D and J segments. Another mechanism is junctional site diversity, occurring at the junction of the variable region gene segments during recombination. Further junctional diversity may occur in the heavy chain junctions due to the insertion of one to several nucleotides at the ends in a template-independent fashion by the enzyme terminal deoxynucleotidyl transferase (TdT). Lastly, the repertoire of antibodies can be further expanded as a result of somatic hypermutation, thus creating changes in the amino acid sequences of the variable region of the Ig, as in a fine-tuning modification resulting in increased antibody affinity for a given antigenic epitope. For additional details on the generation of antibody diversity, we suggest a review published elsewhere (Tonegawa 1983).

Each individual B cell produces antibodies with a single type of variable region sequence. With the exception of the variability resulting from somatic mutation, a mature B cell and its progeny will have the same variable region sequence. Furthermore, they synthesize either κ or λ light chains but not both.

Sequence of rearrangements of immunoglobulin genes
There is a hierarchy of Ig gene recombinations starting first with rearrangement of heavy chain genes, followed by κ and the λ light chain genes. The initial event brings about the joining of a D_H with a J_H segment of the heavy chain gene, followed by a V_H segment combining with this DJ junction. The attempt to form a VDJ joining may be successful, in which case a μ cytoplasmic heavy chain may be synthesized, or may be aberrant, with an incomplete heavy chain being produced. Upon complete heavy chain rearrangement, attempts at light chain gene recombination generally comes for κ genes first. If V_K and J_K are successfully joined in a cell already possessing a complete $V_H D_H J_H$ recombination, a μ, κ surface Ig will result. In case the maternal and paternal κ alleles rearrange aberrantly or are deleted, the cell next attempts to rearrange the λ genes; if effective, this results in a μ, λ surface Ig; if ineffective or aberrant, there is no synthesis of light chain, and the cell remains at the pre-B stage. The flexibility of joining of V_H, D_H and J_H may lead to nonproductive rearrangements relatively frequently and the sequence of rearrangements of heavy and light chain genes is also prone to errors, both of which may result in a sizable portion of B cell precursors incapable of further expansion.

The progress in the understanding of important biological events in B cell development, as a result of the utilization of molecular biological techniques, has been quickly accompanied by procedural applications of practical medical importance. Korsmeyer and co-workers first proposed the analysis of patterns of Ig gene rearrangement as a powerful and sensitive tool to assess clonality in B cell proliferative disorders (Korsmeyer et al 1981). This is now used to determine cell lineage and clonality, to diagnose

B cell neoplasias and monitor therapy, and has also provided insights into mechanisms resulting in malignant transformation in some B cell diseases. An example of the latter is the observation that chromosomal translocations in Burkitt's lymphoma involve the locus containing the c-myc oncogene on chromosome 8 and the genes for either Ig heavy, κ light or λ light chains, on chromosomes 14, 2 and 22, respectively (Klein et al 1983, Croce & Nowell 1985a).

THE ROLE OF T CELLS IN CELLULAR IMMUNE RESPONSES

T cells also derive from hematopoietic stem cells and the precursors of T cells mature in the thymic environment. There are several subtypes of T cells, including those that mediate regulatory functions such as help, as well as those involved in effector functions, such as the lysis of cells bearing antigens on their surface, and the production of lymphokines. Whether a distinct subclass of T cells is involved in suppression alone is not clear. Collectively, T cells are responsible for the cellular immune responses. In order to carry out their functions in immune responses, T cells must be able to recognize a wide range of foreign antigens. Unlike immunoglobulins which are able to recognize free (soluble) antigens, T cells recognize foreign antigens only in the context of their own cells' major histocompatibility complex (MHC) gene prod-ucts—HLA system in humans, H_2 system in mice—in what is termed MHC restric-tion (Zinkernagel & Doherty 1975). CD4 (T4) helper and a minority of CD4 (T4) cytotoxic cells co-recognize an antigen and structures on class II MHC products, whereas CD8 (T8) cytotoxic T cells co-recognize an antigen in conjunction with class I MHC molecules.

Prior to the cloning of the T cell receptor (TcR) genes, this receptor was first identified as a distinct structure present only on T cells (Haskins et al 1983, Acuto & Reinherz 1985). Anticlonotypic monoclonal antibodies were raised against a given T cell clone and shown to be able to differentiate this clone from other T cell clones. These antibodies were used to immunoprecipitate structures from human T cells of approximately 90 kilodaltons (kd), separated under reducing conditions into two components of approximately 50 kd and 40 kd. The larger and more acidic glycoprotein was termed α chain, while the smaller and more basic polypeptide was called β chain. Thus, the intact TcR is a disulfide-linked heterodimer. This heterodimer forms part of a macromolecular complex with the invariant peptides of the CD3 (T3) complex. Upon recognition of an antigen by the TcR, the CD3 (T3) complex is apparently responsible for transducing the signal to the interior of the cell, thus initiating the cellular response. As a result, there is an increase in cytosolic-free calcium and activa-tion of a protein kinase system (Weiss & Stobo 1984). These events lead to a series of steps in which previously silent genes become expressed, such as the ones encoding IL-2 and IL-2 receptors. The production of IL-2 and the expression of IL-2 receptors are critical in terms of determining the magnitude and duration of immune response (Smith 1984). Transfection experiments on mutant T cell lines have shown that a complete T3-TcR complex must be on the cell surface for responses to antigens or anticlonotypic antibodies to occur, and that the components of the T3 complex and the TcR heterodimeric polypeptides co-modulate each other (Ohashi et al 1985).

THE CLONING OF THE T CELL RECEPTOR GENES

Two groups independently isolated cDNA clones from human (Yanagi et al 1984) and murine (Hedrick et al 1984a) sources, that coded for the β chain of the TcR. They first used subtractive hybridization and differential screening to isolate a number of cDNA clones that appeared only in T cells. Some of these cDNA clones were shown to undergo somatic rearrangements in clones of functional T cells and leukemic cells of thymic origin (Hedrick et al 1984a, Toyonaga et al 1984). By comparing the partial protein sequence of the TcR β chain with the deduced amino acid sequence of these cDNAs, it was clear the cDNAs contained the gene coding for the β chain. Moreover, the primary structure of the proteins deduced from the cDNA's sequence revealed significant homology with the products of the Ig and MHC genes (Yanagi et al 1984, Hedrick et al 1984b, Hannun et al 1984). Application of similar techniques and the use of oligonucleotide probes deduced from the partial protein sequence of the TcR α chain led to the isolation of cDNAs encoding the α chain (see Kronenberg et al 1986 and Toyonaga & Mak 1987).

Based on the deduced primary structure on the α and β chain polypeptides of the TcR, these were shown to be composed of a variable (V) and a constant (C) domain connected by a diversity (D) (at least for the β chain) and a joining (J) segment. The overall structure of each chain is very similar to that of a light chain Ig molecule, except that they include an extended transmembrane and cytoplasmic portion. This then led to the concept of an Ig gene superfamily, defined as a group of multigene families and single gene copies related by sequence, suggesting that they have evolved from a common primordial precursor, but not necessarily related in function (Hood et al 1985). Other members of this gene superfamily include Thy-1, CD8 (T8), CD4 (T4), MHC class I, MHC class II, and the poly Ig receptor for polymeric IgA and IgM molecules.

Another T cell specific gene has been cloned and designated γ chain gene (Saito et al 1984). This gene undergoes somatic rearrangement during early stages of T cell development and its function was not known until recently. The fact that most early reports of γ chain gene cDNA sequences indicated they were derived from nonfunctional messages added to the puzzle. However, utilizing antibodies directed against the constant region of human γ chain, γ chain protein could be shown by immunoprecipitation to be present on CD4-, CD8-negative thymocyes from patients with primary immunodeficiency states (Brenner et al 1986), and on approximately 3% of peripheral blood CD4-negative, CD8-positive T cells from normal individuals (Bank et al 1986). These cells have TcR γ chain associated with the T3 peptide but no mature TcR α- or β-chain messages. Soon thereafter, there was a report of functional γ chain cDNAs from athymic nude mouse (Yoshikai et al 1986), and these observations raised a possible role for the γ chain as a component of a hypothetical second TcR, an alternative receptor functioning in some circumstances. To add more evidence in favor of a second T cell receptor, a polypeptide of about 45–50 kd could be co-precipitated with γ chain, and it was tentatively called the δ chain (Brenner et al 1986, Bank et al 1986, Weiss et al 1986). Very recently, there were reports of a constant-like gene located 3' to the V_α genes and 5' to the J_α genes whose deduced amino acid sequence is consistent with a δ polypeptide chain (Chien et al 1987, Takihara et al 1988). The γ–δ heterodimer also forms complexes with CD3 (T3) molecules.

Genomic organization of the T cell receptor genes
Multiple bands were observed when full length α or β chain cDNAs were used to probe germline genomic DNA from fibroblasts (Yanagi et al 1984, Toyonaga et al 1984, Minden et al 1985). DNA from cloned T cells, leukemic T cells or leukemic T cell lines also revealed several bands, although the band patterns were different from those representing germline configuration and from each other. Comparison of DNA from fibroblasts and from leukemic cells from the same patient showed that the differences in band patterns were not due to an inherited restriction fragment length polymorphism. These findings indicated that distinct somatic rearrangement of TcR genes had occurred in different T cell clones (Fig. 5.1).

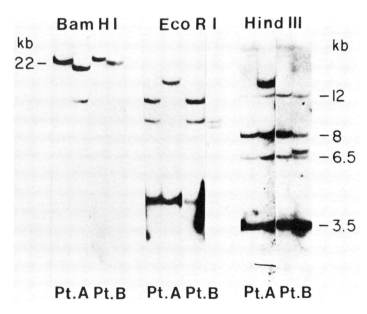

Fig. 5.1 A Southern blot of DNA extracted from the fibroblasts (first lane) and leukemia cells (second lane) of two different patients. The DNA was digested with either BamHl, EcoRl or HindIII, separated by agarose gel electrophoresis, transferred to nitrocellulose, and probed with a constant region probe for TcR β. Rearrangement of the TcR is evident when comparing the leukemic DNA to the fibroblast DNA in both cases and with all three enzymes. The 9.5 kb EcoRl band is due to contamination of the probe with V and J sequences and is not the result of partial digestion.

Organization of the β chain T cell receptor genes
The TcR β genes are mapped to chromosome 7 in man (7q34) and 6 in mouse (Caccia et al 1984, Morton et al 1985). In their germline configuration, these genes are composed of discontinuous genetic segments which bear resemblance to Ig variable, diversity, joining and constant gene elements and are referred to in the same manner (Fig. 5.2). It is estimated that there are approximately 100 V_β gene segments in man, a number considerably smaller than the κ and heavy chain Ig V genes. The V_β genes are distributed in over a dozen families (Toyonaga & Mak 1987). A leader sequence is at the 5' end of each V segment, separated from the rest of the coding sequences by an intron. There are highly conserved heptamer and nonamer sequences,

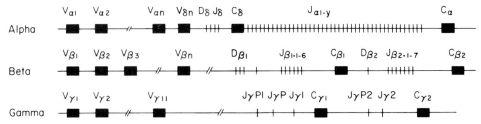

Fig. 5.2   Schematic representation of the genomic organization of the TcR genes. Note the location of the TcR δ genes in the TcR α gene locus.

immediately 3' of the coding sequences, and separated by a non-conserved spacer (Siu et al 1984).

The diversity and joining segments and constant region genes are located in a region of about 20 kb. There are two highly conserved C region genes approximately 10 kb apart, the 5' C gene designated as $C_{\beta1}$ and the 3' C gene as $C_{\beta2}$ (Toyonaga et al 1985). They are also similar in their general organization, with their first two exons coding for most of the extracellular constant domain, the third exon sequences corresponding to part of the transmembrane region, and the last exon containing the sequences coding for the cytoplasmic domain, as well the 3' untranslated region of the β chain message. The introns and the 3' noncoding regions share little similarity to each other, whereas the coding sequences of the two C regions are highly homologous, having only four amino acid differences between them. The lack of homology between the 3' nontranslated sequences has been used to distinguish transcripts from the two C regions. About 4 kb 5' of each C region is a cluster of joining segments. In the human, the $J_{\beta1}$ and the $J_{\beta2}$ clusters (each with 6 functional segments) are upstream of $C_{\beta1}$ and $C_{\beta2}$, respectively. The highly conserved heptamer and nonamer structures, separated by a spacer, are located adjacent to the 5' end of each J segment. A single D segment is found about 650 basepairs (bp) 5' of each J cluster. Each D segment is flanked on its 5' side by a heptamer and a nonamer with a 12-base spacer and on its 3' side by the heptamer and nonamer with a 23-base spacer. The presence of the heptamers and nonamers with their varying spacer sequences satisfies the 12/23 bp rule, whereby recombination occurs only between a pair of Ig or TcR gene segments, one with a 12-nucleotide spacer and the other with a 23-nucleotide spacer, each 12 nucleotides representing a full turn in the DNA helical structure (Fig. 5.3). Considering that each D_β is flanked on its 5' side by a 12-base spacer and on its 3' side by a 23-base spacer, both VJ and DD joining are theoretically possible, potentially expanding the diversity of the J_β gene products. A D_β gene segment can be linked to a V_β gene in all three translational reading frames, a feature not seen in Ig heavy D segments. Somatic hypermutation for increased V region diversification, as seen in Ig genes, has not been detected for TcR V region genes. In view of the similarity of the overall organization of the two C region genes and the associated D and J gene segments, it has been proposed that these tandem structures arose through gene duplication (Toyonaga et al 1985, Kronenberg et al 1986). A comparison of the human and murine TcR β genes show remarkable conservation of the coding regions when one considers that the two species diverged some 70 million years ago.

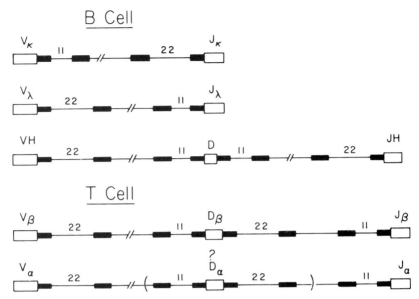

Fig. 5.3   Schematic representation of the heptamer, nonamer and spacer sequences flanking Ig and TcR gene segments.

Organization of the α chain T cell receptor genes
The TcR α locus is on human chromosome 14, in the 14q12 region, with the variable region being proximal and the constant region distal, in relation to the centromere (Caccia et al 1985). The genomic organization of the α chain V gene segments is very similar to that of the β chain and Ig genes. It is estimated that there are approximately 16 V_{α} families in human, containing a total of 70–80 different V region segments. With the use of pulse field gel electrophoresis, it has been possible to obtain a physical macro-restriction map of the entire human α locus which spans close to 1000 kb pairs and includes the V_{α}, J_{α} and C_{α} genes. The V_{α} segments are spread out over 750 kb pairs (Griesser et al 1988). There is only one α constant region in human and mouse, divided into four exons, with the first two encoding the extracellular domain, while the third codes for transmembrane and cytoplasmic portion of the protein. The 3' untranslated sequence occupies its own exon.

The J gene segments have an unusual distribution, occupying a region of approximately 80 kb 5' of the C_{α} region, and appear to be more than 50 individual segments in number. No D_{α} segments have been identified yet.

Organization of γ chain T cell receptor genes
The human TcR γ chain genes are located on the short arm of chromosome 7, in the 7p15 region (Murre et al 1985). There are 11 V_{γ} segments in the human genome (Kimura et al 1987, Forster et al 1987). Five joining gene segments and two constant region genes have been found, arranged as $J_{\gamma 1}$–$C_{\gamma 1}$ and $J_{\gamma 2}$–$C_{\gamma 2}$. Each γ gene is flanked by a heptamer separated from a nonamer by a spacer.

Organization of the δ chain T cell receptor genes
The rather recent description of a constant region gene located within the murine TcR α locus and approximately 85 kb 5' of the C alpha region (Chien et al 1987)

was followed by its human counterpart being found (Takihara et al 1988) which are 80% homologous to each other. The human C_δ does not cross-hybridize to C_α. The C_δ exons span a region of over 5 kb. Two J segments have been found upstream to C_δ with flanking heptamer and nonamer recombinational sequences. A few V_δ segments have been sequenced, and a D_δ gene has also been found (Hata et al 1987, Takihara et al 1988).

Recombination of T cell receptor genes

The recombinational signals flanking the V, D and J segments of the TcR genes are very similar for Ig and TcR genes. Moreover, it has been recently shown that the same recombinase enzyme may be operative in the joining of these gene segments (Yancopoulos et al 1986), and this may explain why in some T cell lines the Ig heavy chain genes are rearranged and in some B cell lines the TcR genes are rearranged. Similarly to what occurs with Ig genes, the first event in TcR β chain gene rearrangement is a DJ joining. This rearrangement can sometimes result in truncated transcripts being expressed, of approximately 1.0 kb for β chain (containing only D, J, C and sequences 5' of the D segment) and 1.3 kb for α chain (consisting of J, C and 5' J germline sequences). These incomplete or non-productive transcripts can be occasionally found in B cells. A final recombination event brings a V region gene adjacent to the DJ or J segments, resulting in the expression of a complete 1.3 or 1.6 kb message from the β and α chain genes, respectively.

The TcR γ and δ chain genes also undergo somatic rearrangement. For the δ genes, analysis of several T cell lines have shown either no transcripts or the presence of transcripts of 2.2, 1.8, 1.5 and 1.2 kb, with the 1.8 and 1.2 kb messages being expressed mainly in thymocytes (Takihara et al 1988). The mechanisms that can produce these four transcripts are not known at this time and possible explanations include alternate splicing, production of transcripts from rearranged and non-rearranged genes, or messages with alternate polyadenylation sites.

REARRANGEMENT OF IMMUNOGLOBULIN AND THE T CELL RECEPTOR GENES IN HEMATOLOGICAL NEOPLASIAS

As a stem cell differentiates into a mature lymphocyte Ig and TcR genes, originally as discontinuous segments in their germline configuration, undergo rearrangements often associated with deletion of segments of DNA, thus changing the location of restriction-endonucleases sites. If appropriate site-specific endonucleases are employed, these changes can be detected in a Southern blot and used to distinguish the rearranged from the germline form of the gene(s) under study. A polyclonal T cell population is expected to contain many different rearrangements of the TcR genes, each yielding a restriction fragment of a different size. Collectively, none of these rearrangements in particular can be seen as a new band on Southern transfers, as a result of a lack of sensitivity of the methods currently used to detect them. However, in a T cell tumor most cells have the same rearrangement, resulting in new single-sized fragment(s) containing the TcR gene used. Since in most instances rearrangements occur in both homologous chromosomes, two new bands are present. Until recently, it was difficult to categorically establish monoclonality in T cell lymphoproliferative processes, since no cell surface phenotypic markers have been identified which can be used to unequivocally demonstrate clonality.

TcR β chain genes have been used to study malignant and non-malignant hematological pathologies, demonstrating that the detection of rearrangements of these genes is a useful marker of T cell lineage (Minden & Mak 1986). The establishment of clonality of malignant cells in cases of T lymphomas or lymphoid leukemias has been possible through the use of TcR chain gene probes, either at presentation or relapse. These studies are particularly useful when morphologically normal T cells are preponderant and there is no clear marker to determine whether one is dealing with a clonal or polyclonal expansion of T lymphocytes. However, one should bear in mind that the clonality of a cell population does not necessarily equate with a malignant phenotype of this clonal population (Davey & Waldmann 1987, Reis & Mak 1987), since benign monoclonal proliferations are known to occur. Also, the occurrence of inherited polymorphism in Ig or TcR genes may be misinterpreted as rearrangements of these genes. Such polymorphisms appear to be rare for Ig heavy and κ light chain genes, and TcR genes. The inclusion of non-lymphoid DNA samples as an internal control is advisable, such as DNA from granulocytes or skin fibroblasts obtained from the same individual whose lymphoid cells are being studied.

In terms of sensitivity, a clonal population comprising as little as 1% of the total cell population can be detected with current hybridization techniques (Arnold et al 1983, Minden & Mak 1986). In practical terms, several million cells yield 10 µg of DNA, enough for Southern blot analysis; therefore, if 1% of these cells represent a clonal population of T cells in this sample, they can be detected as a rearranged band (Fig. 5.4).

After many unsuccessful attempts using TcR α gene probes to detect rearrangements, this has now been possible, with the utilization of J_α probes (Sangster et al 1986). The TcR γ genes can be used to detect clonality, but not to determine cell lineage (Griesser et al 1986a). The recently described TcR δ genes are either deleted or rearranged in all T cell lines or leukemias studied so far (Takihara et al personal communication; M. Minden personal communication).

Once a particular pattern of Ig or TcR gene rearrangement has been determined for a patient's lymphoid neoplasia, this information can be used as a highly sensitive tumor-specific marker, which has improved the ability to identify persisting tumor cells following therapy and that helps in the early detection of a relapse.

The studies discussed below are representative of the studies on the structure of the TcR chain genes in haematological neoplasias, since a thorough listing of papers on this subject is beyond the scope of this publication.

T cell disorders

T cell acute lymphoblastic leukemia (T-ALL)

Several groups have studied the structure of the TcR β chain genes in 127 cases of T-ALL (Aisenberg et al 1985, 1987, Bertness et al 1985, Davey et al 1986b, Flug et al 1985, Hara et al 1987, Kitchingman et al 1985, Minden et al 1985, Norton et al 1988, O'Connor et al 1985b, Pelicci et al 1985, Rabbitts et al 1985a, Tawa et al 1985, 1987, Waldmann et al 1985, Williams et al 1987) (Table 5.1). One or both alleles of the β chain genes were rearranged in all except one of the cases. In the

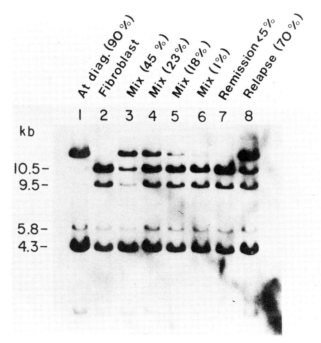

Fig. 5.4 A Southern blot illustrating the sensitivity of the technique for detecting a clonal population. Lane 1 represents a sample obtained at the time of diagnosis and contained >90% blasts. Fibroblast DNA from the same patient is in lane 2. Lanes 3, 4, 5 and 6 represent mixtures of the diagnosis DNA and fibroblast DNA; the % is the % of leukemic DNA in the sample. Lane 7 has a remission sample in which <5% of the cells were identified as blasts. Lane 8 is a relapse sample in which 70% of the cells were blasts. The DNA was cut with EcoRI, separated by agarose gel electrophoresis, transferred to nitrocellulose, and probed with a constant region fragment of TcR β. The band characteristic of the leukemic cells can be seen in the sample consisting of 1% leukemic cells and 99% fibroblasts DNA. The remission sample containing <5% blasts does not have a band characteristic of the leukemic cells; thus, the number of leukemic cells in this sample is <1%.

cases where analysis of cell surface markers was carried out, heterogeneous results were obtained in that no single marker was present in all cases. For example, cells with rearrangement of TcR β genes did not always express the CD3 (T3) cell surface antigen. All 48 cases of T-ALL examined have shown rearrangement of the TcR γ genes (Aisenberg et al 1987, Davey et al 1986, Hara et al 1987, Norton et al 1988, Subar et al 1988, Tawa et al 1987). Davey and co-workers demonstrated rearrangements of the TcR γ genes in all CD2 (T11)-positive leukemias. Three cases of CD7-positive, CD2-negative T-ALL, considered as stem cell or very early pre-T leukemias, were shown by the same group to have the TcR β genes in the germline configuration, whereas the TcR γ genes were rearranged in two of these cases. The TcR δ chain genes were analyzed in 19 cases of T-ALL (Hara et al submitted). There was biallelic rearrangement in 5 out of 7 CD3− and in 4 out of 12 CD3+ samples. In 8 other CD3-positive samples, 3 had a single TcR δ gene allele rearrangement with the other allele showing TcR α rearrangement. In the other 5 CD3+ T-ALL both alleles showed rearrangements of the TcR α genes and deletion of the δ loci. A total of 6 cases from this series were examined for transcription of TcR genes, with 5 expressing TcR δ mRNA; the case without TcR δ mRNA expressed TcR γ and a truncated

Table 5.1   Rearrangement of TcR_β chain genes in leukemia and lymphoma. *Key:* T-ALL, T cell precursor acute lymphoblastic leukemia; ATL, adult T cell leukemia; T-CLL, T cell chronic lymphocytic leukemia; ALL, common non-B, non-T ALL, cALLa+; B-CLL, B-cell chronic lymphocytic leukemia; AIL, angioimmunoblastic lymphadenopathy; AML, acute myeloblastic leukemia. See text for references.

	No of cases	Rearranged TcR_β	Rearranged Ig H C
1. *T cell malignancies*			
T-ALL	127	126	18 (13 not done)
ATL	50	50	1 (6 not done)
T cell lymphoma	56	49	0 (11 not done)
T cell prolymphocytic leukemia	20	20	0 (1 not done)
Sezary syndrome/mycosis fungoides	56	55	1 (39 not done)
T-CLL	33	33	0 (8 not done)
T8 lymphocytosis	17	13	0 (4 not done)
Lymphomatoid papulosis	6	5	not done
2. *B cell and pre-B cell malignancies*			
ALL	77	19	76
Lymphoma	59	6	59
B-CLL	45	5	45
Myeloma	2	0	2
3. *Other hematopoietic malignancies*			
Lennert's lymphoma	6	6	0
Hodgkin's disease	37	4	2 (1 not done)
AIL	12	9	4 (also TcR_β)
AML	68	9	6 (also TcR_β in 2 cases)

α gene rearrangement may take place after rearrangements of the TcR δ genes with concurrent deletion of the rearranged δ genes in T cell differentiation.

Immunoglobulin gene probes were used in 114 of all the cases listed above, studied for the structure of the TcR β genes, and rearrangements of the Ig heavy, but not Ig light chain genes, were detected in 18 instances.

Chronic T cell malignancies

Virtually all cases of chronic T cell malignancies such as T cell chronic lymphocytic leukemic (T-CLL), T cell prolymphocytic leukemia (T-PLL), adult T cell leukemia (ATL), mycosis fungoides and Sezary syndrome that have been analysed showed rearrangement of TcR β chain genes (Aisenberg et al 1985, Baer et al 1985, Bertness et al 1985, Flug et al 1985, Isaacson et al 1985, Minden et al 1985, O'Connor et al 1985, Pelicci et al 1985, Rabbitts et al 1985, Waldmann et al 1985, Weiss et al 1985). In cases of mycosis fungoides the draining lymph nodes were demonstrated to harbor tumor cells. Weiss et al (1985) have shown clonal TcR β gene rearrangement not only in lymph nodes with unambiguous infiltration by mycosis fungoides (MF), but also in lymph nodes of patients with MF thought to contain only benign reactive cells by histological analysis. Aisenberg et al (1987) have reported rearrangements of both TcR β and γ genes in 3 cases of cutaneous T cell lymphoma. In 4 cases of T-CLL, the TcR β genes were rearranged in all of them, and the γ genes did so in three of these samples. As for ATL, which have a phenotype indentical to that of Sezary cells, the TcR β genes were reported to rearrange in 50 of 50 cases.

The TcR γ genes have been found to rearrange in most cases of mature T cell neoplasias (Aisenberg et al 1987, Davey et al 1986, Rabbitts et al 1985b, Matsuoka et al 1988, Subar et al 1988, Quertermous et al 1986).

T cell lymphomas
The TcR β genes were rearranged in most (49 out of 56) of the non-Hodgkin's T cell lymphomas examined (Bertness et al 1985, Flug et al 1985, Griesser et al 1986a,b, Isaacson et al 1985, O'Connor et al 1985, Pelicci et al, 1985, Williams et al 1987). In one study, the TcR β genes were in germline configuration and the TcR γ genes were rearranged in two cases. Of four cases of T-cell lymphoblastic lymphoma studied, the TcR β genes were rearranged in two and in germline configuration in the other two; none of these cases had rearrangements of Ig heavy or light chain genes. Using two genomic J_δ probes, Tkachuk et al (1988) analyzed 14 samples of T cell lymphoma, and found TcR δ gene rearrangement or deletion in 6 cases. In all cases where the TcR δ genes were rearranged , so were the TcR δ and γ genes.

T8 or T_γ lymphocytosis
Seventeen cases of CD8 (T8) γ-lymphocytosis or cytotoxic-suppressor lymphocytosis and neutropenia were studied with TcR β gene probes (Aisenberg et al 1985, Bertness et al 1985, Rambaldi et al 1985, Waldmann et al 1985b). This is a rare disorder with a benign course characterized by lymphocytosis of large granular lymphocytes expressing CD8 and, in most instances, CD3, with receptors for the Fc portion of IgG. Thirteen patients had a clonal population of T cells in their peripheral blood. Based on this, one of the authors has equated T8 lymphocytosis to benign monoclonal gammopathy (Aisenberg et al 1985). The chronic nature of this ailment indicates that the finding of a clonal population does not necessarily indicate the presence of a malignant disease. The fact that not all patients with T8 lymphocytosis have a clonal population may be due to a technical artefact, indicate that the syndrome is heterogeneous, or due to the fact that the disease starts off being polyclonal but a single clone becomes dominant over time. A predominant T cell clonal population has been found in one patient with T4 lymphocytosis (M. Minden 1985, unpublished observation).

Lymphomatoid papulosis
This entity is a chronic disease with a relatively benign course, characterized by repetitive episodes of self-healing papular lesions, which eventually ulcerate and then resolve as scars. The histologic appearance of the lesions, however, is consistent with that of a malignant lymphoma, containing mononuclear cells along with a prominent population of large atypical cells that either have cerebriform nuclei or resemble Reed-Sternberg cells. Tumor tissue from 6 patients with this entity were studied (Weiss et al 1986), with 5 revealing evidence of clonality when analysed with a TcR β gene probe, a result confirmed in 4 samples probed with TcR γ DNA. The 1 patient whose specimen did not show clonality with both the β and γ probes had a scant sub-epidermal infiltrate, with a comparatively low number of atypical cells. Three rearranged bands were detected in 1 patient, suggesting the presence of at least 2 clonal populations in this sample, since rearrangement of both TcR β gene alleles in a monoclonal proliferation would result in only 2 rearranged bands. Varying patterns

of TcR β gene rearrangement were seen in 3 separate specimens from another patient, suggesting that different lesions may contain different T cell clones.

B cell and pre-B cell malignancies

Non-B, non-T acute lymphoblastic leukemia
Specimens from 77 patients with non-B, non-T-ALL analyzed with Ig and TcR β probes have shown rearrangements of Ig heavy chain genes in virtually all cases, and this was considered as evidence of B cell lineage and these leukemias are now considered as precursor B cell ALL, together with pre-B-ALL. However, rearrangement of the TcR β chain genes was found in 19 of these patients and the patterns of rearrangement did not differ significantly from that seen in T cell malignancies (Aisenberg et al 1985, Davey et al 1986, Minden et al 1985, Pelicci et al 1985, Tawa et al 1985). Some recent series have analysed samples of precursor B-ALL with J_H, TcR β and also TcR γ probes. The Ig heavy chain genes were rearranged in 76 of 77 cases, in combination with TcR γ rearrangement in 20 cases and with concurrent TcR γ and β gene rearrangements in another 18 cases. Thus, it seems that TcR γ genes do rearrange in approximately 50% of the cases of precursor B-ALL, confirming that TcR γ gene rearrangement is not a reliable indicator of cell lineage. In most cases of precursor B-ALL with TcR γ gene rearrangement, one allele remains in the germline configuration, whereas in T-ALL both alleles are rearranged (Asou et al 1987, Tawa et al 1987, Williams et al 1987). Norton et al (1988) obtained similar results on analysis of 32 cases of precursor B-ALL, all with rearranged IgH genes, simultaneously with rearrangements of TcR β and γ chain genes in 10 cases, of β genes only in 5, and of γ genes only in 7 cases.

A recent study used J_H, TcR β, γ and 3 TcR α probes to examine 18 cases of T-ALL and 46 of precursor-B-ALL (Hara et al 1987). Rearrangements of the TcR α genes were observed in only 2 of 18 T-ALL, indicating that perhaps the majority of T-ALLs would have rearrangements involving J_α segments located upstream of the probes used. In contrast, TcR α gene rearrangements were observed in 15 out of 46 precursor-B-ALL. Nine of those cases also had both the TcR γ and β genes rearranged, whereas the remaining 6 cases had these genes in the germline disposition. The same group has examined 29 cases of precursor B-cell ALL with all TcR genes, and have found the TcR δ genes to be rearranged in 20 cases (69%), a frequency higher than those for the TcR α (59%), γ (52%) or β genes (31%), and observed that the TcR δ gene seems to be the earliest TcR gene to rearrange, followed by TcR γ and β rearrangement (Hara et al submitted). Therefore, it appears that TcR α and δ chain gene rearrangements are not specific for cells of T lymphoid lineage, and that TcR γ and/or β gene rearrangements do not seem essential for TcR α and δ gene rearrangements, at least in the case of precursor B-cell ALL.

Chronic B cell malignancies
The TcR β genes were found to be rearranged in 5 out of 45 cases of B cell CLL analyzed (Aisenberg et al 1987, Pelicci et al 1985, Waldmann et al 1985). In a few cases, the rearrangement of the TcR β genes is questionable, since it was observed with one restriction enzyme but not confirmed in the same DNA samples digested with other enzymes, thus favoring TcR β gene polymorphism instead of

the conventional rearrangements seen in T cell populations (Aisenberg et al 1987). TcR γ chain gene rearrangements have not been detected in B-CLL.

Non-Hodgkin's lymphoma of B cell type
Rearrangements of TcR genes were seen in approximately 10% of the cases studied (in 6 of 59 cases) (Griesser et al 1986a, b, Pelicci et al 1985, Williams et al 1987). Tkachuk and co-workers (1988) have studied 14 samples of B cell lymphomas and B cell lines and shown the TcR δ genes to be in germline configuration in all cases. In all those samples, at least one IgH allele was rearranged, with or without concurrent TcR β or γ gene rearrangements. Overall, TcR genes have been found to rearrange in about 10% of the chronic B cell neoplasias, a figure higher than the incidence of Ig gene rearrangement in neoplasias of mature T cell origin.

Other hematopoietic malignancies

Other types of lymphomas
This refers to a group of lymphomas including Lennert's lymphoma, Ki 1[+] lymphomas, angioimmunogloblastic lymphadenopathy and Hodgkin's disease, entities in which the presence of a clonal population of cells had not been clearly demonstrated previously.

LENNERT'S LYMPHOMA
Rearrangements of the TcR β chain genes were observed in 6 out of 6 cases of Lennert's lymphoma. There was no rearrangement of Ig genes (Griesser et al 1986a, O'Connor et al 1985). The TcR γ chain genes have also been found to be clonally rearranged in the cases analysed (Griesser et al 1986a). The TcR δ genes have been found to be completely or partially rearranged in 3 out of 5 samples, with suggestion that in 2 cases only 1 allele was rearranged. All 5 cases had TcR β and γ rearrangements (Tkachuk et al, 1988).

Ki 1[+] LYMPHOMA
Griesser et al (1986b) examined 10 cases of this type of lymphoma and found that 4 cases showed rearrangement of TcR β genes only, 3 had rearranged TcR β and Ig heavy chain genes, but not light chain genes, and 3 had both the TcR β and Ig heavy chain genes in the germline configuration. As for the TcR δ genes, they were rearranged in 5 of 11 cases studied, all of them also showing TcR β and γ chain rearrangements and the IgH genes in the germline configuration (Tkachuk et al, 1988).

ANGIOIMMUNOBLASTIC LYMPHADENOPATHY (AIL)
The TcR β genes were rearranged in 9 out of 12 cases analyzed (Bertness et al 1985, Griesser et al 1986b). In addition, Ig heavy chain genes were rearranged in 4 of these 9 cases. One of these samples also had rearrangement of the Ig κ light chain gene.

The finding of TcR β gene rearrangement in AIL and Lennert's lymphomas, where clonal populations of cells comprise a major portion of the lymph node, may be taken as evidence that these are disease processes of T cell origin.

HODGKIN'S DISEASE

Reports of studies of TcR and Ig gene rearrangements in Hodgkin's disease have at times been contradictory. In an analysis of 11 cases, a faint but noticeable band was detected in 4 cases when probed with TcR β chain genes (Bertness et al 1985, Griesser et al 1986b). It is significant that 1 of the cases studied had approximately 50% Reed-Sternberg cells, and no rearrangement was seen in this case. Also, no rearrangements of Ig genes were seen in all cases in these series. Later, Griesser et al (1987a) studied 22 cases of Hodgkin's disease (HD) and found examples of rearrangements of IgH genes alone, TcR γ genes alone, TcR γ and β genes simultaneously, and of germline configuration for IgH and TcR genes. They suggested that Hodgkin's lymphomas may contain clonal lymphoid populations and that different rearrangement patterns may be associated with distinct subclasses of HD. Knowles et al (1986) examined 18 cases of HD and found minor clonal population in 3 of them. Cases with more than 25% RS cells did not show clonal TcR or Ig rearrangements. Their conclusion was that HD is composed predominantly of polyclonal B and T cell populations, that minor B or T cell populations unrelated to RS cells can be occasionally found in HD, and that RS cells do not represent clonal B or T cell expansion. A recent study of 6 cases of HD has shown TcR δ rearrangement in only 1 case (Tkachuk et al, 1988).

In summary, the consensus seems to be that the question of whether a clonal population found, if any, represents the neoplastic cells or a clonal proliferation in response to some antigens is still unanswered.

Acute myeloblastic leukemia (AML)

TcR β chain genes were shown to be rearranged in 3 out of 24 patients with AML studied by Cheng et al (1986). All of these patients expressed myeloid cell surface markers. Interestingly, 2 of the patients were positive for TdT, and 1 of these patients was positive for the T cell surface marker T6. An interesting picture emerged when Seremetis et al (1987) detected a high frequency of TcR β and/or Ig gene rearrangement (60%) in cases of AML expressing TdT. Of 13 TdT$^+$ AML, rearranged TcR β genes only were seen in 4 cases, with rearrangements for IgH chain genes only in 3 cases, and for both TcR β and IgH chain genes in 1 case. Of the 25 TdT$^-$ AML, 1 had rearranged the TcR β genes only, and another had rearranged the IgH genes (frequency lower than 8%). The authors proposed that the close association between TdT expression and TcR β/Ig gene rearrangements in TdT$^+$ AML further suggests a role for TdT in the mechanisms leading to the assembly of diverse Ig or TcR genes. The enzyme TdT was initially considered a lymphoid lineage-associated marker, but the use of more sensitive techniques for detection of this enzyme has shown that approximately 10% of the cases of AML express TdT. From the series reported thus far, it appears that patients with TdT$^+$ AML have a poor prognosis. Preliminary observations indicate that the TcR δ genes may be occasionally rearranged in AML (M. Minden, unpublished observations).

A note of caution is that the finding of rearrangement of TcR β or γ chain genes in non-T cell malignancies raises the question of the specificity of this finding in terms of defining T cell lineage. Analyzes of TcR genes expression by Northern blot may help by showing the mRNA corresponding to those genes to be truncated, reflecting incomplete rearrangement. Thus, with regards to using rearrangements of the

TcR β or γ gene to determine the lineage of a cell population one must exercise caution and take into account additional information such as the structure of the Ig genes and the expression of cell surface markers.

REARRANGEMENT OF BOTH Ig AND TcR GENES IN LYMPHOPROLIFERATIVE DISORDERS

The use of monoclonal antibodies specific for developmental antigens has greatly helped to clearly define the cell lineage and stage of differentiation of most lymphoproliferative disorders. However, this method still fails to detect either clonality or lineage of abnormal cells in some of these disorders. It is difficult to detect clonality in T cell disorders with phenotypic analysis, especially in T cell-rich processes such as Lennert's and large cell anaplastic (Ki 1$^+$) lymphomas. Genotypic analysis with the use of Ig and TcR genes has elucidated the B or T cell origin of most lymphoproliferative disorders but has also revealed complex gene rearrangement patterns in a few cases, in that not only TcR but also Ig genes rearrangement occurs in the same tissues (Table 5.2), thus raising questions about the value and meaning of genotypic studies

Table 5.2   Ig and TcR gene rearrangement patterns in lymphoproliferative disorders. *Key:* AIL, angioimmunoblastic lymphadenopathy; Ki 1, large cell anaplastic Ki 1$^+$ lymphoma; ATL, adult T cell leukemia; HD, Hodgkin's disease.

| | Rearrangement pattern | | | | | | |
| | Ig | | TcR | | | Probable | Examples |
Occurrence	H	L	γ	β	α	lineage	(pathological diagnosis)
Frequent	−	−	+	+	−/N.D.	pre-T or T	T-ALL; T cell lymphoma; Lennert's lymphoma; AIL, Ki 1
	−	−	+	+	+/N.D.	T	ATL; T-CLL; T-ALL, T cell lymphoma; T$_\gamma$-lymphocytosis
	+	−	−	−	−	pre-B	non-T ALL
	+	+	−	−	N.D.	B	B-ALL; B-CLL; B cell lymphoma
	+	+/−	+	−	N.D.	B, pre-B	B-ALL; B-CLL; B cell lymphoma, non-T ALL
Infrequent	+	+/−	−	−	N.D.	B, pre-B	HD
	+	+	+	+	N.D.	B	AIL, B cell lymphoma
	−	−	+	−	N.D.	pre-T(?)	Ki 1, HD
	−	−	+	+	N.D.	pre-T(?)	HD
	+	−	+	+	−/N.D.	pre-T(?)	AIL; Ki 1, T-ALL; non-T ALL
	−	−	−	+	N.D.	T	T cell lymphoma
	+	−	+	+/−	+/N.D.	pre-B/pre-T	non-T ALL; B cell lymphoma

for definition of lineage of these few cases. For example, TcR and Ig genes rearrangements have been demonstrated in AML (Cheng et al 1986, Seremetis et al 1987), forcing one to consider the issue of lineage promiscuity.

From those series reporting simultaneous rearrangements of TcR and Ig genes, it is clear that the frequency of bigenotype is higher in B than in T cell lymphoproliferative disorders, and this is valid for disorders of either mature or immature lymphoid phenotypes. Also, these inappropriate rearrangements are seen more in immature than in mature lymphoid neoplasias. In addition, there are differences in the patterns of rearrangements, with usually only one Ig heavy chain allele rearranging in T cell disorders, with the Ig light chain genes remaining unrearranged. In B cell disorders, the tendency is clearly for only one TcR β or γ gene allele to rearrange, as opposed to biallelic rearrangements seen in T cell neoplasias.

A possible explanation for the crosslineage rearrangements is the presence of both B and T cells clonal expansions. This is unlikely, however, for the malignant cells in B cell leukemias are immunocytochemically of pure B cell phenotype. Also, the equal intensity of the rearranged TcR and Ig gene bands on Southern blot autoradiography suggests that these rearrangements occur in a cell population of equal size. The concept of lineage promiscuity (Greaves et al 1986), with respect to Ig and TcR gene rearrangement in the same lymphocyte, is then attractive. The most likely explanation for the phenomenon of lineage promiscuity at the gene level is the accessibility of the TcR and the Ig gene loci to the recombinase enzyme operative in facilitating recombination of discontinuous subunits of these genes (Yancopoulos et al 1986). These inappropriate rearrangements only involve recombination of a D with a J segment (the first event in recombination), but not of a V segment with an assembled DJ recombinant (the second step in a complete recombination process). Thus far, complete (VDJ) rearrangement of the TcR β chain genes in B cell neoplasias, or of IgH chain genes in T cell tumors have not been reported. Furthermore, no full length RNA transcripts corresponding to the gene rearrangements described above have been detected. Therefore, one should assume that neither TcR γ gene rearrangement nor incomplete DJ joining of TcR β or IgH gene segments are indicative of lineage commitment. The occurrence of these promiscuous rearrangements during tumor progression, rather than during developmental differentiation programming, is another possibility. The finding of incomplete IgH and TcR gene rearrangement in some cases of AML supports this hypothesis.

The occurrence of rearrangements of both TcR and Ig genes is substantially higher in lymphoproliferative disorders whose lineage is difficult to ascertain on the basis of histological or immunological analysis. These include Ki 1$^+$ lymphomas, AIL/AIL-like lymphomas and non-T ALL (Table 5.2). A high proportion of tumor cells with rearrangement of both IgH and TcR genes were detected in samples if Ki 1$^+$ lymphomas and AIL (Griesser et al 1986b). In most of these cases, the TcR γ genes were more often rearranged, with no apparent bias towards rearrangements of either their IgH or TcR β chain genes in these same cells. For those cases, it is possible that the malignant transformation occurred in a lymphoid procursor cell that became frozen at a stage of differentiation prior to commitment to either B or T cell lineage. In some cases of AIL and Ki 1$^+$ lymphomas there was rearrangement of the TcR β, γ and δ chain genes, with the Ig heavy and light chain genes remaining in the germline configuration, thus indicating T cell origin. The T cell phenotype was confirmed by immunochemistry in most of these cases.

An interesting, and perhaps the most heterogeneous, group of lymphoproliferative disorders in terms of their immunogenotype is that of non-T ALL. A large proportion of non-T ALL have shown rearrangement not only of the IgH genes but also of the TcR genes (Asou et al 1987, Hara et al 1987, Tawa et al 1985). In some cases of precursor B cell ALL, IgH as well as any combination of TcR δ, α and γ chain gene rearrangement occurs, with or without TcR β chain gene rearrangement, even if the leukemic population expresses only cytoplasmic Ig μ chains (Hara et al 1987, Norton et al 1988, Tawa et al 1985).

The issue of explaining the dual genotype of some lymphoid tumors is still unresolved, and considerations have been given as to whether this represents a normal or an abnormal feature of lymphoid differentiation pathways. A few studies have reported IgH chain gene rearrangement and expression in mouse thymocytes and T lymphocytes (Kemp et al 1980, Kurosawa et al 1981). This phenomenon may have some functional significance or may identify a subpopulation of bipotent lymphoid cells, with properties of both B and T cells. However, the bigenotypic tumors examined maintain a pure B or T cell phenotype, making this explanation unlikely. Griesser and co-workers have proposed that the complex Ig and TcR gene rearrangement patterns may reflect a clonal population originating from an undifferentiated hematopoietic cell that underwent rearrangement of these genes prior to lineage commitment. As an alternative, the dual genotype may reflect a stage in lymphoid differentiation in which a committed B or T cell maintains the potential for lineage switch, with the fidelity of the immunophenotyping then reflecting the final lineage commitment of the cell, and the dual genotypic markers remaining as an irreversible footprint of the previous commitment (Pelicci et al 1985). Still another possibility is that the dual genotype may reflect the simultaneous activation in T and B cells of common molecular mechanisms regulating the rearrangement of the Ig and TcR loci.

Alternatively, the concurrent rearrangement of the TcR and Ig genes in immature B leukemias may represent events that are not part of the normal B cell differentiation pathway, and the high incidence of dual genotype in precursor B cell leukemias may result from the lack of signals present in more mature cells that terminate gene rearrangements (Davey et al 1986b). It is possible that the recombinases responsible for facilitating Ig and TcR gene rearrangements may remain active until an effective stop signal (mature Ig or TcR molecules) is produced, resulting in suppression of the recombinase(s) or closing of open chromatin sites. If a complete mRNA leading to the production of Ig products is not present in a precursor B cell, the recombinase(s) may remain active, with ensuing activation of both Ig and TcR genes; if a transforming event occurs at this stage, it could result in the clonal expansion of a population of cells with dual rearrangements. On the other hand, the dual genotype could be present in cells destinated to a dead-end, as it is the case with numerous thymocytes whose fate is cell death, perhaps as a consequence of defective gene rearrangements. If such cells are the target of transforming events, they could originate a bigenotypic clone of tumor cells and escape cell death. Another possibility is that bigenotypia results from a transformation-related event and reflects the derangement of the genetic machinery or of the program regulating differentiation in the neoplastic cells.

INVOLVEMENT OF T CELL RECEPTOR GENES IN CHROMOSOMAL TRANSLOCATIONS

Recurrent chromosomal translocations occur in a number of tumors. Some of them have been studied at the molecular genetic level, such as the ones involving chromosomes 9 and 22 in chronic myeloid leukemia (Gale & Cannani 1985) and the translocations involving chromosome 8 (where the c-myc oncogene is located) and either chromosome 2, 14 or 22 (containing the Ig light κ, heavy and light λ genes, respectively) in Burkitt's lymphoma (Klein 1983, Croce & Nowell 1985). Recurrent translocations have also been observed in some T cell processes including those involving the 7q33 and 7p13 regions of the TcR β chain (Hecht et al 1985, Isobe et al 1985, Morton et al 1985) and γ chain genes, respectively (see Table 5.3). The most frequent

Table 5.3 Translocations involving T cell receptor genes

Disease	Translocation	Loci involved	References
Pre-T (T cell)	t(1;14)(p32;q11)	L-myc?-TcR$_\alpha$ N-ras?-TcR$_\alpha$ src-2?-TcR$_\alpha$	Kurtzberg et al (1985)
	t(8;14)(q24;q11)	c-myc-TcR$_\alpha$	Williams et al (1984), Mathieu-Mahul et al (1985), Erikson et al (1986), Shima et al (1986)
	t(10;14)(q23;q11)	TdT?-TcR$_\alpha$ onc?-TcR$_\alpha$	Dube et al (1986) Kagan et al (1987)
	t(11;14)(p13;q11)	Wilm's-TcR$_\alpha$ onc?-TcR$_\alpha$	Williams et al (1984), Sadamori et al (1985), Erikson et al (1985), Lewis et al (1985)
	t(12;14)(q24;q11)	onc?-TcR$_\alpha$	Sadamori et al (1985)
	inv(14)(q11;q32)	IgH-TcR$_\alpha$	Zech et al (1984), Baer et al (1985), Denny et al (1986a)
	t(14;14)(q11;q32)	IgH?-TcR$_\alpha$	Shah-Reddy et al (1982), Sadamori et al (1985)
		akt?-TcR$_\alpha$ onc?-TcR$_\alpha$	
	t(7;9)(q34;q33)	TcR$_\beta$-abl?	Hecht et al (1984), Smith et al (1986)
Pre-B (B cell) leukemia/lymphoma	inv(14)(q11;132)	IgH-TcR$_\alpha$	Denny et al (1986a)
Ataxia-telangectasia	inv(7)(p13;q33)	TcR$_\gamma$?-TcR$_\beta$?	Hecht et al (1975)
	t(7;14)(p13;q11)	TcR$_\gamma$?-TcR$_\alpha$?	Welch et al (1975)
	t(7;14)(q34;q11)	TcR$_\beta$?-TcR$_\alpha$?	Kaiser-McCaw et al (1975)
	inv(14)(q11;q32)	TcR$_\alpha$?-IgH?	Aurias et al (1980)
	t(14;14)(q11;q32)	TcR$_\alpha$?-IgH?	Scheres et al (1980), Taylor et al (1982), Kohn et al (1982), Fukuhara et al (1983), Battey et al (1983)

translocations, however, involve the region of 14q11 to 14q13, the region containing the TcR α (and δ) genes. For example, three such translocations are: two reciprocal translocations between 14q12 and 8q24 (Shima et al 1986) and between 11p13 and 14q12 (Williams et al 1984, Lewis et al 1985), and an inversion involving 14q11 and 14q32 (Williams et al 1984; Hecht et al 1984, Zech et al 1984, Croce et al 1985, Baer et al 1985, Denny et al 1986b). Some of these translocations will be briefly discussed.

In the t(8;14)(q24;q12) studied, the breakpoint is between V_α and C_α, with the translocation involving the region of the J_α segments, and results in the C_α gene being translocated to a region immediately 3' of the c-myc oncogene. It is possible that activation of the c-myc gene by TcR α gene elements occurs in a manner similar to the activation of this oncogene in Burkitt's lymphoma. As for the t(11;14)(p13;q11), the exact nature of the gene involved in the p13 region is not known. This locus has been implicated in the development of Wilm's tumor, and it is possible that either this Wilm's tumor-associated gene or another as yet unidentified gene is involved in the malignant transformation, as a result of its altered structure or expression by its translocation into the TcR α chain locus.

Another translocation, t(10;14)(q24,q11), has been reported in some cases of T-ALL and high grade T cell lymphomas (Dube et al 1986, Hecht et al 1985). Kagan et al (1987) have found that the breakpoint on chromosome 10 is distal to the TdT gene, and that the C_α gene was translocated to chromosome 10, with the V_α gene segments remaining on the 14q- chromosome. They suggested that a proto-oncogene is located proximal to the breakpoint at 10q24, and proposed the name TCL3 to this putative proto-oncogene, whose deregulation would lead to T cell leukemia or lymphoma.

The inv(14)(q11;q32) has been detected in lymphomas and chronic T-CLL, virus-associated T cell leukemias and in T cell monoclonal proliferations in individuals with ataxia-telangectasia (references on Table 5.3). Two breakpoints exist on the long arm of the inv(14) chromosome. The telomeric breakpoint creates a fused structure in which an Ig V_H gene segment joins a TcR J_α segment (Denny et al 1986a). This V_H–$J_\alpha C_\alpha$ joining is productive, resulting in the formation of a hybrid gene, part Ig and part TcR, transcribed into mRNA with a completely open reading frame. This telomeric joining has been seen in T cell disorder and in at least one case of B-ALL. The centromeric breakpoint of inv(14) involves gene segments different from those that constitute the joining site at the telomeric breakpoint (Baer et al 1987). A proto-oncogene is not known to be involved in this inversion, and it is tempting to speculate that the gene products resulting from this inversion may play a role in oncogenesis. However, this inversion is not seen only in tumor cells, and is occasionally detected in stimulated normal T cells and in T cells from patients with ataxia-telangectasia (Kirsh et al 1985).

ACKNOWLEDGEMENTS

We are grateful to Diana Quon for preparing this manuscript. HG is now at the Institute of Pathology, Christian Albrecht University, Kiel, Federal Republic of Germany. MDR is at Sunnybrook Medical Center, Toronto, Canada.

REFERENCES

Acuto O, Reinherz E L 1985 New England Journal of Medicine 312: 1100–1111
Aisenberg A C, Krontiris T G, Mak T W, Wilkes B M 1985 New England Journal of Medicine 313: 529–533
Aisenberg A C, Wilkes B M, Jacobson J O 1987 Journal of Clinical Investigation 80: 1209–1214
Asou N, Matsuoka M, Hattori T et al 1987 Blood 69: 968–970
Arnold A, Cossman J, Bakhshi A, Jaffe E S, Waldmann T A, Korsmeyer S J 1983 New England Journal of Medicine 309: 1593–1599
Aurias A, Dutrillaux B, Buriot D, Lejeune J 1980 Mutation Research 69: 369–374
Baer R, Chen K-C, Smith S D, Rabbits T H 1985 Cell 43: 705–713
Baer R, Forster A, Rabbitts T M 1987 Cell 50: 97–105
Bank I, DePinho R A, Brenner M B, Cassimeris J, Alt F W, Chess L 1986 Nature 322: 179–181
Battey J, Moulding C, Taub R et al 1983 Cell 34: 779–787
Bertness V, Kirsh I, Hollis G, Johnson B, Bunn P A Jr 1985 New England Journal of Medicine 313: 534–538
Brenner M B, McLean J, Dialynas D P et al 1986 Nature 322: 145–148
Caccia N, Kronenberg M, Saxe D et al 1984 Cell 37: 1091–1099
Caccia N, Bruns G A, Kirsch I R., Hollis G E, Bertness V, Mak T W 1985 Journal of Experimental Medicine 161: 1255–1260

Cheng G, Minden M D, Mak T W, McCulloch E A 1986 Journal of Experimental Medicine 163: 414–424

Chien Y H, Iwashima M, Kaplan K B, Elliott J F, Davis M M 1987 Nature 327: 677–682

Croce C, Nowell P C 1985 Blood 65: 1–7

Croce C M, Tsujimoto Y, Erikson J, Nowell P 1984 Laboratory Investigation 51: 258–267

Croce C M, Isobe M, Palumbo A et al 1985 Science 227: 1044–1047

Davey M P, Waldmann T A 1986 New England Journal of Medicine 315: 509–511

Davey M P, Bongiovanni K F, Kaulfersch W et al 1986 Proceedings of the National Academy of Sciences USA 83: 8759–8763

Denny C T, Hollis G F, Hecht F et al 1986a Science 234: 197–200

Denny C T, Yoshikai Y, Mak T W, Smith S D, Hollis G F, Kirsch I R 1986b Nature 320: 549–551

Dube I D, Raimondi S C, Pi D, Kalousek D K 1986 Blood 67: 1181–1184

Erikson J, Williams D L, Finan J, Nowell P C, Croce C M 1985 Science 229: 784–786

Flug F, Pelicci P-G, Bonetti F, Knowles H D M, Dalla-Favera R 1985 Proceedings of the National Academy of Sciences USA 82: 3460–3465

Forster A, Hucks S, Ghanem N, Lefranc M-P, Rabbitts T H 1987 European Molecular Biology Organization Journal 6: 1945–1950

Fukuhara S, Hinuma Y, Gotoh Y-L, Uchino H 1983 Blood 61: 205–207

Gale, R P, Cannani E 1985 British Journal of Haematology 60: 395–408

Greaves M F, Chan L C, Furley A J W, Watt S M, Molgaard H V 1986 Blood 67: 1–11

Griesser H, Feller A, Lennert K et al 1986a Blood 68: 592–594

Griesser H, Feller A, Lennert K, Minden M D, Mak T W 1986b Journal of Clinical Investigation 78: 1179–1184

Griesser H, Feller A C, Mak T W, Lennert K 1987 International Journal of Cancer 40: 157–160

Griesser H, Tkachuk D, Mak T W 1988 Blood (submitted)

Griesser H, Champagne E, Tkachuk D et al 1988 European Journal of Immunology 18: 641–644

Hannum C H, Kappler J W, Trowbridge I S, Marrack P, Freed J H 1984 Nature 312: 65–68

Hara J, Benedict S H, Mak T W, Gelfand E W 1987 Journal of Clinical Investigation 80: 1770–1774

Hara J, Benedict S H, Champagne E et al Proceedings of the National Academy of Sciences USA (submitted)

Haskins K, Kubo R, White J, Pigeon M, Kappler J, Marrack P 1983 Journal of Experimental Medicine 157: 1149–1169

Hata S, Brenner M B, Krangel M S 1987 Science 238: 678–681

Hecht F, Kaiser-McCaw B, Peakman D, Robinson A 1975 Nature 255: 243–244

Hecht F, Morgan R, Hecht B K-M, Smith S D 1984 Science 226: 1445–1447

Hecht F, Morgan R, Gemmill R M, Hecht B K-M, Smith S D 1985 New England Journal of Medicine 313: 758–759

Hedrick S M, Cohen C I, Nielsen E A, Davis M M 1984a Nature 308: 149–153

Hedrick S M, Nielsen E A, Kavaler J, Cohen D I, Davis M M 1984b Nature 309: 153–158

Hood L, Kronenberg M, Hunkapiller T 1985 Cell 40: 225–226

Isaacson P G, O'Connor N T, Spencer J et al 1985 Lancet 2: 688–691

Isobe M, Erikson J, Emanuel B S, Nowell P C, Croce C M 1985 Science 228: 580–582

Kagan J, Finan J, Letopsky J, Emmanuel C B, Nowell P C, Croce C M 1987 Proceedings of the National Academy of Sciences USA 84: 4543–4546

Kaiser-McCaw B, Hecht F, Harnden D G, Teplitz R L 1975 Proceedings of the National Academy of Sciences USA 72: 2071–2075

Kemp D J, Wilson A, Harris A W, Shortman K 1980 Nature 286: 168–170

Kimura N, Du R-P, Mak T W 1987 European Journal of Immunology 17: 375–378

Kirsch I R, Brown J A, Lawrence J, Korsmeyer S J, Morton C C 1985 Cancer Genetics and Cytogenetics 18: 159–171

Kitchingman G R, Rovigatti U, Mauer M A, Melvin S, Murphy S B, Stass S 1985 Blood 65: 725–729

Klein G 1983 Cell 32: 311–315

Knowles H D M, Neri A, Pelicci P-G et al 1986 Proceedings of the National Academy of Sciences USA 83: 7942–7946

Kohn P H, Whang-Peng J, Levis W R 1982 Cancer Genetics and Cytogenetics 6: 289–302

Korsmeyer S J, Hieter P A, Ravetch J V, Poplack D G, Waldmann T A, Leder P 1981 Proceedings of the National Academy of Sciences USA 78: 7096–7100

Kronenberg M, Siu G, Hood L, Shastri N 1986 Annual Reviews of Immunology 4: 529–591

Kurosawa Y, von Boehmer H, Hass W, Sakano H, Trauneker A, Tonegawa S 1981 Nature 290: 565–570

Kurtzberg J, Gibner S, Hershfield M S 1985 Journal of Experimental Medicine 162: 1561–1565

Lewis W H, Michaelopoulos E E, Williams D L, Minden M D, Mak T W 1985 Nature 317: 544–546

Mathieu-Mahul D, Caubet J F, Bernheim A et al 1985 European Molecular Biology Organisation Journal 4: 3427–3431

Matsuoka M, Hagiya M, Hattori T et al 1988 Leukemia 2: 84–90
Minden M D, Mak T W 1986 Blood 68: 327–336
Minden M D, Toyonaga B, Ha K, Yanagi Y, Chan B, Gelfand E, Mak T 1985 Proceedings of the National Academy Sciences USA 82: 1224–1227
Morton C C, Duby A D, Eddy R L, Shows T B, Seidman J G 1985 Science 228: 582–585
Murre C, Waldmann R A, Morton C C et al 1985 Nature 316: 549–551
Norton J D, Campana D, Hoffbrand A V et al 1988 Leukemia 2: 27–34
O'Connor N T J, Weatherall D J, Feller A C et al 1985 Lancet I: 1295–1297
Ohashi P S, Mak T W, Van den Elsen P et al 1985 Nature 315: 606–610
Pelicci P-G, Knowles H D M, Dalla-Favera R 1985 Journal of Experimental Medicine 162: 1015–1024
Quertermous T, Musse C, Dialynas D et al 1985 Science 231: 252–257
Rabbitts T H, Stinson A, Forster A, Foroni L et al 1985a European Molecular Biology Organization Journal 4: 2217–2224
Rabbitts T H, Lefranc M P, Stinson M A et al 1985b European Molecular Biology Organization Journal 4: 1461–1465
Rambaldi A, Pelicci P-G, Allavena P et al 1985 Journal of Experimental Medicine 162: 2156–2162
Reis M D, Mak T W 1987 Blood Reviews 1: 89–96
Sadamori N, Kusano M, Nishino K et al 1985 Cancer Genetics 17: 279–282
Saito H, Kranz D, Takagaki Y, Hayday A, Eisen H, Tonegawa S 1984 Nature 312: 36–40
Sangster R N, Minowada J, Suciu-Foca N, Minden M, Mak T W 1986 Journal of Experimental Medicine 163: 1494–1508
Scheres J M J C, Hustinx T W J, Weemaes C M R 1980 Journal of Pediatrics 97: 440–441
Seremetis S V, Pelicci P-G, Tabilio A et al 1987 Journal of Experimental Medicine 165: 1703–1712
Shah-Reddy I, Mayeda K, Mirchandani I, Koppitch F C 1982 Cancer 49: 75–79
Shima M, LeBeau M M, McKeithan T W et al 1986 Proceedings of the National Academy of Sciences USA 83: 3439–3443
Siu G, Clark S, Yoshikai Y et al 1984 Cell 37: 393–401
Smith K 1984 Annual Reviews of Immunology 2: 319–334
Smith S D, Morgan R, Link M P, McFall P, Hecht F 1986a Blood 67: 650–656
Smith S D, Link M P, Trela M et al 1986b New England Journal of Medicine 315: 195–196
Subar M, Pellici P-G, Neri A et al 1988 Leukemia 2: 19–26
Takihara Y, Champagne E, Griesser H et al 1988 European Journal of Immunology 18: 283–287
Tawa A, Hozumi N, Minden M, Mak T W, Gelfand E W 1985 New England Journal of Medicine 313: 1033–1037
Tawa A, Benedict S M, Hara J, Hozumi N, Gelfand E W 1987 Blood 70: 1933–1939
Taylor A M R 1982 In: Bridges BA, Harnden G (eds) Ataxia-telangiectasia: A cellular and molecular link between cancer, neuropathology and immune deficiency Wiley, New York p 53–81
Tkachuk D C, Griesser H, Takihara Y et al 1988 Blood 72: 353–357
Tonegawa S 1983 Nature 302: 575–581
Toyonaga B, Mak T W 1987 Annual Reviews of Immunology 5: 585–620
Toyonaga B, Yanagi Y, Suciu-Foca N, Minden M, Mak T W 1984 Nature 311: 385–388
Toyonaga B, Yoshikai Y, Vadasz B, Chin B, Mak T W 1985 Proceedings of the National Academy of Sciences USA 82: 8624–8628
Waldmann T A 1987 In: Stamatoyannopoulos G, Nieuhuis A W, Leder P, Mojerus P W (eds) Molecular basis of blood diseases Saunders, Philadelphia p 245–270
Waldmann T A, Davis M M, Bongiovanni K F, Korsmeyer S J 1985a New England Journal of Medicine 313: 775–783
Weiss A, Stobo J D 1984 Journal of Experimental Medicine 160: 1284–1299
Weiss A, Newton M, Crommie D 1986 Proceedings of the National Academy of Sciences USA 83: 693–700
Weiss L M, Hu E, Wood G S, Moulds C, Clearly M L, Warnke R, Sklar J 1985 New England Journal of Medicine 313: 539–544
Weiss L M, Wood G S, Trela M, Warnke R A, Sklar J 1986 New England Journal of Medicine 315: 475–479
Welch J, Lee C L Y, Beatty-De Sana J W et al 1975 Nature 255: 241–242
Williams D L, Look A T, Melvin S L et al 1984 Cell 36: 101–109
Williams M E, Innes D J, Borowitz M J et al 1987 Blood 69: 79–86
Yanagi Y, Yoshikai Y, Leggett K, Clark S P, Aleksander I, Mak T W 1984 Nature 309: 143–149
Yancopoulos G D, Blackwell T K, Suh H, Hood L, Alt F W 1986 Cell 44: 251–259
Yoshikai Y, Reis M, Mak T W 1986 Nature 324: 482–485
Zech L, Gahrton G, Hammarstrom L et al 1984 Nature 309: 858–860
Zinkernagel R M, Doherty P C 1975 Journal of Experimental Medicine 141: 1427–1437

6. Molecular basis of B- and T-cell neoplasia

G. Russo   F. G. Haluska   M. Isobe   C. M. Croce

INTRODUCTION

Most human hematological neoplasias exhibit non-random chromosomal alterations (Yunis 1983). These alterations are represented by chromosomal translocations, inversions, deletions and trisomies. The first consistent cytogenetic alteration in a human malignancy was observed by Nowell & Hungerford (1960), who described the presence of a minute marker in the cells of a patient with chronic myelogenous leukemia (CML), termed the Philadelphia chromosome (Ph'). The Philadelphia chromosome was subsequently identified as the $22q^-$ resulting from a reciprocal t(9;22)(q34;q11) chromosomal translocation, a hallmark of nearly all CMLs. In 1972 Manolov & Manolova (1972) described the presence of a marker chromosome 14 in a patient with Burkitt lymphoma that was shown later to be the result of another reciprocal chromosomal translocation, t(8;14)(q24;q32), which is present in approximately 80% of Burkitt's lymphomas (Zech et al 1976). Since then, many other cytogenetic studies have focused on hematological neoplasias, and the reclassification of these neoplasias has made possible a better correlation between specific chromosomal alterations and different hematopoietic malignancies.

Another advance in the understanding of human neoplasias was the identification of a relatively small set of normal cellular genes, called cellular proto-oncogenes, that are homologs of retroviral oncogenes (Bishop 1987). These oncogenes are believed to serve as substrates for many of the somatic alterations responsible for malignant transformation. The molecular cloning and the advent of techniques like in situ hybridization, somatic cell hybrids, and high resolution chromosome banding made possible the mapping of genes to specific regions of chromosomes. Very interestingly, some of the oncogenes were mapped to points where chromosomal alterations frequently occur in human hematopoietic neoplasia. Therefore, c-*myc* was mapped to chromosome 8q24 (Dalla-Favera et al 1982) and c-*abl* to chromosome 9q34 (Heisterkamp et al 1983). Thus arose the possibility that these oncogenes could be directly involved in human neoplasia.

In addition, the finding that immunoglobulin (Ig) and T-cell receptors (TCRs) are encoded by genes that undergo somatic rearrangements (Tonegawa 1983, Hedrick et al 1984, Yanagi et al 1984), and the further mapping of these genes on human chromosomes to the same locations involved in the aforementioned human neoplastic translocations made possible a further definition of these genetic alterations in hematopoietic malignancies.

In this review we will discuss and summarize the molecular aspects of chromosomal translocations, with special emphasis on B- and T-cell malignancy.

Table 6.1 Comparison of features of endemic and sporadic Burkitt's lymphomas

	Endemic	Sporadic
Geographic location	Equatorial Africa	Europe and North America
Age	Children	Young adults
Organ involved	Jaw	Marrow and abdomen
EBV presence	+	−
IgM secretion	−	+
Recombinase-mediated translocation	+	−
Isotype switch-mediated translocation	−	+

B-CELL NEOPLASIA

Burkitt lymphoma

Burkitt lymphoma is a neoplasm of B-cell lineage that strikes children and young adults. It is a fast-growing and very aggressive tumor (Ziegler et al 1981). Two types of Burkitt lymphoma are known: endemic and sporadic. Differences in the two forms of tumors at the epidemiological, immunological and molecular levels are presented in Table 6.1 Histologically, the two types of tumors show minor differences, and the hallmark of the two forms is the involvement of the distal end of the long arm of chromosome 8q24->qter. In approximately 75% of the cases this segment translocates to the long arm of chromosome 14q32, the locus where the immunoglobulin heavy chain (IgH) maps (Croce et al 1979). In 16% of the cases the 8q24->qter band translocates to band 22q11, the location of the λ-chain of Ig (Erikson et al 1981), and in the remaining 9% the segment is translocated to band 2p11 where the κ-chain resides (McBride et al 1982). These translocations are illustrated in Figure 6.1 Somatic cell genetic analysis of the breakpoints and the molecular cloning of these translocations later revealed that two genes involved in these chromosomal rearrangements were c-*myc* and the Ig locus (Dalla-Favera et al 1983, Croce et al 1983, Erikson et al 1983).

Molecular analysis has been successfully conducted in sporadic and in endemic cases. The breakpoints on chromosomes 8 and 14 are quite heterogeneous. Breakpoints in the IgH locus are found within the D_H segment (Haluska et al 1987a), J_H segments (Haluska et al 1986), and in the S_μ (Gelman et al 1983), S_γ (Hamlyn et al 1984), and Sα (Showe et al 1985) regions. In the variant translocations t(2;8) and t(8;22), breaks occur in V_κ (Erikson et al 1983) or J_κ (Lipp & Hartl 1986) or 5′ of C_λ on chromosome 22 (Croce et al 1983). Heterogeneity in the breakpoints is also observed on the c-*myc* side. In fact, c-*myc* can be translocated far 5′ of the c-*myc* locus (Haluska et al 1986, Haluska et al 1987a), upstream of the first exon (Hamlyn & Rabbitts 1983, Wiman et al 1984), within the first intron (Gelman et al 1983, Showe et al 1985), or at a variable distance 3′ of the coding region (Croce et al 1983, Erikson et al 1983). In this last case, c-*myc* remains on chromosome 8, and a region 3′ of the break is translocated to chromosome 2 or chromosome 22 (thus the term 'variant translocation') (see Fig. 6.1). As a consequence of the translocation, the c-*myc* oncogene fails to respond to its normal mechanism of control and is transcribed constitutively

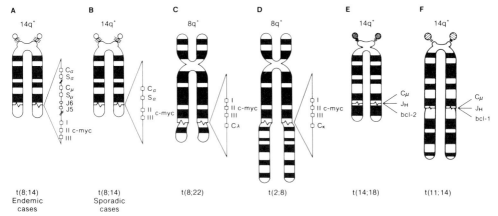

Fig. 6.1 Chromosome translocations observed more frequently in B-cell neoplasia. The configurations of the immunoglobulin genes and c-*myc*, *bcl*-2, *bcl*-1 as revealed by molecular cloning studies are illustrated. The 14q$^+$ chromosome resulting from the t(8;14) in endemic (A) and sporadic (B) cases in Burkitt's lymphoma is illustrated. (C) and (D) represent the 8q$^+$ chromosome as observed in the variant translocations in Burkitt's lymphoma. (E) shows the 14q$^+$ found in follicular lymphoma where the *bcl*-2 locus (chr. 18) is translocated to the IgH locus. (F) represents the 14q$^+$ from B-ALL where the *bcl*-1 locus (chr. 11) is translocated to the IgH. C, S and J indicate constant, switch and joining regions of the immunoglobulins.

at a high level (Croce et al 1983, Erikson et al 1983). This probably results from the juxtaposition of the c-*myc* oncogene to one of the genetic elements present in the immunoglobulin loci (enhancers) or enhancer-like elements capable of activating *in cis* at a considerable distance.

Follicular lymphoma

Follicular lymphoma is one of the most frequent hematopoietic neoplasias in humans. Cytogenetically, 80% of the cases carry a t(14;18)(q32;q21) translocation (Yunis 1983, Fukhhara et al 1979) (Fig. 6.1). By screening a genomic library from a cell line derived from a patient with a pre-B-cell leukemia carrying two chromosomal translocations, a t(8;14)(q24;q32) and a t(14;18)(q32;q21), Tsujimoto and associates were able to isolate genomic clones that encompassed both breakpoints using a J_H probe (Tsujimoto et al 1984a). Rearrangements were detected in approximately 75% of human follicular lymphomas by using probes originated from the chromosome 18 site (Tsujimoto et al 1985a). The locus defined by these probes was named *bcl*-2 (B-cell lymphoma/leukemia 2). Furthermore, probes derived from segments of DNA near the breakpoint were used to detect an mRNA of 5.5 kb.

The *bcl*-2 gene has since been characterized at a more detailed level in humans and in mice (Tsujimoto & Croce 1986, Negrini et al 1987). At the genomic level, *bcl*-2 is composed of three exons, with an untranslated first exon, a facultative 220 bp intron I, but an enormous 370 kb intron II (Seto et al 1988). Breakpoints usually occur in approximately 90% of the cases in the 3′ portion of the gene and rarely in the 5′ portion of the gene (Tsujimoto et al 1987a). At the transcriptional level, *bcl*-2 is composed of three messages (8.5, 5.5 and 3.5 kb) generated by differential splicing and polyadenylation (Tsujimoto & Croce 1986). Expression is tissue-specific in mouse adult tissue; spleen and thymus express the highest level of *bcl*-2 transcript (Negrini et al 1987). Two proteins, one of 239 amino acids (named *bcl*-2 α) and one of 205 amino acids (named bcl-2 β), are encoded by these transcripts (Tsujimoto et al 1987b). The two proteins differ at their carboxy terminals. Antiserum raised against the bcl-2 protein immunoprecipitates a protein that is associated with the cell membrane, which might suggest the involvement of the bcl-2 protein in the signal transmission during B-cell proliferation.

Translocations in follicular lymphoma appear to deregulate bcl-2 expression, probably with the same mechanism of cis-activation described for the Burkitt lymphoma. Both the breakpoints in the 5' or in the 3' end of the bcl-2 locus leave the gene intact, as in the myc case where the exons coding for the myc protein are never altered by the translocation.

B-CLL and B-ALL

In approximately 10% of B-CLL, a t(11;14)(q13;q32) chromosomal translocation has been found (Van Den Berghe et al 1984) (Fig. 6.1). Using the same strategy previously described for the isolation of bcl-2, a new region on chromosome 11 was isolated and characterized (Tsujimoto et al 1984b). This region was called bcl-1 (B-cell leukemia/lymphoma 1). This translocation has been observed in some non-Hodgkin lymphomas and sometimes in multiple myeloma.

Another site of importance on chromosome 11 is band 11q23. The band 11q23 is associated with a remarkable variety of translocations, such as the t(11;14)(q23;q32) in B-ALL and the t(4;11)(q21;q23). The same band appears to be involved also in translocations of other acute non-lymphoid leukemia (Shows et al 1987). No chromosomal translocation in this region has been cloned to date.

T-CELL NEOPLASIA

Molecular genetics of T-cell leukemia/lymphoma

Lymphatic neoplasms involving T-cells are considerably less common than their B-cell counterparts. However, chromosomal translocations are present in these patients as well. The molecular cloning of the genes coding for T-cell receptors and the mapping of these genes has made it possible to isolate and characterize translocation breakpoints and possibly the genes or oncogenes that are involved in T-cell leukemogenesis. We and others have mapped the genes coding for TCRα and β to bands 14q11 (Croce et al 1985) and 7q35 (Isobe et al 1985), respectively. TCRγ maps to 7p15 (Murre et al 1985). And recently, TCRδ has been localized within TCRα at 14q11 (Chien et al 1987; Isobe et al 1988). Each of these loci has recently been recognized as a 'hot spot' in chromosomal translocations involving T-cell malignancies. In a recent report from Raimondi et al (1988), more than 50% of the chromosomal abnormalities in T-cell malignancies have been mapped to regions involving TCRs.

One of the most interesting findings in the organization of the genes coding for molecules involved in the formation of TCRs has been the recent linkage of the Tα and Tδ loci in mouse and human on band 14q11. The orientation on chromosome 14 of these receptors is centromere VαJδCδJαCα (Fig. 6.2). It appears that while only a few Jδ are present, a large number (>28) of Jα are present spanning over 80 kb from the constant region (see Fig. 6.2). The extraordinary length of the Jα region and the presence of the Jδ segments upstream of Jα makes this region highly active during T-cell differentiation as V-D-J joining proceeds. This activity can result

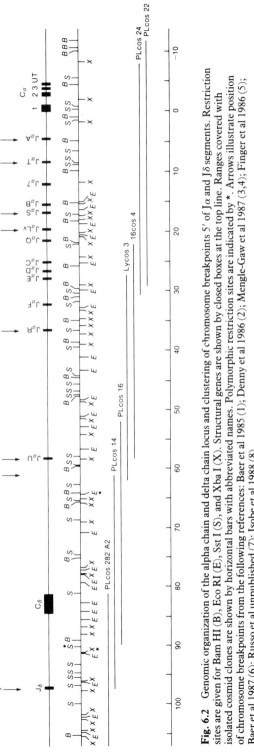

Fig. 6.2 Genomic organization of the alpha chain and delta chain locus and clustering of chromosome breakpoints 5′ of Jα and Jδ segments. Restriction sites are given for Bam HI (B), Eco RI (E), Sst I (S), and Xba I (X). Structural genes are shown by closed boxes at the top line. Ranges covered with isolated cosmid clones are shown by horizontal bars with abbreviated names. Polymorphic restriction sites are indicated by *. Arrows illustrate position of chromosome breakpoints from the following references: Baer et al 1985 (1); Denny et al 1986 (2); Mengle-Gaw et al 1987 (3,4); Finger et al 1986 (5); Baer et al 1987 (6); Russo et al unpublished (7); Isobe et al 1988 (8).

in mistakes during T-cell differentiation leading to translocations. The consequence of translocation is the activation of genes that are able to deregulate the normal growth program of T-cells (see following pages for a more detailed discussion). Furthermore, the presence of a consistent number of J segments has until now made the characterization of many translocations involving the T α/δ locus difficult.

Translocations involving c-myc

To date some chromosomal translocations have been characterized involving Tα and presumably Tδ. The first observation that the Tα locus could be involved in chromosomal translocations involving c-*myc* was made using somatic cell genetics and *in situ* hybridization. Analyzing somatic cell hybrids between tumor cells from a patient with T-ALL carrying a t(8;14)(q24;q11) and murine partners, Erikson et al (1986) showed that the translocation split the Tα locus, leaving the Vα on the 14q$^-$ and translocating the Cα locus 3$'$ of the c-*myc* on the 8q$^+$ chromosome. By molecular cloning of a similar translocation in a cell line, SKW3, derived from a patient with a T-CLL, Finger et al (1986) showed that the breakpoint on chromosome 8 mapped to a position 3 kb 3$'$ of c-*myc* while the chromosome 14 breakpoint occurred 36 kb 5$'$ of Cα. Furthermore, since human c-*myc* transcripts were expressed only in hybrids containing the 8q$^+$ chromosome but not in hybrids containing the normal chromosome 8, Erikson et al (1986) concluded that the translocation of the Cα locus 3$'$ to the c-*myc* oncogene can result in its transcriptional deregulation.

The recent finding that Tδ is situated between Vα and Cα suggests its possible involvement in translocations as well. In the somatic cell hybrids obtained from a patient with T-ALL previously described, containing the 8q$^+$, a unique rearrangement involving a Jδ segment has been shown to segregate with this chromosome, suggesting that the translocation had involved the Tδ locus (Isobe et al 1988).

Significantly, the T-cells demonstrating such involvement are of immature phenotype. This observation is in agreement with the finding of the expression of TCRδ in early T-cells. In the case of SKW3 where the translocation involves the Tα locus, the cells are of more mature phenotype (Sangster et al 1986). The observation of a correlation between phenotype and TCR involved in the chromosome translocation allows us to predict TCRδ involvement in T-cell leukemia/lymphoma of a more immature phenotype and TCRα and/or TCRβ in more mature T-cell malignancies.

Translocations involving 14q32 (tc1-1)

Translocations involving band 14q11 have been described in many T-cell leukemia/lymphoma cases. Most of these rearrangements involve chromosome 14q32, either in a t(14;14)(q11;q32) chromosomal translocation or in an inv(14) (q11;q32). This alteration is found in 60% of T-PLL (Brito-Babapulle et al 1987), in 80% of a series of T-CLL described separately by Ueshima et al (1984) and Zech et al (1986), and in a large number of cases with ATL (Sadamori et al 1985).

Another interesting observation comes from the study of patients with ataxia-telangiectasia (AT). AT is an immunodeficiency of B- and T-cells associated with cerebellar ataxia, oculocutaneous-telangiectasias, and deficient DNA repair following exposure to ionizing radiation. Patients with AT are prone to develop cancer, especially of the lymphatic tissue. Among these patients, T-cell leukemias appear to be preponderant.

Another characteristic of this disease is the elevated number of chromosomal translocations when non-malignant T-cells of these patients are analyzed. A frequency of chromosomal translocations 40 times higher than expected is observed, particularly involving 7p13, 7q35, 14q11 and 14q32. The high incidence of chromosomal abnormalities involving the cytogenetic loci of the T-cell receptors (with the exception of 14q32) is probably due to the high number of mistakes occurring during physiological rearrangements of TCRs. However, pre-leukemic clonal expansion of cells carrying abnormalities in 14q32 has been documented in many of the cases prior to the development of the overt malignancy (Taylor & Butterworth 1986). In this respect, AT represents a good model to study how a T-cell clone carrying a specific chromosomal translocation evolves into a full-blown leukemia. Even if we still lack a precise correlation between cytogenetics, morphologic data and phenotype of T-cell malignancy, we will attempt in the following sections to review some of the relevant data that has recently been gathered on the molecular characterization of these types of tumors.

The 14q32 chromosomal abnormality has been subject to many controversial arguments. Since the IgH locus maps to the 14q32 band, many investigators have suggested that this alteration could involve a recombination between IgH locus and $T\alpha$ locus. Instead, we proposed that a possible oncogene, tcl-1 (Fig. 6.3), could be on 14q32,

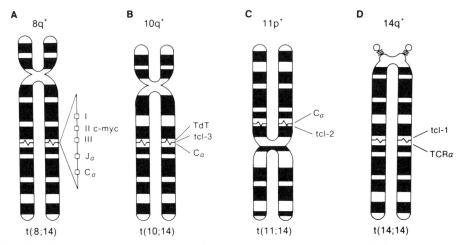

Fig. 6.3 Chromosome translocations observed more frequently in T-cell neoplasia. (A) Schematic representation of the $8q^+$ resulting from juxtaposition of TCRα to 3′ myc. (B), (C), (D) Schematic representation of putative oncogenes tcl-1, tcl-2, tcl-3 and relevant chromosome markers as explained in the text. In (D), the t(14;14) chromosome translocation is diagrammed. Cα indicates the constant region of the TCRα chain.

since it was unlikely that the gene implicated in the majority of these translocations involving T-cells was the IgH locus. The first molecular cloning of inv(14)(q11;q32) in a cell line SupT1 seemed to favor the hypothesis of a recombination between $T\alpha$ and IgH locus. In this cell line, in fact, Baer et al (1985) described an abnormal recombination which occurred between a variable region of IgH and a joining region from TCRα. Subsequent reports from the same group and from our laboratory analyzing other chromosomal translocations in T-cells have shown more recently that all these breakpoints on 14q32 are centromeric to the IgH locus. Mengle-Gaw et al (1987) described two molecular cloning experiments from two patients with T-CLL carrying a t(14;14)(q11;q32) translocation and an inv(14)(q11;q32) inversion in which the breakpoint was proximal to the J_H locus. Baer et al (1987) reported the same results by analysis of a malignant clone carrying a t(14;14)(q11;q32) translocation in a patient with T-cell leukemia and AT. We reported a case of a t(7;14)(q35;q32) translocation in a patient with T-ALL and AT carrying a breakpoint that was not only proximal to the J_H locus but mapped centromeric to D14S1, a polymorphic locus lying on band 14q32.2, while the IgH locus is on 14q32.3 (Russo et al 1988). In the same area, another breakpoint from a patient with a t(14;14)(q11;q32) translocation has been recently cloned and characterized (Russo, unpublished results). Fine mapping of these latter two breakpoints using high resolution chromosome banding has finely located these two breaks at band 14q32.1. None of these five breaks appears to be linked at the DNA sequence level (Russo, personal observation), so that this area does not appear to be closely clustered as in the case of c-*myc* in endemic Burkitt lymphoma or c-*abl* in CML. It is however, important to note that an oncogene *akt*-1, has been mapped on 14q32 (Testa et al 1985).

Translocations involving other loci (tcl-2, tcl-3)

Two additional chromosomal translocations observed in T-cell malignancies are the t(11;14)(p13;q11) translocation and the t(10;14)(q24;q11) translocation (Fig. 6.3). In both translocations a split between Vα and Cα region has been described; we assigned the terms *tcl*-2 and *tcl*-3 to the loci on 11p13 and 10q24 (Erikson et al 1985, Kagan et al 1987).

In the cell line SupT1, the same cell line carrying the inv(14)(q11;q32) inversion described above, Reynolds et al (1987) described another t(7;9)(q34;q34.3) translocation. Molecular cloning of the breakpoint showed that TCRB was joined to DNA of chromosome 9. Using a probe from chromosome 9q34.3, these authors were able to show that other T-cell tumors possessed DNA rearrangements near the band 9q34.3. They were able to detect multiple transcripts in SupT1 RNA and small amount of larger transcripts in T-cells lacking the chromosomal translocation. The band 9q34.3 is also the band where c-*abl* maps, but the data presented by Reynolds and co-workers seems to exclude the involvement of the c-*abl* in this translocation and proposes the existence of a new oncogene on sub-band 9q34.3.

Mechanisms of chromosomal translocations

A molecular analysis of the translocation breakpoints described above has led us to formulate some hypotheses about the mechanisms underlying the translocations.

The first observation was made by Tsujimoto et al (1985b) when the t(11;14)(q13;q32) was analyzed. They observed the presence on chromosome 11 surrounding the breakpoint of signal sequences that are believed to mediate V-D-J recombination in the immunoglobulin and TCR genes. These signal sequences consist of a heptamer-nonamer: 7 conserved nucleotides immediately abutting the variable (V), diversity (D) or joining (J) regions, then a non-conserved spacer of 12 or 23 nucleotides followed by a 9 nucleotide conserved segment. A characteristic feature of normal V-D-J joining is that at the site of joining nucleotides may be added, substituted or deleted. Additional nucleotides are called N regions; their addition is believed to be mediated by the enzyme terminal deoxynucleotidyl transferase (Desiderio et al 1984). Hope et al (1986) recently reported that the recombinase exhibits specific endonucleocytic activity that cleaves Ig sequences at CCA and TGG motifs.

Recent examination of many chromosome translocation breakpoints at Ig or TCR loci reveals that both Ig and T-cell malignancies share many common features:

1. These breakpoints usually lie immediately 5′ to J segments or sometimes to D segments where recombination in these genes normally occurs.

2. Analysis of the normal sequences from the other site of the breakpoints usually reveals that signal sequences homologus to heptamer-nonamer or heptamers alone are consistently found (see Haluska et al 1987b for review).

3. Existence of extranucleotides are usually found at the translocation breakpoints.

4. CCA and TG motifs have been found on the breakpoint sites.

All of these phenomena strongly suggest that the translocations either in T-cells or B-cells occur through the mistaken operation of the immunoglobulin or TCR recombinase.

In other cases like sporadic Burkitt lymphoma, the chromosomal translocation occurs usually in the Ig switch sequences (Hamlyn et al 1983, Showe et al 1985). In this case, it has been proposed that the translocation is mediated by a mistaken operation of the enzymes that catalyze Ig isotype switching.

CONCLUSIONS

We have summarized the molecular findings associated with some of the cytogenetic data known on human T- and B-cell neoplasias. Three features have been clearly elucidated in the recent past: first, the Ig locus and TCR genes are involved in genetic lesions in lymphatic neoplasia; second, putative oncogenes can be activated by their juxtaposition to the aforementioned Ig and TCR genes through elements activating *in cis* or through other mechanisms; third, the same enzymatic mechanisms that normally operate in B- and T-cells can lead to mistakes and then to chromosomal translocations.

Furthermore, we are convinced that the molecular characterization of B- and T-cell neoplasia can enable us to define a better classification in the near future of these tumors in view not only of their morphological features but also in view of the underlying genetic lesions.

REFERENCES

Baer R, Chen K C, Smith S D et al 1985 Cell 43: 705–713
Baer R, Heppel A, Taylor A M R et al 1987 Proceedings of the National Academy of Science USA 84: 9069–9073
Bishop J M 1987 Science 235: 305–310
Brito-Babapulle V, Pomfres M, Matutes E et al 1987 Blood 70: 926–931
Chien Y, Iwashima M, Kaplan K B et al 1987 Nature 327: 677–682
Croce C M, Shander M, Martinis J et al 1979 Proceedings of the National Academy of Science USA 76: 3416–3419
Croce C M, Thierfelder W, Erikson J et al 1983 Proceedings of the National Academy of Science USA 80: 6922–6929
Croce C M, Isobe M, Palumbo A et al 1985 Science 227: 1044–1047
Dalla-Favera R, Bregni M, Erikson J et al 1982 Proceedings of the National Academy of Science USA 79: 7824–7827
Dalla-Favera R, Martinotti S, Gallo R C et al 1983 Science 219: 963–967
Denny C T, Hollis G F, Hecht F et al 1986 Science 234: 197–200
Desiderio S V, Yancopoulos G D, Paskind M et al 1984 Nature 311: 752–755

Erikson J, Martinis J, Croce C M 1981 Nature 294: 173–175
Erikson J, Nishikura K, ar-Rushdi A et al 1983 Proceedings of the National Academy of Science USA 80: 7581–7585
Erikson J, Williams D L, Finan J et al 1985 Science 229: 784–786
Erikson J, Finger L, Sun L et al 1986 Science 232: 884–886
Finger L R, Harvey R C, Moore R C A et al 1986 Science 234: 982–985
Fukuhara S, Rowley J D, Variakojis D et al 1979 Cancer Research 39: 3118–3124
Gelman E P, Psallidopoulos M S, Papas T, Dalla-Favera R 1983 Nature 306: 799–803
Haluska F G, Finver S, Tsujimoto Y et al 1986 Nature 324: 158–161
Haluska F G, Tsujimoto Y, Croce C M 1987a Proceedings of the National Academy of Science USA 84: 6835–6839
Haluska F G, Tsujimoto Y, Croce C M 1987b Trends in Genetics 3: 11–15
Hamlyn P H, Rabbitts T H 1983 Nature 304: 135–139
Hedrick S M, Nielsen E A, Kavaler J et al 1984 Nature 308: 153–158
Heisterkamp N, Stephenson J R, Groffen J et al 1983 Nature 306: 239–242
Hope T J, Aguilero R J, Minic M E et al 1986 Science 231: 1141–1144
Isobe M, Erikson J, Emanuel B S et al 1985 Science 228: 580–582
Isobe M, Russo G, Haluska F G, Croce C M 1988 Proceedings of the National Academy of Science USA 85: 3933–3937
Kagan J, Finan J, Letofsky J et al 1987 Proceedings of the National Academy of Science USA 84: 4543–4546
Lipp M, Hartl P 1986 Current Topics in Microbiological Immunology 132: 162–168
McBride D W, Heiter P A, Hollis G F et al 1982 Journal Experimental Medicine 155: 1480–1485
Manolov G, Manolova Y 1972 Nature 237: 33–34
Mengle-Gaw L, Willard H F, Smith C I E et al 1987 EMBO Journal 6: 2273–2280
Murre C, Waldmann R A, Morton C C et al 1985 Nature 316: 549–552
Negrini M, Silini E, Kozak C, Tsujimoto Y, Croce C M 1987 Cell 49: 455–463
Nowell P C, Hungerford D A 1960 Science 132: 1497
Raimondi S C, Behm F G, Pui C H et al 1988 Blood 70 (sup 1): A683 (abstract)
Reynolds T C, Smith C D, Sklar S 1987 Cell 50:107–117
Russo G, Isobe M, Pegoraro L et al 1988 Cell 53: 137–144
Sadamori N, Kusano M, Nishino K et al 1985 Cancer Genetic Cytogenetics 17: 279–282
Sangster R N, Minowada J, Sciu Foca N et al 1986 Journal Experimental Medicine 163: 1491–1508
Seto M, Jaeger U, Hockett R D et al 1988 EMBO Journal 7: 123–131
Showe L C, Ballantine M, Nishikura K et al 1985 Molecular and Cellular Biology 5: 501–508
Shows T B, Davis L M, Qiw S et al 1987 Symposia on Quantitative Biology LI: 867–877
Taylor A M R, Butterworth S V 1986 International Journal of Cancer 37: 511–516
Testa J R, Huebner K, Croce C M et al 1985 Cytogenetic Cellular Genetics 40: 761 (abstract)
Tonegawa S 1983 Nature 302: 575–581
Tsujimoto Y, Finger L, Yunis J et al 1984a Science 226: 1097–1098
Tsujimoto Y, Yunis J, Onorato-Showe L et al 1984b Science 224: 1403–1406
Tsujimoto Y, Cossman J, Jaffe E et al 1985a Science 228: 1440–1443
Tsujimoto Y, Jaffe E, Cossman J et al 1985b Nature 315: 340–343
Tsujimoto Y, Croce C M 1986 Proceedings of the National Academy of Science USA 83: 5214–5218
Tsujimoto Y, Bashir M M, Givol I et al 1987a Proceedings of the National Academy of Science USA 84: 1379–1331
Tsujimoto Y, Ikegaki N, Croce C M 1987b Oncogene 2: 3–7
Ueshima Y, Rowley J D, Variakojis D et al 1984 Blood 63: 1028–1031
Van Den Berghe H, Vermaelen K, Louwagie A et al 1984 Cancer Genetic Cytogenetics 11: 381–387
Wiman K G, Clarkson B, Hayday A C et al 1984 Proceedings of the National Academy of Science USA 81: 6798–6802
Yanagi Y, Yoshikai Y, Legget K et al 1984 Nature 308: 145–152
Yunis J J 1983 Science 221: 227–236
Zech L, Haglund U, Nilsson K et al 1976 International Journal of Cancer 17: 47–56
Zech L, Godal T, Hammarstrom L et al 1986 Cancer Genetic Cytogenetics 21: 67–72
Ziegler J L, Miner R C, Rosenbaum E 1981 New England Journal of Medicine 305: 735–745

7. Chronic myeloid leukemia: pathogenesis and management

J. M. Goldman

INTRODUCTION

The term chronic myeloid leukaemia (CML) describes a specific form of leukaemia characterized by progressive splenomegaly, leucocytosis, anaemia, marrow hypercellularity and the finding in most cases of the specific chromosomal abnormality, the Philadelphia (Ph) chromosome, in all dividing cells of the myeloid series and in some B lymphocytes. Between 5 and 10% of patients with CML have variant features. For example some patients have a disease that resembles Ph-positive CML but their leukaemic cells are cytogenetically normal, so-called Ph-negative CML. A second category of patients with atypical CML have a disease that superficially resembles CML but lacks the Ph chromosome and shows increased numbers of relatively mature monocytes in the peripheral blood, a finding not characteristic of Ph-positive CML. Such patients are usually classified as chronic myelomonocytic leukaemia, a category currently included in the French-American-British classification of the myelodysplastic syndromes. A third category of atypical patients are the rare children with juvenile CML, a disease characterized by leucocytosis, lymphadenopathy, rashes, usually normal leukaemic cell cytogenetics and poor response to therapy. Finally very rare patients have chronic neutrophilic leukaemia, a form of chronic leukaemia with splenomegaly and the presence in the blood of increased numbers of morphologically normal mature neutrophils. The marrow cytogenetics are usually normal. Unlike Ph-positive CML, the neutrophil alkaline phosphatase is raised or normal.

Recent molecular studies have added to our understanding of the nature of the changes that may take place at the stem cell level in Ph-positive CML (reviewed by Gale & Cannani 1985, Goldman 1987, Dreazen et al 1988, Gale & Goldman 1988, Groffen & Heisterkamp 1988, Pendergast & Witte 1988). It is now well established that the reciprocal translocation t(9;22) results in formation of a chimeric BCR-ABL gene which gives rise to the BCR-ABL fusion protein, P210, that presumably plays some role in perturbing stem cell kinetics.

Ph-positive CML is characteristically a biphasic or triphasic disease. Many patients at diagnosis are asymptomatic or have only relatively mild complaints; if the proportion of blast cells in their blood and marrow is relatively low and the clinical response to standard cytotoxic drugs is good, they are classified as having 'chronic' or 'stable' phase disease. After a variable period of time (median 3–4 years) such chronic phase disease may undergo an abrupt alteration usually associated with increasing numbers of blast cells in the blood and marrow. Survival after onset of blastic transformation is usually only a matter of months. However, a substantial proportion of patients with CML have a disease that passes more insidiously from chronic phase to blastic phase. This intermediate phase may be marked by splenomegaly or leucocytosis resistant to cytotoxic drugs, increasing thrombocytosis or by gradually increasing blast numbers that have not yet reached the somewhat arbitrary criteria for transformation. It is referred to as the accelerated phase.

MOLECULAR BIOLOGY

The ABL proto-oncogene

The ABL proto-oncogene is the cellular homologue of the transforming sequence, v-*abl*, that characterizes the Abelson mutant of the Moloney murine leukaemia virus, an acutely transforming retrovirus capable of inducing B-cell lymphomas in selected mouse strains. The ABL gene in man is located on chromosome 9 at band q34 and spans about 215 kbp. There are two alternative exons at the 5' end (designated Ib and Ia) followed by a common set of ten 3' exons which are transcribed as two major species of mRNA, measuring 6 and 7 kbp respectively. The normal function of the ABL gene product is unknown.

In 95% of patients with Ph-positive CML the ABL gene is translocated to the Ph chromosome. Studies designed to localize the breakpoint at genomic level showed that it varied widely in different patients. The breaks were always 5' of ABL exon II (the first common exon) and occurred usually in the long intron between exons Ib and Ia but occasionally in either of the flanking introns (Fig. 7.1). This means

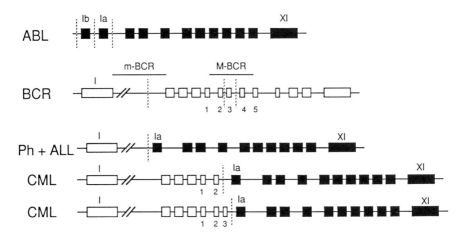

Fig. 7.1 Schematic representation of the BCR and ABL genes. The figure shows known exons indicated as boxes and introns as lines. The arabic numerals below the BCR gene exons identify the exons within the breakpoint cluster region (Groffen et al 1984). Representative positions for breakpoints in CML and Ph-positive ALL are shown as vertical dashed lines. The proposed new nomenclature (M-BCR and m-BCR) for the breakpoints is explained in the text. The two different breakpoints in M-BCR give rise to the two chimeric genes with slightly different linkages characteristic of CML and the breakpoint in m-BCR gives rise to the fused gene that characterizes Ph+, BCR−, ALL. (Reproduced from Gale & Goldman 1988 with permission of the publishers).

that the ten 3' exons of ABL are always translocated to the Ph chromosome, usually but not always in association with exon Ia and occasionally with exon Ib also.

The BCR gene

Whereas the breakpoint in or 5' of the ABL oncogene on chromosome 9 varies considerably between different patients, the breakpoints on chromosome 22 are restricted to a relatively short (5.8 kbp) sequence of genomic DNA at band q11 the breakpoint cluster region (*bcr*) (Groffen et al 1984) or more recently the major breakpoint cluster region (M-BCR) (Gale & Goldman 1988). The M-BCR forms part of the BCR (PHL) gene that spans more than 70 kbp of DNA and consists of about 20 exons encoding 1271 amino acids. As with ABL, the function of the normal BCR gene is unknown. In Ph-positive CML breaks occur at varying positions in the introns between exons 2 and 3 or exons 3 and 4 of the M-BCR. This results in formation of a chimeric gene of which the upstream portion consists of varying numbers of BCR-derived exons and the downstream portion of exons derived from the ABL gene (Fig. 7.1).

Ph-positive CML

The consistency of these genomic changes in Ph-positive CML provides evidence but in no way proof of their importance in the pathogenesis of the chronic phase of the disease. Further confirmatory evidence comes from study of the gene product. Leukaemic cells from patients with Ph-positive CML have a unique mRNA of 8.0 kb size which is the transcription product of the chimeric gene (Gale et al 1984). This in turn is translated as a protein of 210 kDa (P210) which has the ability to phosphorylate other proteins on tyrosine residues (Konopka et al 1984). The normal ABL gene product lacks such tyrosine kinase activity and one may speculate therefore that the juxtaposition of BCR with ABL sequences in the Ph chromosome leads to expression of a fused protein in which the 'dormant' kinase domain has been activated by some mechanism the details of which are not yet established. Presumably this activation results in constitutive ability of the P210 to phosphorylate a target substrate in an excessive or otherwise inappropriate manner.

The precise temporal relationship of the formation of the BCR-ABL chimeric gene to the pathogenesis of chronic phase CML is unclear. It is possible for example that clonal changes precede the acquisition of the Ph chromosome in some cases, a conclusion which if confirmed would suggest that undetermined genomic changes must also precede and predispose to acquisition of the BCR-ABL chimeric gene. Once chronic phase disease is established, there is some preliminary evidence that patients with breakpoints placed downstream in the M-BCR may be more likely to enter early transformation than those with breakpoints placed more upstream (Schaefer-Rego et al 1987). Conversely there is no evidence that patients with unduly prolonged survival have unique forms of the BCR-ABL gene. A number of groups have studied the possibility that further genomic changes might occur in the BCR-ABL gene at the time of (or just preceding) haematological transformation. In general the pattern of abnormal restriction fragments recognized on Southern analysis of DNA collected in chronic phase remains unchanged in transformation and identification of the P210 is if anything facilitated. These observations make it improbable, but by no means exclude the possibility, that further acquired changes within BCR-ABL underlie transformation in the majority of cases. Conversely changes at the DNA level involving other known oncogenes, including RAS, MYC and P53, have been reported in individual patients in transformation. Such findings are consistent with the notion that the acquisition of the BCR-ABL chimeric gene underlies chronic phase CML but that other acquired oncogene changes, which may be very variable between patients, are essential for expression of the fully transformed phenotype.

Ph-negative CML

About 5% of patients with a form of leukaemia that resembles more or less closely Ph-positive CML have a normal karyotype in their leukaemic cells, so called Ph-negative CML. The precise classification of these patients is still controversial and some investigators believe that they are designated more correctly as examples of the myelodysplastic syndrome. It seems clear nonetheless that a proportion of patients with Ph-negative CML have a disease that is totally indistinguishable on clinical and haematological criteria from Ph-positive CML (other than by cytogenetics). A high proportion of these Ph-negative patients have the same molecular changes as patients with Ph-positive CML—namely translocation of ABL to a morphologically normal chromosome 22, formation of a chimeric BCR-ABL and expression of the 8.0 kb mRNA and P210$^{BCR-ABL}$ (Morris et al 1986, Ganesan et al 1986, Dreazen et al 1987). There are three important points that stem from these observations: first, the finding of a chimeric BCR-ABL gene in some patients with Ph-negative CML suggests that this lesion, rather than the Ph translocation per se, is central to the pathogenesis of the chronic phase; secondly, it begs the important question of what sort of mechanism could cause the translocation of a relatively short sequence of genomic DNA and its accurately placed 'interstitial insertion' into chromosome 22; and thirdly, the fact that not all patients with Ph-negative CML have a chimeric BCR-ABL gene in their leukaemic cells focuses attention on the fact that there must be other ways of generating a similar (or identical) haematological phenotype.

Ph-positive acute leukaemia

It has been known for some years that an abnormal chromosome 22 indistinguishable by conventional methods from the Ph chromosome of CML could be identified in about 2% of children with acute lymphoblastic leukaemia (ALL), in 17–25% of adults with ALL and in 1–2% of patients with acute myeloid leukaemia (AML) (Catovsky 1979). Recent studies of patients with Ph-positive ALL have revealed that ABL is translocated to the Ph chromosome, as in Ph-positive CML, in all cases. About half these patients have breakpoints in the M-BCR (BCR+); these patients express an 8.0 kb mRNA and the P210$^{BCR-ABL}$ (Fig. 7.1). The other half of the patients show no evidence of DNA rearrangement in the M-BCR (BCR−). They have however a breakpoint in the first (large) intron of the BCR gene (the so-called minor breakpoint cluster region, m-BCR) with formation of a BCR-ABL chimeric gene analogous to but substantially smaller than the BCR-ABL gene of Ph-positive CML (Hermans et al 1987). The fusion protein characteristic of Ph+, BCR− ALL is 190 (or 185) kDa (P190) (Kurzrock et al 1987a, Chan et al 1987, Clark et al 1987). Thus patients with Ph-positive ALL all have an activated ABL oncogene but activation can occur by one of two distinct methods, both of which involve the BCR gene. There is no evidence that these differing genomic events correlate with clinical or prognostic differences in individual patients.

Patients with Ph-positive AML are extremely rare and have been studied less comprehensively than those with Ph-positive ALL. It appears however that the same molecular heterogeneity may be present—there are be examples of Ph-positive AML with breakpoints in the m-BCR and P190 expression (Kurzrock et al 1987b) as well as cases of true AML (as distinct from CML in myeloid transformation) with breakpoints in the M-BCR and P210 expression. Study of the molecular lesions in Ph-positive acute leukaemia again underscores the point that either variant of the BCR-ABL chimeric gene can activate the ABL protein and thereby establish the 'transformed' phenotype but other unknown genomic events must determine the target cell for this malignant transformation.

COMPLETE REMISSION IN Ph-POSITIVE CML

Normal haemopoiesis in man is believed to depend on the presence in the marrow of a population of haemopoietic stem cells which are termed pluripotential because they can apparently differentiate along either myeloid or lymphoid lineages. Several lines of evidence suggest that CML is the disease par excellence of the pluripotential stem cell (reviewed by Greaves 1982 and Goldman & Lu 1982). For example the Ph chromosome is found mainly in the progeny of myeloid progenitor cells in the marrow but also in cells of B and occasionally T lineage. The findings that CML in transformation can manifest predominantly myeloid or lymphoid features, and that the lymphoid features, though usually showing a pre-B phenotype, may on occasion be characteristic of the T lineage, are consistent with the notion that the target cell for transformation was itself pluripotential or was descended from a leukaemic cell with such potential. Moreover study of the distribution of isoenzyme types in females with CML who are heterozygous for glucose-6-phosphate dehydrogenase as well as study of the distribution of apparently clonal chromosomal abnormalities in patients who are somatic mosaics provide evidence that the disease was of clonal origin, at least in the cases studied, and therefore was presumably derived from a single pluripotential stem cell.

The molecular mechanism by which the normal kinetics of the pluripotential stem cell may be perturbed by formation of the $P210^{BCR-ABL}$ fusion protein has been discussed above. However, it must be mentioned parenthetically that there are other views concerning the basic defect in CML. The Sloan Kettering group have proposed that the fundamental kinetic disturbance is discordant maturation rather than unregulated proliferation at the stem cell level (Strife & Clarkson 1988). According to this concept the earliest committed CML progenitors have a *reduced* proliferative capacity and the more mature progenitors as a consequence undergo increased numbers of divisions which results in expansion of the total leukaemic cell population.

The above theory notwithstanding, the simplest interpretation of the sequence of events underlying the clinical manifestations of CML is to assume that the acquisition in a haemopoietic stem cell of the BCR-ABL fusion protein leads to steady expansion of the Ph-positive stem cell compartment associated with increased proliferation in the committed granulocytic series and to a lesser extent in the other myeloid lineages. This presumably results in suppression of the Ph-negative (putatively normal) haemopoietic stem cells but there is no evidence that they are in fact destroyed. It is indeed impossible in most cases to demonstrate cytogenetically normal myeloid cells in newly diagnosed patients using standard techniques but this is readily explained on two bases: such residual normal stem cells may be in 'profound' Go and therefore difficult to induce to divide in short term culture; equally relevant is the enormous extent to which such normal stem cells will be outnumbered by the leukaemic stem cells and their proliferating progeny. If this view of the biology of CML is correct, it means that complete remission should be obtainable at least in principle in every patient, as it seems to be in acute leukaemia, and that failure to do so reflects our inability to recognize and exploit critical differences between normal and leukaemic stem cells. The developing knowledge of the molecular changes in CML, referred to above, suggests that methods for selectively suppressing leukaemic cell proliferation may be available in the not too distant future.

MANAGEMENT OF CHRONIC PHASE

Although the prognosis for individual newly diagnosed patients has not changed substantially in comparison with 10 years ago, the number of therapeutic options has increased pari passu in some cases with the sophistication of the patient. Increasingly patients will expect from their physicians a frank explanation of prognosis and of the reasons for choosing a particular therapeutic strategy. Such decisions must therefore be based on a careful consideration of the clinical features in any given case. The main areas of uncertainty are easily defined: when to start treatment; which cytotoxic drugs to use; whether to use α-interferon, whether and when to undertake bone marrow transplantation; and how to advise the younger patient in relation to fertility and pregnancy. Some of these questions are considered below.

General strategy for managing chronic phase disease

Ten or 20 years ago it was possible to start treatment for newly diagnosed patient with CML with busulphan without too much deliberation. Indeed it was still possible at that time to conceal from the patient details of diagnosis and prognosis on the grounds that the clinical course was inexorable and nothing was to be gained by worrying the patient. Such is no longer the case. The first priority for the physician after CML is diagnosed is to explain to the patient the diagnosis in as much detail as seems necessary. Some general view of prognosis may be included in this discussion. This is particularly important if treatment by bone marrow transplantation is an option.

Once a decision has been taken to treat the patient, the choice lies between busulphan, hydroxyurea and α-interferon. To some extent the choice between busulphan and hydroxyurea can be dictated by the patient. For those who like the idea of intermittent therapy and are untroubled by the certainty of infertility, busulphan has much to recommend it; conversely for younger patients concerned about loss of fertility or for those who have no objection to taking drugs on a daily basis, hydroxyurea is more suitable. If α-interferon is under study in a particular centre, then an individual patient may be encouraged to enter the study and may welcome the fact that he or she is being treated with an experimental drug. Some patients may ask for treatment with α-interferon without being entered into a controlled study. It is reasonable to accede to this request but the patient should understand clearly that the ability to restore partial or even complete Ph-negative haemopoiesis does not guarantee that life will thereby be prolonged.

If the patient is relatively young (less than 45 years), then treatment by bone marrow transplantation should be considered whether or not the patient has an HLA-identical sibling (see below). If a suitable donor is identified, one can say with certainty that transplant should be carried out at some time before the onset of acceleration or transformation, but the optimal timing within the chronic phase is extremely difficult to define. One possible compromise, suitable especially for patients who fall within a relatively good prognostic category (Sokal et al 1985), would be to administer α-interferon for 12–18 months but then to proceed directly to transplant if no cytogenetic improvement is obtained; if however Ph-negative haemopoiesis is restored, transplant could reasonably be further delayed.

When to start treatment
Although opinions are divided as to whether to initiate treatment automatically soon after diagnosis and having done so whether it is useful to maintain the leucocyte count in or near the normal range, no clinical study has been designed to address these questions and it remains uncertain whether or not 'aggressive' or 'meticulous' control of chronic phase disease should be attempted. Conversely there is no doubt that treatment should be initiated promptly for patients with symptoms or in whom the early onset of symptoms can be anticipated.

Role of leucapheresis
The peripheral blood of patients with untreated CML contains very large numbers of committed myeloid progenitor cells and by implication stem cells also. This assumption has been amply proved by the demonstration that cryopreserved autologous buffy coat cells can restore haemopoiesis in patients subjected to 'supralethal' whole body irradiation (Haines et al 1984). Thus in ideal circumstances it is possible to argue that all newly diagnosed patients should have buffy coat cells collected and stored before initiation of chemotherapy. Such stored cells could serve a number of purposes:

1. They could be used to restore haemopoiesis in the rare patient who develops marrow aplasia after treatment with busulphan;
2. They could be used to restore haemopoiesis in the event of graft failure following allogeneic marrow transplantation; or
3. They could be used for autografting after high dose chemotherapy administered in chronic phase (Marcus & Goldman 1986) or in transformation.

Since each of these indications involves an unusual clinical situation, the case for routinely cryopreserving peripheral blood stem cells is weak if facilities are not readily available or if this would mean substantial delay in initiation of needed treatment.

Cytotoxic drugs
There have been no major recent advances in the use of cytotoxic drugs in the management of chronic phase disease. Studies were carried out in the late 1970s to assess the possible merits of giving busulphan at high dosage (50, 100 or 150 mg) in a single dose at 4–12 week intervals based on the level of the leucocytosis (Douglas et al 1978, Vicariot et al 1979). This method is convenient for the patient but seems to offer no advantage over more conventional low dose administration.

A multi-centre study organized by the Medical Research Council in the UK compared the use of busulphan in standard dosage with that of busulphan together with 6-thioguanine. The final analysis of this study has not yet been published but preliminary results showed clearly that whereas control of the leucocyte count was achieved more rapidly with the two drug combination than with busulphan alone, the risk of hepatic toxicity was increased by treatment with 6-thioguanine and no other important advantage for the combination was identified.

In 1982 the Denver group reported a non-randomized study comparing busulphan with hydroxyurea as principal cytotoxic agents for CML in chronic phase (Bolin et al 1982). In this relatively small study hydroxyurea was associated with superior median survival (35 vs. 69 months). The study requires confirmation in larger prospectively randomized comparisons of the two agents. In the meantime it is notable that hydroxyurea seems to be replacing busulphan as drug of choice for newly diagnosed patients in many countries.

Interferons

Since 1982 a number of interferon (IFN) molecules, both natural and recombinant, have been used to treat patients with CML (Table 7.1). Their precise mechanism

Table 7.1   The various types and sources of interferons

Natural interferons	
Leukocyte interferon	IFN-α(Le)
Lymphoblastoid interferon	IFN-alpha-N1 (Burroughs Wellcome Co.)
Fibroblast interferon	IFN-β
Immune interferon	IFN-γ
Recombinant interferons	
alpha-2	IFN-alpha-2b (Schering Corporation)
alpha-A	IFN-alpha-2a (Roche Laboratories)
alpha-2arg	IFN-alpha-2c (Boehringer Ingelheim Ltd.)
alpha-1	rIFN-α1
alpha-D	rIFN-αD
beta	rIFN-β
gamma	rIFN-γ

of action is unknown but they probably bind to specific surface receptors which are then internalized and thereafter directly or indirectly influence the probability of cell division and differentiation. Alpha and beta IFNs appear to use the same surface receptor and probably act by inhibiting proliferation of leukaemic progenitor cells. Cells sensitive to IFN show a marked increase in 2′,5′ oligoadenylate synthetase after binding of IFN to the surface receptor. IFNs may also regulate the expression of some oncogenes. For example expression of MYC in Daudi cells and of HRAS in mouse NIH-3T3 cells are both reduced by exposure to IFN. It would be tempting to speculate that IFNs act in CML by selectively suppressing proliferation of cells expressing the BCR-ABL chimeric gene, but there is at present no evidence that the growth of CML cells is inhibited to a greater extent than that of their normal counterparts.

In 1983 Talpaz and colleagues reported the results of treating 7 patients with CML in chronic phase with natural α-IFN. Five of the patients achieved complete haematological remission with some reduction in the proportion of Ph-positive marrow metaphases in each case. Results of treating a further series of patients with recombinant human α IFN-2a were reported more recently by the same group (Talpaz et al 1986).

Seventeen patients were treated with IFN at a dose of 5 mega units/m² daily. Twelve patients achieved complete haematological remission, 3 showed partial restoration of Ph-negativity and 4 showed complete though transient restoration of 100% Ph-negativity. Similar good haematological responses were reported recently by the Italian and German Cooperative Groups but the proportion of patients who achieved a reduction in the proportion of Ph-positive marrow metaphases was lower and no patient achieved 100% Ph-negativity (Niederle et al 1987, Morra et al 1987). Recent evidence suggests that patients who enter transformation during or after treatment with α-IFN are more likely to have lymphoid blast crises than patients treated by other means. Whether this is due to the ability of α-IFN to precipitate lymphoid transformation or to reduce the probability of myeloid transformation is unclear. Indeed the trend 'favouring' lymphoid transformations is not statistically significant.

The toxicity of treatment with α-IFN is not inconsiderable. The dosage required for control of CML is higher than that required for treatment of hairy cell leukaemia and most patients experience flu-like symptoms for the first few weeks of treatment. Somnolence and undue suppression of platelet counts may occur. Administration is inconvenient in comparison with other cytotoxic drugs because IFN must be given by subcutaneous injection. All these problems would be acceptable if the use of IFN to control the leucocyte count and when possible to restore Ph-negative haemopoiesis were associated with prolongation of survival.

Autografting in chronic phase
Pilot studies have been performed at the Hammersmith Hospital in London in which patients still in the chronic phase were treated with high dose chemotherapy followed by transfusion of reconstituted buffy coat cells that had been collected and cryo-preserved at diagnosis (Marcus & Goldman 1986). The objective of this study was to reduce the size of the leukaemic stem cell pool and possibly to induce Ph-negativity by a mechanism still poorly understood. Preliminary results of autografting in chronic phase for 11 patients showed that the procedure is relatively safe. Ten patients were restored to chronic phase haemopoiesis and 5 required no further treatment for a median period of 10 months post-autografting. One of these patients was restored to durable Ph-negative haemopoiesis after autografting with Ph-positive stem cells (Brito-Babapulle et al 1987). Another patient however failed to sustain haemopoiesis after autografting and now requires long term platelet support. In general the results of this somewhat speculative clinical study cannot yet be fully evaluated.

An equally promising approach to induction of Ph-negativity for patients with Ph-positive CML involves attempts to purge marrow cells in vitro before autografting. There is evidence that in vitro purging can be achieved by use of the alkylating agent 4-hydroperoxycyclophosphamide (Degliantoni et al 1985) but an alternative approach might exploit the fact that Ph-negative cells appear to have a proliferative advantage over leukaemic progenitors in various liquid and Dexter-type culture systems (Coulombel et al 1983).

Pregnancy
For the haematologist specializing in management of patients with leukaemia it is not uncommon to encounter a patient in the first trimester of pregnancy in whom CML has been established as a result of the blood test performed at her first

antenatal visit. Such patients were formerly advised that termination of pregnancy was advisable but this approach is probably not necessary and may be harmful. The use of cytotoxic drugs should be avoided if the pregnancy is allowed to continue. A proportion of patients will require no treatment even though the leucocyte count is in the range of 100–200 × $10^9/l$. Other patients may be managed by blood transfusion alone. For the patient requiring treatment leucapheresis carried out weekly or 2-weekly is very effective. The leucocyte count typically falls by as much as 50% following a 2-hour procedure but rises thereafter. Leucapheresis appears however to be effective in the longer term, presumably as a result of the selective removal of immature myeloid cells. Radiotherapy to the spleen with suitable shielding of the gravid uterus has been recommended but is inherently less safe for the fetus. In the last trimester of pregnancy the use of hydroxyurea is probably safe for the fetus and treatment with cytotoxic drugs to reduce excessive thrombocytosis is desirable.

A related problem is the question of pregnancy for the younger female who has not yet conceived or indeed is not yet married. In both cases it may be wise to avoid administration of busulphan. In the former case a married woman need not automatically be discouraged from pregnancy if she and her husband both desire it. The techniques of oocyte or embryo cryopreservation may develop sufficiently within the next decade to offer practical benefit for patients requiring treatment with conventional agents or by bone marrow transplantation.

MANAGEMENT OF ACCELERATED PHASE AND BLASTIC TRANSFORMATION

The management of patients whose disease has progressed beyond chronic phase remains unsatisfactory and therefore controversial. For patients with features of accelerated disease considerable benefit may still be obtained by switching cytotoxic drugs, for example from busulphan to hydroxyurea, or by splenectomy. For the patient in overt blastic transformation, full characterization of the predominating blast cell population may provide valuable information on which to base therapy.

Survival in transformation

Kantarjian and colleagues at the MD Anderson Hospital in Houston have recently reported results of analysing survival in 242 patients with CML in blastic transformation treated during the period 1970 to 1986 (Kantarjian et al 1987). The blast cell population could be characterized in 153 patients, of whom 96 (63%) had myeloid transformations, 31 (20%) lymphoid transformations and 26 (17%) were undifferentiated. Of 192 evaluable patients, 114 (60%) had cytogenetic evidence of clonal evolution, usually a double Ph, isochromosome 17 and/or trisomy 8. The patients were treated with a variety of different cytotoxic drug regimens, as would be expected in view of the timespan of the study. The overall median survival was 18 weeks, a value not greatly different from the 12 weeks reported in a similar study from a multi-centre cooperative group (Coleman et al 1980). In the Houston study complete haematological remission was achieved in 44 (23%) of the 195 patients who were evaluable. The major determinants associated with short survival were anaemia, thrombocytopenia, myeloid or undifferentiated blast morphology and cytogenetic evolution.

Chemotherapy

On the basis of their study Kantarjian et al (1987) were unable to make firm recommendations for the management of CML in transformation. For patients in myeloid transformation the combination of mithramycin and hydroxyurea has proved valuable on occasion. Koller & Miller (1986) treated 9 patients (6 myeloid, 2 lymphoblastic and 1 undifferentiated) with mithramycin (plicamycin) at a dose of 25 μg/kg on alternate days for 3 weeks combined with daily hydroxyurea at doses up to 4 g. All 6 patients with myeloid transformation were restored to chronic phase disease without any intervening period of pancytopenia. The authors reported that mithramycin caused the circulating leukaemic blast cells from the patients who responded to differentiate into granulocytes in vitro. They noted also that mithramycin causes HL60 cells to differentiate in vitro. They suggested therefore that the two drug combination acted by inducing blast cell differentiation in vivo, although other mechanisms cannot be excluded. These encouraging preliminary results justify further study of this two drug combination, but the same high response rate in myeloid transformation has not yet been confirmed by other centres.

For patients in lymphoid transformation it seems logical to initiate treatment with the same chemotherapy protocol as is locally in use for the treatment of adult acute lymphoblastic leukaemia. If haematological remission is achieved, 'maintenance' chemotherapy can then be continued in accordance with the protocol. Prophylaxis of CNS disease should be undertaken with intrathecal methotrexate but cranial irradiation is not definitely justified.

Autografting

A number of studies were performed in the late 1970s and early 1980s in which patients in transformation were treated with high dose chemotherapy or chemoradiotherapy followed by infusion of previously cryopreserved blood- or marrow-derived stem cells. Though haematological reconstitution was usually rapid and patients were in most cases restored to 'second' chronic phase, the duration of such second chronic phase was characteristically short (median 12 weeks) and overall survival for most patients was only marginally prolonged, if at all (Haines et al 1984). There was however a small proportion of patients in whom the longer duration of second chronic phase seemed to justify a second autograft procedure (and on rare occasions a third procedure); these patients undoubtedly had some prolongation of life in comparison with more conventional methods of treatment. In summary autografting in transformation cannot be recommended as routine treatment of CML in transformation.

BONE MARROW TRANSPLANTATION

Cytoreductive regimens

The administration of chemoradiotherapy before transplantation for the patient receiving (allogeneic) marrow from an HLA-identical sibling has two objectives—to eradicate leukaemia and to induce a degree of immune suppression that will permit the donor marrow stem cells to engraft. Recent evidence suggests that CML may still be cured even when occasional leukaemic cells can be identified after transplant. Moreover the presence of T lymphocytes in the donor marrow inoculum may be important both to facilitate engraftment and to effect cure of the leukaemia (see below).

The initial attempts to treat patients with CML by allogeneic marrow transplantation were directed mainly at patients whose disease had already progressed beyond chronic phase (Doney et al 1978, 1981). The standard conditioning involved the use of cyclophosphamide (usually 60 mg/kg × 2 doses) followed by total body irradiation (TBI), usually 10 Gy. The results were for the most part unsatisfactory. When attention was turned to transplantation for patients still in the chronic phase, similar protocols were adopted (Curtis & Messner 1982, Clift et al 1982, Goldman et al 1982, Champlin et al 1982, Speck et al 1982). Thus for example the Seattle group has in general made use of cyclophosphamide and TBI, either single dose or fractionated (Clift et al 1982, Thomas et al 1986), and we at the Hammersmith Hospital in London have used cyclophosphamide followed by fractionated TBI (2 Gy fractions twice daily for 5 or 6 doses) (Goldman et al 1982, 1986). At the Sloan Kettering Cancer Center in New York the standard protocol comprises cyclophosphamide with hyperfractionated TBI—the radiotherapy is given as 120 cGy 3 times daily to a total dose of 1320 or 1440 cGy (Cunningham et al 1987). A variety of different radiotherapy schedules is in use.

There is indeed no clear evidence that radiotherapy forms an essential component of conditioning for patients undergoing allogeneic BMT for CML. The Baltimore group has accumulated extensive experience with the use of busulphan (usually 4 mg/kg daily × 4 days) followed by cyclophosphamide (usually 60 mg/kg daily for 4 days) (Santos et al 1985, Tutschka et al 1987). Although this combination may be unduly toxic for patients who have already received substantial doses of busulphan before transplantation, it is certainly an effective schedule for conditioning for patients with acute leukaemia and success with its use in CML casts doubt on the necessity for including TBI in the conditioning schedule.

Timing of transplantation for patients with HLA-identical siblings

It is now well established that the results of allogeneic BMT are optimal if the transplant is performed in the chronic phase (Table 7.2). In the 1970s a number of attempts

Table 7.2 Actuarial results of allogeneic BMT using HLA-identical sibling donors according to phase of CML at the time of transplant. Results are based in part of data analysed by the International Bone Marrow Transplant Registry (Speck et al 1984, Goldman et al 1988). Values are means ± 95% confidence intervals.

	Actuarial probability (%) at 4 years		
Phase of CML	Survival	Relapse	Leukaemia-free survival
Chronic phase	55 ± 10	12 ± 10	45 ± 10
Accelerated phase	25 ± 15	50 ± 20	20 ± 15
Blastic transformation	12 ± 15	60 ± 20	12 ± 15

were made, mainly in Seattle, to treat by BMT patients already in blastic transformation (Doney et al 1978, 1981). The majority of patients died of transplant-related complications, mainly graft-versus-host disease (GVHD), pneumonitis or infections, and most who survived suffered relapse of their leukaemia. A small number of these patients did however become long-term survivors. A recent analysis of results from Seattle showed that the probability of leukaemia-free survival 4 years after BMT in transformation was 15% (Thomas et al 1986); the equivalent figure based on data reported to the International Bone Marrow Transplant Registry (IBMTR) is 12%

(Speck et al 1984). This means in practice that a transplant undertaken for a patient in transformation is highly likely to fail but is not entirely hopeless and is thus very logical from the patient's point of view.

It appeared at one stage that results of allografting for patients in acceleration would be substantially better than those achieved for patients in transformation (McGlave et al 1982). More recent results suggest however that if followed for longer periods the majority of patients transplanted in transformation will relapse (Speck et al 1984, Thomas et al 1986). The most recent analysis reported by the IBMTR showed a probability of relapse at 4 years of 55% and of survival of 32%.

The results of BMT using HLA-identical sibling donors for patients with CML in chronic phase who were in general under the age of 50 have now been reported from a large number of individual centres. Two relatively large series of patients have been reported from Seattle (Thomas et al 1986) and the Hammersmith Hospital (Goldman et al 1986); the largest number of patients has been analysed from data reported to the IBMTR (Speck et al 1984, Goldman et al 1985). The most recent report from the IBMTR (Goldman et al 1988) shows that the probability of survival and of relapse are 55% and 19% respectively at 4 years post-transplant. It should be noted however that this analysis includes recent patients who received T cell depleted donor marrow cells. If these patients are excluded from the analysis, the probability of relapse is 9% and the probability of leukaemia-free survival 47%. These results agree relatively well with those reported from Seattle (Thomas et al 1986), where the actuarial probabilities of survival and of relapse were 49% and 20% respectively. Relapse for the purpose of these analyses includes haematological and clinical relapses but excludes relapses that are 'cytogenetic only' (see below).

Once it is agreed that the results of transplant are optimal if the procedure is carried out during the chronic phase, the question arises as to when within the chronic phase the procedure should be undertaken. Data from Seattle show that there exists a significant inverse relationship between the duration of disease before transplant and the probability of surviving the procedure (Thomas et al 1986). If confirmed, this would provide some support for the view that transplant for eligible patients should be performed as soon as possible after diagnosis. However, an analysis performed on 405 patients in chronic phase by the IBMTR failed to establish a relationship between disease duration and survival post-transplant (Goldman et al 1988).

Sokal and his colleagues have performed retrospective analyses on relatively large numbers of patients in the age group that might be eligible for transplantation (less than 45 years) and established a small number of factors definable at diagnosis that appear to be related to survival in multivariate analysis (Sokal et al 1985). These factors are patient sex, spleen size, haematocrit, platelet count and % of circulating blast cells. Using these factors an equation was constructed whereby patients were divided into three prognostic categories with median survivals ranging from $2\frac{1}{2}$–$5\frac{1}{2}$ years (Fig. 7.2). Using information of this type, one can then estimate the probability of survival at 1, 2 or 3 years for an individual patient. For example a man with a large spleen and a high platelet count at diagnosis might be expected to survive for a shorter period than a woman with an impalpable spleen and a platelet count below $600 \times 10^9/l$. At the Hammersmith Hospital we have been impressed by the prognostic value of another feature—the amount of chemotherapy required to control chronic phase disease within the first year of diagnosis (Wareham et al 1982).

Whatever prognostic features one uses, clearly that prognosis for individual patients does differ and such differences can if desired be taken into account when formulating a treatment policy. This approach has been taken further by Segel et al (1986). They constructed a mathematical model that exploited the prognostic categories defined by Sokal and took into account calculated risks of marrow transplantation at different ages in an attempt to balance the risks in an individual patient of transformation on the one hand against transplant-related mortality on the other. Such an approach is of considerable theoretical interest but the conclusions reached are frequently over-ridden in the clinic by rather more practical considerations, in particular the preferences on the patient.

Use of T-cell depletion to prevent GVHD

Interest has focused for some years on the possibility that the incidence and severity of GVHD might be reduced if T cells could be removed from or inactivated in the donor marrow before transfusion to the patient. Various techniques have been explored for this purpose. The most commonly used and also the most convenient method is to incubate donor marrow with anti-T lymphocyte monoclonal antibodies (McAbs) which fix human or rabbit complement and lyse T cells in vitro or by a combination of actions in vitro and in vivo. The Royal Free Hospital group in London has used McAbs with CD3 and CD8 activities (Prentice et al 1984). The CT-2 McAb used by the UCLA transplant group has CD2 activity (Mitsuyasu et al 1986). Much experience worldwide has been gained with the use of Campath-1, a McAb active against incompletely defined antigens on T and B cells and on some monocytes which fixes human complement avidly in vitro (Waldmann et al 1984, Apperley et al 1986a, b, 1988, Heit et al 1986, Papa et al 1986, Hale et al 1988). Other techniques for elimination of T cells include soybean lectin agglutination in conjunction with E-rosette formation and counterflow elutriation (Cunningham et al 1987, de Witte et al 1986). In general, study of the proportion of T cell remaining after marrow is treated by one or other of these techniques shows a T cell reduction in excess of 99%.

It became clear from early studies using T depleted donor marrow that the incidence and severity of GVHD were reduced. It became clear also that the risk of graft failure— either primary graft failure with little or no evidence of engraftment at any stage or of late graft failure with a preceding period of normal or near normal engraftment— was increased. The major problem associated with the use of T depleted marrow cells for patients with CML is however the substantial increase in risk of relapse (Goldman et al 1988; Apperley et al, 1988) (Fig. 7.3). This effect seems to be independent of the method employed for T cell depletion. It applies both to patients allografted in chronic phase and to patients allografted in later phases of their disease. In a recent report from Seattle 100% of patients transplanted in accelerated phase with T depleted donor marrow who survived long enough had in fact relapsed (Clift et al 1987); this contrasts with an actuarial risk of relapse (Table 7.2) of 55% for patients in acceleration transplanted with unmanipulated donor marrow (Speck et al 1984). The increased risk of relapse associated with T depleted donor marrow is seen also in patients allografted for acute leukaemia; the magnitude of the difference between recipients of T depleted marrow and historical controls is however less impressive.

The possible mechanisms by which T cells may protect against relapse and therefore

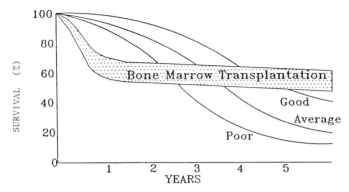

Fig. 7.2 Probability of survival for patients under the age of 45 years allografted in chronic phase with marrow from HLA-identical sibling donors. The transplant survival curve has been superimposed on survival curves for patients in the three prognostic categories defined by Sokal et al (1985) on the assumption that they received conventional therapy. (Reproduced from Champlin et al 1988 with permission of the authors and publishers.)

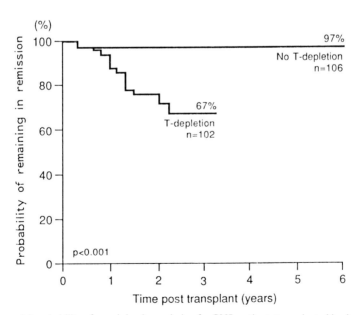

Fig. 7.3 Actuarial probability of remaining in remission for CML patients transplanted in chronic phase with marrow from HLA-identical sibling donors according to whether or not donor marrow was depleted in vitro of T cells. The data were collected from 8 transplant centres in Europe and North America. Patients who died without evidence of relapse were censored from the analysis at the date of death. (Reproduced from Apperley et al 1988 with permission of the authors and publishers.)

presumably contribute to cure have been mentioned above but they remain essentially unknown. A specific immunological mechanism might be involved but one might speculate that this is rendered less probable by the substantial disparity in relapse rate between recipients of T depleted and recipients of syngeneic marrow.

The problem of graft failure seems to be related to survival in the host of radio-resistant immunologically competent cells which, in the absence of T cells of donor origin, are capable of mediating graft rejection (Butturini et al 1986). Preliminary evidence suggests that the problem of graft rejection can be reduced or eliminated merely by increasing the immune suppression pre-transplant (Patterson et al 1986). The problem of relapse is more intractable (Table 7.3). It is possible that this could

Table 7.3   Possible approaches to reducing relapse for recipients of T-depleted donor marrow cells. *Key:* LAK, lymphokine activated killer cells; IFN, interferon; IL-3, interleukin-3.

1. Intensify conditioning
2. Partial T cell depletion, e.g. 90%
3. Selective T cell depletion, e.g. CD8
4. Fresh donor T cells post-BMT
5. Irradiated donor T cells post BMT
6. Donor LAK cells post BMT
7. Alpha-IFN post BMT
8. GM-CSF or IL-3 post BMT
9. Other lymphokines post BMT
10. Other methods

be overcome by increasing the intensity of anti-leukaemic treatment pre-transplant or by adding back T lymphocytes or their biological products post-transplant. The concept of giving additional anti-leukaemic therapy to the patient post-transplant is intrinsically unattractive. Perhaps the best hope for the future is the possibility (by no means a certainty) of distinguishing the T cell subpopulations that mediate GVHD from those that mediate a graft-versus-leukaemia effect. It would then be possible to address the problem of selective elimination of the former.

Graft-versus-leukaemia (GVL) effect

There is experimental evidence from animal model systems that graft-versus-host disease (GVHD) may exert an anti-tumour or anti-leukaemic effect (Truitt et al 1986). In the clinical setting there is evidence that patients with acute leukaemia who undergo allogeneic BMT and sustain acute or acute and chronic GVHD may have a lower probability of relapse than comparable patients without GVHD (Weiden et al 1979, 1981, Butturini et al 1987). It is assumed that T lymphocytes in the donor marrow are capable of mediating GVHD on the one hand and a GVL effect on the other (Gale & Reisner 1986). Whether the same sub-population of T cells mediate these two diverse effects is not known. A similar trend is seen in patients allografted with HLA-identical donor marrow for CML in chronic phase but the overall relapse rate is low and the 'benefit' of GVHD is not statistically significant. These clinical data do however cast doubt on the notion that the only component of the transplant procedure critical for cure is the chemoradiotherapy and that the graft functions only as haemopoietic 'rescue'.

The concept that a GVL effect plays an important role in the cure of leukaemia after allografting for CML in chronic phase gains further support from the results of T cell depleted transplants (discussed in more detail above). Thus results of a series of studies have now been reported in which patients in chronic phase were transplanted with donor marrow cells that had been depleted in vitro of T lymphocytes by different methods. In every study the probability of relapse in patients receiving T depleted marrow cells was higher, usually very significantly so, than in comparable patients who received unmanipulated marrow cells.

Using published clinical data it is possible to some extent to separate the anti-leukaemic effects of GVL and of GVHD, both putatively mediated by T lymphocytes of donor origin (Butturini & Gale 1987). Thus for the sake of argument if one estimates that the actuarial probability of relapse at 4 years for patients in chronic phase allografted with unmanipulated marrow is 10%, for patients allografted with syngeneic marrow is 25% and for patients allografted with T depleted marrow is 50%, the contribution towards cure of the T cell component of the graft must be 40%, of which the non-syngeneic component must be 15% (Table 7.2). This can be broken down further if one accepts that there is as difference in probability of relapse in recipients of unmanipulated marrow cells according to whether the patient does or does not sustain GVHD, e.g. 5 versus 15%. In this case the difference between the relapse rates in these two patient categories (10%) may be computed as the anti-leukaemic contribution of GVHD and the difference between relapse rates for syngeneic transplants and that for non-GVHD allogeneic transplants (25–15 = 10%) may be computed as the anti-leukaemic contribution of the GVL effect.

The mechanisms by which T lymphocytes exert a GVL effect remain highly speculative (Butturini & Gale 1987). If significant antigen disparities between donor and recipient exist outside the major histocompatibility complex, as are thought to underlie the pathogenesis of GVHD, they could be the basis also for an attack by donor T lymphocytes against host leukaemia cells. Alternatively the effects of T lymphocytes could be less specific. They are capable of producing a variety of lymphokines, including haemopoietic growth factors, interferons, transforming growth factors and tumour necrosis factors. Any of these could be active in eradicating residual leukaemic cells already damaged by chemoradiotherapy. Another possible mechanism by which T cells could influence survival of leukaemia cells relates to the tempo and extent of engraftment of normal donor stem cells. If for example the number of sites in the bone marrow where stem cells could replicate was limited and if there were competition between normal donor and host leukaemic stem cells for these sites, then the removal of any factor that favoured proliferation of normal cells (such as might be produced by normal T cells) would give a proliferative advantage to the residual leukaemia (Hale et al 1988, Butturini & Gale 1987).

Age at transplant

It is a general observation that the degree of morbidity and mortality following BMT for leukaemia is related to the age of the patient and CML in this regard is no exception. Data reported by the IBMTR and from Seattle show clearly that mortality post-transplant is lower in patients under the age of 20 than in older patients (Thomas et al 1986, Goldman et al 1988). There is some uncertainty however as to the extent to which this age-related risk is truly a continuum. In some reports patients in the age ranges 20–30, 30–40 and 40–50 fare equally well post-transplant.

Use of alternative donors
Initial transplants in CML in transformation were carried out with identical twin donors. The majority of patients relapsed post-transplant but occasional patients became long-term survivors and were apparently cured. This led to studies of the value of syngeneic BMT carried out for patients still in the chronic phase (Fefer et al 1979, 1982, Goldman et al 1981, Jones et al 1987). In the absence of GVHD the morbidity and mortality associated with the procedure is low but occasional patients died of idiopathic or CMV-associated pneumonitis post-transplant. The probability of relapse after syngeneic BMT seems rather variable. Based on experience obtained in Seattle (Fefer et al 1979, 1982, Thomas et al 1986) and the Hammersmith Hospital (Jones et al 1987) the risk of relapse is no different from that following HLA-identical sibling transplants for comparable patients. Others however have found that the risk is higher (Table 7.2) (International Bone Marrow Transplant Registry 1987). It may or may not be relevant that patients in Seattle and at the Hammersmith Hospital have in general received high dose busulphan in addition to cyclophosphamide and total body irradiation as conditioning pre-transplant.

The great majority of transplants for CML have been carried out with unmanipulated marrow from HLA-identical sibling donors. In this situation engraftment occurs in >95% of cases. The incidence of GVHD for patients allografted in chronic phase ranges from 40–80% and GVHD alone or associated with interstitial pneumonitis is the major cause of death. Only a relatively small number of transplants have been performed for leukaemia including CML using with partially mismatched family donors (Beatty et al 1985, Hows et al 1986). It seems in general that results obtained with one-antigen mismatched donors may be very similar to those obtained with totally HLA-identical sibling donors; conversely disparity at more than one HLA antigen is associated with an increased risk of severe GVHD and an increased risk of graft failure.

A small number of transplants have been performed in which the donor was an HLA-matched unrelated volunteer (Goldman et al 1987, McGlave et al 1987). DNA typing techniques were used in some cases to confirm donor/recipient identity at DR and DQ loci (Bidwell et al 1987). It is too early to draw firm conclusions but it is at least possible that the use of such donors will yield results similar to those achievable with HLA-identical siblings.

RELAPSE AFTER BONE MARROW TRANSPLANTATION

The definition of relapse and the interpretation of the finding of Ph-positive marrow metaphases after allogeneic marrow transplantation are complex. For practical purposes it may be assumed that patients transplanted in accelerated or transformed phases usually show, if they relapse, the same haematological features as were present before transplant. The cytogenetic pattern may however be the same as that seen pre-transplant or may show evidence of further evolution with acquisition of further cytogenetic changes characteristic of transformation (Cooperative Study Group 1988, Przepiorka & Thomas 1988).

Relapse after transplantation in chronic phase

Although relapse after transplantation in chronic phase seems to be relatively uncommon (see above), the figure might be higher if the definition was more stringent. There are in general three possible patterns of relapse (Table 7.4). It has been known

Table 7.4   Patterns of relapse after allogeneic BMT for CML in chronic phase

1. *Cytogenetic relapse*
   The finding of a low proportion of Ph-positive metaphases in the marrow at varying intervals after BMT. The proportion may then fall (transient relapse), persist essentially unchanged (cytogenetic relapse) or proceed to haematological relapse.

2. *Haematological relapse*
   The finding of haematological features of CML, e.g. leucocytosis, thrombocytosis, basophilia, eosinophilia, etc., together with Ph-positive marrow metaphases.

3. *Blastic phase relapse*
   The finding of haematological features of blastic transformation without a recognized preceding phase of relapse to chronic phase.

for some years that occasional patients having a low proportion of Ph-positive marrow metaphases identified at various intervals after transplantation do not necessarily proceed to clinical relapse (Thomas et al 1986, Goldman et al 1986, Apperley et al 1986b). A more systematic study was reported recently from the European Cooperative Study Group on Chromosomes in Transplanted Patients (1988). The investigators analysed chromosomal findings in 100 patients allografted in various phase of CML at different centres in Europe. Of the 76 patients transplanted in chronic phase, there were 6 haematological (or 'clinical') relapses. In 5 cases the cytogenetic features at relapse were similar to the findings pre-transplant, in that the patient was either 100% Ph-positive or a Ph-positive/negative chimera. In 1 case additional chromosomal changes, notably 46,XX,Ph,t(4;5)del(13)(17) were present. This of course raises the possibility that the patient might have been in occult transformation at the time of transplant.

The European Group was able to identify an additional 22 patients who had occasional detection of Ph-positive metaphases at different interval post-transplant. None of these patients had progressed to haematological relapse at the time of the report and they therefore satisfied the criteria (Table 7.4) for cytogenetic relapse. In these patients the Ph chromosome was observed in 1–30% of metaphases, usually less than 10%. There were three groups, those with Ph-positive metaphases observed only within the first 90 days post-transplant (n = 10), those with Ph-positive metaphases both before and after 90 days (n = 5) and those in whom Ph-positive metaphases appeared only after 90 days (n = 7). Of these 22 patients, 13 satisfied the criteria for transient cytogenetic relapse; 9 had at least one Ph-positive metaphase at the most recent cytogenetic examination.

The same general pattern was observed in patients allografted with unmanipulated donor marrow cells at the Hammersmith Hospital (Arthur et al 1988). Haematological relapses were extremely rare though 1 patient relapsed to chronic phase disease and another directly to blastic transformation. Transient cytogenetic relapses were seen in 2 other patients. Two patients showed Ph-negative metaphases of donor origin at 18 months and 3 years post transplant. In 1 patient a Ph-negative clonal abnormality was seen on 2 consecutive marrow examinations more than 3 years post-transplant. The pattern of relapses was however quite different in patients who received T-depleted donor marrow cells. The finding of Ph-positive metaphases at the first marrow examination post-transplant was relatively common and the majority of these patients progressed to haematological relapse.

In both studies the techniques of cytogenetic analyses would have favoured the development of metaphases in cells of myeloid lineage but the possibility that some Ph+ metaphases were in fact lymphoid cannot be entirely excluded. Furthermore we do not know whether or not the Ph+ cells identified were representative of a population with the ability to replicate extensively. These points notwithstanding, it seems likely that undefined factors operate for months or years after transplantation to suppress resurgence of Ph+ haemopoiesis.

Relapse in cells of donor origin
Two cases have now been reported in which leukaemia relapsed after transplantation in cells with the sex chromosomal complement of the donor who was of opposite sex to the patient (Marmont et al 1984, Smith et al 1985). The mechanism by which this may occur is totally unknown but one may speculate on the various possible explanations. It could be for example that a marrow microenvironmental influence induced leukaemia first in the patient's own cells and subsequently after transplant in donor cells; alternatively a transforming sequence of DNA may have been transferred from host to donor cells at the time of the transplant. It is worth noting that both these patients relapsed in donor cells after preceding episodes of blast cell transformation. This means that the transfer of genetic material must have induced in donor cells both the standard t(9;22) and the additional genomic changes underlying the transformation in these patients.

CONCLUSIONS

Though there has been no definite improvement in the management of chronic phase disease in recent years, it now seems possible that α-IFN or the combination of γ-IFN together with α-IFN could lead to clinical benefit for selected patients. It now seems very probable that allogeneic bone marrow transplantation cures a proportion of patients eligible for the procedure but the mortality associated with transplantation is still daunting. It is to be hoped that newer techniques, possibly autografting in association with a marrow purging stem or possibly approaches based on our new understanding of molecular events in CML, may lead to further therapeutic progress in the 1990s.

REFERENCES

Apperley J F, Rassool F, Parreira A et al 1986a American Journal of Haematology 22: 199–204
Apperley J F, Jones L, Hale G et al 1986b Bone Marrow Transplantation 1: 53–68
Apperley J F, Mauro F, Goldman J M et al 1988 British Journal of Haematology 69: 239–245
Arthur C K, Apperley J F, Guo A-P, Rassool F, Goldman J M 1988 Blood 71: 1179–1186
Beatty P G, Clift R A, Mickleson E M et al 1985 New England Journal of Medicine 313: 765–771
Bidwell J L, Bradley B, Jarrold E A et al 1987 Molecular Immunology 24: 513–522
Bolin R W, Robinson W A, Sutherland J, Hamman R F 1982 Cancer 50: 1683–1686

Brito-Babapulle F, Apperley J F, Rassool F, Guo A-P, Dowding C, Goldman J M 1987 Leukemia Research 11: 1115–1117
Butturini A, Gale R P 1987 Bone Marrow Transplantation 2: 351–354
Butturini A, Seeger R C, Gale R P 1986 Blood 68: 954–956
Butturini A, Bortin M M, Gale R P 1987 Bone Marrow Transplantation 2: 233–242
Catovsky D 1979 British Journal of Haematology 42: 493–498
Champlin R, Ho W, Arenson E, Gale R P 1982 Blood 60: 1038–1041
Champlin R E, Goldman J M, Gale R P 1988 Seminars in Hematology 25: 74–80
Chan L C, Karhi K K, Rayter S I et al 1987 Nature 325: 635–637
Clark S S, McLaughlin J, Crist W M, Champlin R, Witte O N 1987 Science 235: 85–88
Clift R A, Thomas E D, Buckner C D et al 1982 Lancet ii: 621–623
Clift R A, Martin P J, Fisher L, Buckner C D, Thomas E D 1987 Blood 70 (Supplement 1): 291 (abstract no. 1019)
Coleman M, Silver R T, Pajak T F et al 1980 Blood 55: 29–36
Cooperative Study Group on Chromosomes in Transplanted Patients 1988 European Journal of Haematology 40: 50–57
Coulombel L, Kalousek D K, Eaves C J et al 1983 New England Journal of Medicine 306: 1493–1498
Cunningham I, Castro-Malaspina H, Flomenberg N et al 1987 In: Gale R P, Champlin R E (eds) Progress in bone marrow transplantation. Liss, New York, p 359–363
Curtis J E, Messner H A 1982 Canadian Medical Association Journal 126: 649–655
Degliantoni G, Mangoni L, Rizzoli V 1985 Blood 65: 753–757
De Witte T, Hoogenhout J, De Pauw B et al 1986 Blood 67: 1302–1308
Doney K, Buckner C D, Sale G E et al 1978 Experimental Hematology 6: 738–747
Doney K, Buckner C D, Thomas E D et al 1981 Experimental Hematology 9: 966–971
Douglas I D C, Wiltshaw E 1978 British Journal of Haematology 40: 59–64
Dreazen O, Klisak I, Rassool F, Goldman J M, Sparkes R S, Gale R P 1987 Lancet i: 1402–1405
Dreazen O, Cannani E, Gale R P 1988 Seminars in Hematology 25: 35–49
Fefer A, Cheever M, Thomas E D et al 1979 New England Journal of Medicine 300: 333–337
Fefer A, Cheever M D, Greenberg P D et al 1982 New England Journal of Medicine 306: 63–68
Gale R P, Cannani E 1984 Proceedings of the National Academy of Sciences USA 81: 5648–5652
Gale R P, Cannani E 1985 British Journal of Haematology 60: 395–408
Gale R P, Goldman J M 1988 Leukemia 2: 231–324
Gale R P, Reisner Y 1986 Lancet i: 1468–1470
Ganesan T, Rassool F, Guo A-P et al 1986 Blood 68: 957–960
Goldman J M 1987 British Journal of Haematology 66: 435–436
Goldman J M, Lu D-P 1982 Seminars in Hematology 19: 24–256
Goldman J M, Johnson S A, Catovsky D et al 1981 Transplantation 31: 140–141
Goldman J M, Baughan A S J, McCarthy D M et al 1982 Lancet ii: 623–625
Goldman J M, Bortin M M, Champlin R E et al 1985 Lancet ii: 1295
Goldman J M, Apperley J F, Jones L et al 1986 New England Journal of Medicine 314: 202–207
Goldman J M, Apperley J F, Mackinnon S et al 1987 Blood 70 (Supplement 1): 294 (abstract no. 1032)
Goldman J M, Gale R P, Horowitz M M et al 1988 Annals of Internal Medicine 108: 806–814
Greaves M F 1982 In: Shaw M T (ed) Chronic granulocytic leukaemia. Praeger, Eastbourne, p 15–47
Groffen J, Heisterkamp N 1987 Clinical Haematology 1(4)
Groffen J, Stephenson J R, Heisterkamp N et al 1984 Cell 36: 93–99
Haines M E, Goldman J M, Worsley A M et al 1984 British Journal of Haematology 58: 711–722
Hale G, Cobbold S, Waldmann H for Campath-1 users 1988 Transplantation 45: 753–758
Heit W, Bunjes D, Wiesneth et al 1986 British Journal of Hematology 64: 479–486
Hermans A, Heisterkamp N, von Lindern M et al 1987 Cell 51: 33–40
Hows J M, Yin J L, Marsh J et al 1986 Blood 68: 1322–1328
International Bone Marrow Transplant Registry 1987 Personal communication
Jones L, Thein S L, Jeffreys A J, Apperley J F, Catovsky D, Goldman J M 1987 European Journal of Haematology 39: 144–147
Kantarjian H M, Keating M J, Talpaz M et al 1987 American Journal of Medicine 83: 445–454
Koller C A, Miller D M 1986 New England Journal of Medicine 315: 1433–1438
Konopka J B, Watanabe S M, Witte O 1984 Cell 37: 1035–1042
Kurzrock R, Shtalrid M, Romero P et al 1987a Nature 325: 631–633
Kurzrock R, Shtalrid M, Gutterman J U et al 1987b Blood 70: 1584–1588
McGlave P B, Arthur D C, Kim T H, Ramsay N K C, Hurd D D, Kersey J 1982 Lancet i: 665–668
McGlave P B, Scott E, Ramsay N et al 1987 Blood 70: 877–881
Maraninchi D, Gluckman E, Blaise D et al 1987 Lancet ii: 175–178

Marcus R E, Goldman J M 1986 Clinics in Haematology 15: 235–247
Marmont A, Frassoni F, Bacigalupo A et al 1984 New England Journal of Medicine 310: 903–906
Mitsuyasu R T, Champlin R E, Gale R P et al 1986 Annals of Internal Medicine 105: 20–26
Morra E, Alimena G, Lazzarino M et al 1987 New Trends Therapy of Leukaemia and Lymphoma 2: 75–82
Morris C M, Reeve A E, Fitzgerald P H, Hollings P E, Beard M E J, Heaton D C 1986 Nature 320: 281–283
Niederle N, Kloke O, May D, Becher R, Osieka A, Schmidt C G 1987 Investigational New Drugs 5: 19–25
Papa G, Arcese W, Mauro F R et al 1986 Leukemia Research 10: 1469–1475
Patterson H G, Blacklock H A, Brenner M K et al 1986 British Journal of Haematology 63: 221–230
Pendergast A M, Witte O N (1987) Clinical Haematology 1:4 (in press)
Prentice H G, Blacklock H A, Janossy G et al 1984 Lancet i: 472–475
Przepiorka D, Thomas E D 1988 Bone Marrow Transplantation 3: 113–119
Santos G W, Tutschka P J, Brookmeyer R et al 1985 New England Journal of Medicine 309: 1347–1353
Schaefer-Rego K, Dudek H, Popenoe D et al 1987 Blood 70: 448–455
Segel G B, Simon W, Lichtman M A 1986 Blood 68: 1055–1064
Smith J L, Heerema N A, Provisor A J 1985 British Journal of Haematology 60: 415–422
Sokal J E, Baccarani M, Tura S et al 1985 Blood 66: 1352–1357
Speck B, Gratwohl A, Nissen C et al 1982 Blut 45: 237–242
Speck B, Bortin M M, Champlin R et al 1984 Lancet i: 665–668
Strife A, Clarkson B 1988 Seminars in Hematology 25: 1–19
Talpaz M, McCredie K B, Mavligit G M, Gutterman J U 1983 Blood 62: 689–692
Talpaz M, Kantarjian, McCredie K, Trujillo J M, Keating M J, Gutterman J U 1986 New England Journal of Medicine 314: 1065–1069
Thomas E D, Clift R A, Fefer A et al 1986 Annals of Internal Medicine 104: 155–163
Truitt R L, Shih C Y, Lefever A V 1986 Transplantation 41: 301–310
Tutschka P J, Copelan E A, Klein J P 1987 Blood 70: 1382–1388
Vicariot M, Goldman J M, Catovsky D, Galton D A G 1979 European Journal of Cancer 15: 559–563
Waldmann H, Polliak A, Hale G 1984 Lancet ii: 483–486
Wareham N J, Johnson S A, Goldman J M 1982 Cancer Chemotherapy and Pharmacology 8: 205–210
Weiden P L, Flournoy N, Thomas E D et al 1979 New England Journal of Medicine 300: 1068–1073
Weiden P L, Sullivan K M, Flournoy N D et al 1981 New England Journal of Medicine 304: 1529–1533
Zaccaria A, Rosti G, Testoni M et al 1987 Cancer Genetics and Cytogenetics 25: 5–13

8. Recent advances in bone marrow transplantation in the treatment of leukaemia

H. G. Prentice   M. K. Brenner

INTRODUCTION AND GENERAL APPLICATIONS OF BMT

The major application of bone marrow transplantation (BMT) continues to be in the treatment of haematological malignancies. Whilst this might remain so for some years to come, we believe that BMT will ultimately be superseded by other methods of treatment and in the future principal haematological indications for BMT will be the correction of congenital disorders such as thalassaemia (major) and sickle cell disease. In this setting the 'transplant' might be used as a mechanism for obtaining corrective gene transfer (Thomas 1986).

Since the last edition of Recent Advances in Haematology there have been changes in the practice of bone marrow transplantation, some of which have resulted in genuine advances. In this chapter we will deal first with the benefits, and drawbacks, of T cell depletion compared to conventional immunosuppressive drugs used for the prevention of graft versus host disease after BMT. The next section describes the problems of graft failure, immune reconstitution and the issue of graft versus leukaemia (GvL) and describes how biological response modifiers may help to overcome these difficulties. Next we discuss the current indications for and results of BMT in leukaemia and finally the use of matched unrelated donors and the exponentially expanding use of autologous BMT in the treatment of selected haematological malignancies is outlined in the final section.

Regrettably, the results of allogeneic BMT for leukaemia have not shown any substantial improvement during the last decade (Gratwohl et al 1988) although modest gains can reasonably be anticipated from current studies.

Selection of patients for bone marrow transplantation

Bone marrow transplantation (BMT) includes the use of donor (allogeneic or syngeneic) marrow or autologous marrow (ABMT). In general, donor marrow is preferred where the disease involves either marrow derived cells or the marrow compartment, whilst an autologous source is preferable where the marrow compartment is disease free and an allogeneic effect is not required. In current practice, the major exception to this rule is the use of ABMT in haematological and other malignancies where a reasonable assumption can be made that the marrow can be rendered free of disease either by treatment of the patient or of the marrow in vitro (see p. 169). Our current and future suggestions of diseases appropriate to donor or autologous BMT are detailed in Table 8.1.

In each disease category patient selection and the timing of BMT are critical. At present we have no lower age limit for BMT but the upper limit in most centres for allogeneic BMT is 40–50 years and for syngeneic or autologous transplantation

Table 8.1   Marrow source. *Key:* – not indicated; + beneficial in selected cases; (+) not with curative intent; ± benefit unclear at present; ** except in the context of gene insertion; (0) no information available as yet; ALL, acute lymphoblastic leukaemia; AML, acute myeloblastic leukaemia; CML, chronic myeloid leukaemia; CLL, chronic lymphocytic leukaemia; MM, multiple myeloma; SCID, severe combined immune deficiency; LFA, leukocyte functional antigen.

Indication	Donor	Autologous
Marrow aplasia	+	–
		(except where stem cells previously stored)
Haematological malignancies		
ALL	+	+
AML	+	±
CML	+	(+)
CLL	+	(0)
MM	+	(+)
Lymphoma	±	+
Other malignancies (including paediatric)	±	±
Congenital marrow deficiencies		
Erythroid:		
Thalassaemia or enzyme defects	+	– **
Myeloid, e.g. chronic granulomatous disease	+	–
Megakaryocytes:		
Bernard Soulier	+	–
Lymphoid, e.g. SCID	+	– **
LFA-1 def.	+	–
Mixed, e.g. Wiskott-Aldrich	+	–
Inborn errors of metabolism (macrophage dependent)	+	– **

50–60 years of age. Children with life-threatening immunodeficiency diseases or with mucopolysaccharide storage disorders should be transplanted as soon as possible after birth to avoid lethal opportunistic infection or irreversible organ damage (especially neurological). In many cases children will lack a major histocompatibility complex (MHC) identical sibling and instead may receive an HLA mismatched family donor transplant. This source is likely to be replaced, in the future, by the use of HLA matched unrelated donor marrow. Our views on the optimal timing of allogeneic or autologous BMT in the treatment of haematological malignancies are listed in Table 8.2. It must be emphasised that these are our own views and that no consensus exists. We also list options but, of course, these will change with alterations in prognosis based upon conventional chemotherapy.

It must be emphasised that Table 8.2 lists the optimal and not the exclusive timing for transplantation and does not suggest that the BMT cannot produce cure in other settings. Indeed the indication for transplant is most clear in patients with advanced disease who are incurable by conventional treatment, even though their probability of cure with BMT is low. Overall, however, the return (added years of life free of disease) with our limited resources is likely to be greatest where patients with poor prognosis with conventional treatment are selected for early transplantation.

PREVENTION AND TREATMENT OF GvHD

The efficiency of graft versus host disease (GvHD) prophylactic techniques were assessed in animal experiments prior to their introduction into human allogeneic BMT.

Table 8.2   Optimal timing of BMT. *Key*: (+) not with curative intent.

Disease	Sub-type	Age	Karyotype	WBC	Transplant/ remission timing Allogeneic	Autologous
ALL	Common	2–15	Normal/hyperdiploid	<100	2nd	2nd
			Hypodiploid/any structural rearrangement	>100	1st	1st
		15–20	Normal/hyperdiploid Any structural rearrangement		2nd	1st
				>50	1st	1st
		20–60*		>20	1st	1st
	T cell	<20		<50	2nd	? 1st
		20–50/60*			1st	1st
	B cell	<50/60*			1st	1st
	Null	<20			2nd	1st
		20–50			1st	1st
AML	Any	<50/60*			1st	1st
CGL	–				1st	(+)
CLL	–	<50/60*			Responding disease	–
Myeloma	–	<50/60*			Plateau phase	(+)
Lymphoma	Intermediate/ high grade	<50/60*			2nd	? 1st/2nd
Hodgkin's disease	–	<50/60*			2nd	2nd

*Up to 60 years with autografts or syngeneic graft.

There are two major approaches in current use, post-transplant immunosuppression by drugs and T cell depletion (TCD) of donor marrow.

Post-transplant immunosuppression
With post-transplant immunosuppression, the strategy is to block activation, recruitment and division of the alloreactive T cells present in the donor graft. The first, and until recently, most widely used immunosuppressive agent was methotrexate (MTX) tested in mice (Uphoff 1958), dogs (Storb et al 1970) and then introduced by the Seattle team into clinical use (Thomas et al 1975). In man the merits of this drug are still debated since clinical trials have produced conflicting results (Herzig et al 1982, Sullivan et al 1985). The combination of MTX with steroids with or without additional anti-thymocyte globulin (ATG) has proved particularly effective in prevention of GvHD (Filipovich et al 1985). Indeed MTX + steroids are apparently the treatment associated with the best leukaemia-free survival (LFS) in ALL allografts performed in 1st complete remission (Barrett et al 1988), although in theory immune reconstitution may be impaired and the risk of infection correspondingly increased.

The use of Cyclosporin A (CSA) (Borel et al 1976) for GvHD prophylaxis was hailed as a major breakthrough (Powles et al 1978): some of this promise has been fulfilled. Although several studies reported to the International Bone Marrow Transplant Registry (IBMTR) show no apparent reduction in the frequency of acute GvHD (Bortin 1987, Deeg et al 1987) they demonstrate a reduction in the severity of the condition and an improved leukaemia free survival (Gratwohl et al 1986). Toxicity, predominantly to kidneys and liver (Lindholm et al 1986), is not an insurmountable problem where drug levels are carefully controlled. Of more concern is the increasing evidence that CSA might directly or indirectly interfere with the effectors of the graft versus leukaemia (GvL) phenomenon (Weiden et al 1978) and thereby increase the risk of relapse (Ringden et al 1988, Barrett et al 1988).

The combination of the two immunosuppressive agents MTX and CSA, has led to an impressive reduction in the risk and severity of GvHD (Storb et al 1985). Where BMT is undertaken for non-malignant conditions this combination might be optimal, although there is concern about the exacerbation of MTX induced mucositis due to the effects of CSA on renal function. Recent retrospective analysis of relapse risk following BMT for AML in 1st complete remission from Seattle shows a relative (to MTX) relapse risk of 2.31 (Clift et al 1987) and the IBMTR (Gale 1987) also suggests that this effective immunosuppressive combination — like CSA alone — might lead to a reduced GvL effect in allogeneic BMT and increased relapse rates. No controlled studies have as yet been reported.

T lymphocyte depletion
As GvHD is caused by alloreactive T cells in the donor graft, removal of these cells prior to BMT should prevent GvHD. This prediction was confirmed in animal models (Dicke et al 1968) and the original pre-clinical studies were followed by studies in which the incubation of conventional (rabbit) anti-human lymphocyte serum with donor marrow by the Munich group (Rodt et al 1981) gave promising results. The use of plant lectins to concentrate marrow repopulating cells combined with sheep red cells (E) rosetting to deplete T lymphocytes was pioneered at the Sloane-Kettering Hospital (Reisner et al 1980, Reisner et al 1981). This highly efficient method of T cell depletion is still used by this and a few other centres but its disadvantage is the time and labour required. By 1975 the preparation of monoclonal antibodies from mouse (and later rat) hybridoma cell lines was established (Kohler & Milstein 1975). These antibodies have predominantly been T cell specific and were originally used for in vitro coating alone (OKT3) (Prentice et al 1982, Filipovich et al 1982) — and subsequently with in vitro lysis mediated by complement obtained from rabbit serum (Blacklock et al 1983, Prentice et al 1984). A widely used alternative approach to MAb purging has involved treatment of marrow with Campath 1M, an IgM rat monoclonal antibody which reacts not only with T lymphocytes but with B cells, monocytes and some natural killer cells. This antibody is lytic with human complement (Hale et al 1983) resulting in excellent T lymphocyte depletion (Hale et al 1988). Other effective methods of T cell depletion include physical separation, such as discontinuous albumin gradients (Dicke & Van Bekkum 1978) and counterflow electrophoresis (de Witte et al 1986), or the use of magnetic beads (Treleaven & Kemshead 1985) coupled to anti-T cell monoclonal antibodies. One method emerging as highly convenient is the use of immunotoxins (Filipovitch et al 1984). Most of these techniques reliably remove close to 2 logs of T lymphocytes, with Campath being slightly more effective (3 logs) and the lectin method most effective (3–4 logs) (Personal communication R. O'Reilly).

That T cell depletion can significantly reduce (Prentice et al 1984) or even totally prevent acute and chronic GvHD in HLA matched human allogeneic marrow transplantation is now widely accepted and we will not deal with this issue further. Of more interest are the complex biological consequences of T cell depletion which have emerged in recent years. These issues include the altered pattern of immune reconstitution compared with that of unmanipulated BM, the increased risk of graft failure either due to primary resistance or delayed rejection (Patterson et al 1986, Martin et al 1985) and the partial loss of the graft versus leukaemia effect (Weiden et al 1978) in some (Apperley et al 1986, Pollard et al 1986, Mitsuyasu et al 1986) but not all studies (Prentice et al 1988b, Prentice et al 1988a).

OVERCOMING THE PROBLEMS OF CONVENTIONAL AND T CELL DEPLETED BMT

Graft failure

Following the pioneering development work in BMT by Thomas and Santos, it is now clearly established that graft failure is uncommon following infusion of unmanipulated BM into recipients treated with immunosuppressive/antileukaemic conditioning of high dose cyclophosphamide combined either with total body irradiation (TBI) or high dose busulphan. In an analysis of the European experience, the risk of graft failure has been approximately 1% for patients with haematological malignancy, although this risk is substantially higher in BMT for severe aplastic anaemia (SAA) or thalassaemia major.

It was predicted from animal studies that TCD would lead to an increased risk of graft failure, an event which was confirmed in early clinical practice (Patterson et al 1986). It must be assumed that part of the reason for the relatively low risk of graft rejection in BMT for leukaemia relates to the immunosuppressed state of the recipient, due both to the disease itself and to the treatment received and that it is not due exclusively to the conditioning immediately pre-BMT. Of at least equal importance, however, is the immunosuppressive role of the donor marrow derived T lymphocytes. Numerous reports now document an increased risk of primary graft failure or of graft rejection when the only change in procedure has been the removal of T lymphocytes from the donor marrow inoculum. A major supportive role of T lymphocytes in engraftment, unrelated to their immunological role, is untenable given that normal myelopoiesis occurs in the context of congenital total T cell deficiency.

Our own collaborative studies showed that the risk of rejection could be as high as 60% (Patterson et al 1986), while others found a rejection rate of 64% (Martin et al 1985). Where single fraction fast dose rate TBI was used the incidence was, and remains, around 4% (Prentice et al 1988b). Cyclosporin A has reduced the risk of rejection in the large Campath collaborative studies from 19 to 11%. The risk of rejection was directly correlated with the degree of HLA disparity in these studies (Hale et al 1988). Consensus now exists that to reduce this high risk of graft rejection compensation must be made in the form of improved immunosuppressive conditioning. This can take the form of radiobiologically enhanced total body irradiation (TBI) (Patterson et al 1986, Martin et al 1985, Prentice et al 1988b), increased chemotherapy (see pp. 167–169) or more selective and less toxic immunological measures. In this context the treatment of recipients pre-transplant with conventional antithymocyte globulin (ATG) (O'Reilly et al 1986) or monoclonal antibodies directed against immune system cells (Fischer et al 1986, Cobbold et al 1986, Prentice et al 1988c) has produced encouraging results (see pp. 167–169).

With fast dose rate single fraction TBI our own studies show a graft failure rate using HLA identical siblings of <5%, and we are optimistic that the addition of the specific immunological methods currently used in our unrelated donor programme to the HLA identical sibling TCD studies can reduce this risk further.

Delayed immune reconstitution

Following BMT there is a delay in recovery of both cell mediated and humoral immunity. As a consequence there is a high incidence of infection, and this immunoparesis may also contribute to an increased risk of leukaemia recurrence when BMT is undertaken for malignant disease (Witherspoon et al 1982). A number of factors are responsible for post-transplant immunodeficiency (Witherspoon et al 1984). After conventional BMT, one of the most important is probably the combination of GvHD and the immunosuppressive (I/S) drugs used for the prevention and treatment of this complication. T cell depletion of donor marrow prevents significant GvHD and thereby obviates any requirement for I/S drugs (Prentice et al 1984, O'Reilly et al 1986). Thus even though mature T-cells have been removed from the donor graft, T cell depletion could permit more rapid immune recovery. However, although there are clear differences in the pattern of immune recovery between recipients of TCD and non-TCD marrow, in neither group does full reconstitution occur in less than 1 year. Moreover recipients of autografts or syngeneic allografts (who have no GvHD/GvHD prophylaxis) still show a moderate degree of post-transplant immunodeficiency (Baumgartner et al 1988, Reittie et al 1988a,b), emphasising the importance of other factors in delaying immune recovery. These include the damaging effects of conditioning on host thymus and other lymphoid organs (see section on antigen presenting cells) and the immunosuppressive effects of intercurrent viral infections. When donor and recipient are MHC mismatched, failure of MHC restricted interactions between donor lymphocytes and residual host antigen presenting cells in thymus and lymph nodes may also contribute.

Immune reconstitution after conventional BMT

These patients all receive prophylactic I/S drugs for some months after the BMT and when GvHD occurs the I/S regimen is intensified. Although it is difficult to distinguish the effects of GvHD from the effects of the more intensive I/S given as treatment, it is clear that patients with chronic GvHD have a more severe and more prolonged immunoparesis than patients without this complication (Witherspoon et al 1984).

T CELL RECOVERY

T cells after BMT are both phenotypically and functionally abnormal. CD4 (helper) cell numbers remain sub-normal for up to 2 years but CD8 (suppressor/cytotoxic) T cells recover much more rapidly, reaching supranormal levels within the first 2–3 months. The CD4 to CD8 ratio is therefore markedly deranged (Favrot et al 1983). Within the first 3–6 months T cells have two other phenotypic abnormalities. Many have activation markers — including Class II MHC antigens — and CD8, Leu 7 double positive cells are present which may represent activated cytotoxic effector cells. Proliferative responses to recall antigens (such as Candida albicans) are minimal for the first 6–12 months and responsiveness to mitogens, such as PHA and Con-A, is also severely impaired. Helper function — measured by the ability to induce immunoglobulin production by B cells in the presence of pokeweed mitogen — begins to appear after about 3–6 months (Lum et al 1981, Pahwa et al 1982). This functional T cell defect after conventional bone marrow transplantation is associated with production of lower levels than normal of Interleukin 2 (IL2). The addition of exogenous IL2 to in vitro cultures restores many of the proliferative defects, although helper function remains depressed (Welte et al 1984). Impairment of IL2 production does not occur after T cell depleted BMT (see below).

There are in vivo correlates of the T cell paresis detected in vitro; it is, for example, generally impossible to elicit delayed type hypersensitivity responses to recall antigens within the first 6–12 months post-BMT.

RECOVERY OF MHC UNRESTRICTED CYTOTOXIC CELLS (NATURAL KILLER CELLS AND EFFECTORS OF ANTIBODY DEPENDENT CELL MEDIATED CYTOTOXICITY)

Cells positive for natural killer (NK) cell markers Leu 7 and CD16 appear in the peripheral blood within 30 days of BMT and have near normal activity against targets such as K562 (Lopez et al 1980). The kinetics of ADCC recovery are similar, but this pattern of regeneration of both types of effector function is modified after T cell depleted BMT (see below).

B CELLS

B cell numbers in peripheral blood are normal by 3–6 months after BMT (Witherspoon et al 1981) but the proportion of surface IgM positive cells is increased (Elfenbein et al 1982). In vitro functional abnormalities in Ig synthesis disappear by about 6 months post-transplant but serum immunoglobulin levels, particularly those of IgA and IgG_4, may remain depressed for 2–3 years (Witherspoon et al 1981).

ACCESSORY/ANTIGEN PRESENTING CELLS

Monocytes are detected early (less than 6 weeks) after BMT and examination of specialised skin antigen presenting cells (Langerhans cells) shows that host cells are gradually replaced with Langerhans cells of donor origin during the first 6 months post-BMT (Perreault et al 1984). Similar processes are thought to occur in the thymus and the lymphoid organs. However, more detailed examination of APC recovery has indicated that defects in important subsets persisting long term after BMT may contribute to immunodeficiency (Reittie et al 1988b): this aspect is discussed under the section 'Antigen presenting cells after T cell depleted marrow transplantation'.

Immune reconstitution after T cell depleted BMT

T CELLS

Recovery of CD4 positive cells is slow and normal levels are not reached until 6 months or more have passed (Janossy et al 1986). As after conventional BMT, CD8 positive cells recover more rapidly, but there is no overshoot to supranormal levels so that the CD4 to CD8 ratio is not generally below 0.4. Most CD8 cells are DR negative. Few functional studies of T cells have been reported after T cell depleted marrow transplantation, but the capacity to proliferate after lectin stimulation may recover more rapidly than after conventional BMT and near normal helper activity for B cells is seen by 6–8 weeks (Wimperis et al 1987a). However, much of this helper function may be generated by CD4 negative large granular lymphocytes (Brenner et al 1986b) (see below).

Perhaps the major difference between T cell recovery after conventional and T depleted BMT is in the pattern of IL2 production. After conventional BMT, T cells fails to secrete normal levels of IL2 even after stimulation; in contrast after TCD-BMT, CD3 positive T cells *spontaneously* secrete high levels of this growth factor (Brenner et al 1986b, Welte et al 1987). Although spontaneous secretion is relatively short lived and has ceased by 3–4 months post-BMT, it suggests a number of possible therapeutic manoeuvres which could improve the outcome of TCD-BMT (see Techniques for improving post-transplant immunity p 161).

RECOVERY OF MHC UNRESTRICTED CYTOTOXICITY

CD16 and CD8 positive cells with large granular lymphocyte morphology and NK activity reach normal levels within 3–4 weeks of TCD-BMT (Rooney et al 1986, Leger et al 1987, Welte et al 1987). These cells are not only active against the standard NK cell target K562 (see conventional BMT) but also against virus infected and malignant target cells. LGL after TCD-BMT therefore behave like exogenously generated lymphokine activated killer (LAK) cells. Activation occurs in the absence of any detectable stimulus, such as viral infection or graft versus host disease, and may follow LGL recognition of host alloantigens. However, activation is also seen following autografting when alloantigen stimulation cannot be present and so may be predominantly a consequence of abnormalities in NK regulation by a regenerating immune system (Reittie et al 1988a). Whatever mechanism generates activation, the process is continued by paracrine/autocrine secretion of lymphokines, since for the first 2–3 months after TCD-BMT patient lymphocytes spontaneously secrete cytokines capable of recruiting/maintaining LAK function, including gamma IFN and IL2 (Brenner et al 1986b, Keever et al 1987, Welte et al 1987). After this time circulating LAK cells are no longer seen and spontaneous secretion of cytokines ceases. Activated LGL after TCD-BMT also secrete B cell growth and differentiation factors and so provide helper function to regenerating B cells (Brenner et al 1986b).

B CELL RECOVERY

As after conventional transplantation, circulating B cell numbers after TCD-BMT are normal by 6 months. Phenotypically, however, it has been reported that a high proportion of the B cells are CD5 positive (Ault et al 1985). This marker is usually restricted to T cells, but is found on B-CLL cells and on a sub-population of fetal and adult B cells in tonsil and spleen. Not all groups have found circulating CD5 positive B cells after TCD-BMT and the significance of the observation is not yet clear (Drexler et al 1987). However, it is generally agreed that B cell function after TCD-BMT is impaired for up to one year, with poor response to both T dependent and independent mitogens. Paradoxically, serum immunoglobulin levels — including IgA — recover more rapidly than after conventional BMT and do not fall below the lower level of normal (Brenner et al 1986a).

ACCESSORY AND ANTIGEN PRESENTING CELLS

Although study of monocyte and Langerhans cell recovery after conventional trans-plantation appear to show rapid reconstitution, more detailed examination has shown that defects of important APC subsets may persist for a long period. A small proportion of circulating monocytes in normal individuals have the morphology and phenotype of 'true' antigen presenting cells; they have prominent cytoplasmic veils, contorted nuclei, multiple mitochondria and prominent endoplasmic reticulum. These cells are non-phagocytic and express high levels of Class II MHC antigens. They are positive for dendritic cell markers but negative for conventional monocyte antigens. The cells are extremely efficient at presenting soluble protein antigen and at stimulating in mixed lymphocyte cultures. After TCD-BMT, antigen presenting cells with this struc-ture and phenotype rapidly reappear in peripheral blood, and Y chromosome probes in sex mismatched donor and recipient pairs have shown the cells to be of donor origin. However, this particular APC subset disappears from the circulation by 3 months, at which time antigen presentation in the recipient is severely impaired. These specialised APC do not reappear until 1 year or more has passed (Reittie et al 1988b). As yet recovery has only been examined in TD-BMT recipients; but as the observed delay is likely to be a consequence of damage by pre-transplant condition-ing to the lymphoid architecture important for APC growth and differentiation, one would predict that similar defects would occur after conventional BMT. APC defects may therefore make a significant contribution to post-transplant immunodeficiency.

Techniques for improving post-transplant immunity

One approach to reducing the risk of infection and relapse after BMT is to boost immune recovery. Promotion of humoral recovery should reduce mortality from infec-tion while it should be possible to reduce the risk of relapse and latent virus reactivation by augmenting donor effector cells with activity against malignant and virus infected target cells.

HUMORAL IMMUNITY

Many of the infections after BMT could be prevented or modified by circulating antibodies. In animals it has been possible to immunise marrow donors and adoptively transfer antibody secreting B cells to the recipient, in whom they produce protective levels of specific antibody. Similar adoptive transfer techniques have now been shown to be effective in man. Thus, after conventional BMT, immunisation of the donor 1 week pre-BMT allows antibody transfer to the recipient (Saxon et al 1986). A similar pattern of transfer occurs even if the marrow is first depleted of T cells, although here the titre and duration of response in the recipient are increased if *both* donor and patient are immunised pre-transplant (Wimperis et al 1986). Combined immunisation also leads to memory B cell development, so that the recipient can mount a high titre secondary response to antigen challenge as little as 3 months after BMT (Wimperis et al 1987b). This technique allows transfer of antibody to protein recall antigens including hepatitis B, and the possibility of transferring immunity to gram negative organisms such as *Pseudomonas* spp. is currently under investigation (Cryz et al 1987). But the organism for which adoptive transfer of a protective response would be most desirable is cytomegalovirus, since this is the most common cause of death due to infection after BMT. Although attempts are being made to produce appropriate sub-unit vaccines, these are not yet available. However, the results obtained in adoptive transfer studies would suggest an alternative way of protecting recipients against interstitial pneumonitis, the most severe manifestation of CMV reactivation. If antibody has any protective role then one would predict that after T depleted BMT, CMV seropositive recipients of CMV seropositive donors would have a higher titre of protective antibody and hence a lower incidence of CMV pneumonitis than the CMV positive recipients of marrow from CMV negative donors. Observations of the incidence of CMV pneumonitis in the two groups supports this prediction. CMV seropositive recipients of CMV seropositive marrow had a death rate of 3% from CMV interstitial pneumonitis while 41% of the CMV seropositive recipients of CMV seronegative marrow died from the same complication (Grob et al 1987). Contrasting results have been obtained in studies of recipients following *conventional* transplantation, where a seropositive donor appears to convey an increased risk of pneumonitis (Ringden et al 1987). The explanation for this difference is unclear, but one possibility is that recipients of conventional grafts generally receive buffy coat material which contains neutrophils, while recipients of TCD-BMT are given only the mononuclear cell fractions of marrow. Recent evidence suggests that infectious CMV particles are much more readily recovered from neutrophils than from lymphocytes (Saltzman et al 1988). It is suggested that after conventional BMT, transfer of infectious donor strain CMV particles takes place, thereby negating the putative benefits of adoptive transfer of immunity.

Transfer of immunity does not always produce beneficial effects. When a recipient who is blood group A or B is given marrow from a donor who is group O then within 10–21 days of the procedure, donor lymphocytes secrete high titre anti-A or B, producing severe haemolysis in the recipient (Hazlehurst et al 1986). This effect is regularly seen after TCD-BMT but is not reported to occur after conventional BMT unless CSA is used as GvHD prophylaxis (Hows et al 1986).

IMMUNISATION AFTER BMT

Although it is possible to adoptively transfer immunity at the time of transplantation, deliberate immunisation for the first year *after* the transplant is generally unsuccessful, perhaps in part due to the absence of APC subsets (Wimperis et al 1987b). After this time, injection of killed vaccines usually produces modest titres of neutralising antibody, except in patients with chronic (c)GvHD. As a result of these observations we would suggest that the administration of live vaccines should be avoided for 2 years after BMT or for even longer in the presence of cGvHD. In addition, patients with chronic GvHD are generally unable to mount antibody responses to pneumococcal polysaccharide and have a high incidence of pneumococcal septicaemia. They should therefore receive continuous appropriate antibiotic prophylaxis.

CELL MEDIATED IMMUNITY

In clinical medicine, identification of an abnormality associated with a deficiency state is usually followed by attempts to correct the abnormality by replacement therapy. Thus it would be expected that identification of a defect in IL2 production after conventional BMT (p. 159) would by now have been followed by attempts to restore function by the administration of recombinant human IL2. The constraint, of course, has been that the dominant action of IL2 would be to increase the number and activity of alloreactive donor T lymphocytes and thereby accelerate and exacerbate graft versus host disease. Although precisely such an effect has been demonstrated in animal models, these same studies also show that IL2 need not induce GvHD if donor marrow is first depleted of T cells (Malkovsky et al 1986). Recipients of TCD-BMT might then be expected to benefit from IL2 infusion. In vitro, IL2 acts on cells obtained after TCD-BMT to further promote NK effector function and to increase the generation and function of LAK cells with activity against virus infected and malignant target cells (Leger et al 1987). Preclinical studies of the effects of IL2 following T cell depleted allografts in monkeys are currently underway, and phase I trials of IL2 have been undertaken in patients following autologous BMT for AML. Continuous infusion of IL2 produces in vivo effects which match its in vitro activity, so that NK and LAK cytotoxicity are enhanced, lymphocyte interferon-gamma secretion is increased by 1–3 logs and TNF alpha is produced (Heslop et al 1988). The IL2 induced secondary cytokines TNF and IFN-γ have three effects. First, they increase mature neutrophil oxidative metabolism and thereby augment killing of microorganisms: secondly, they inhibit myeloid progenitor growth, and finally, IFN-γ and TNF in combination inhibit the growth and survival of myeloid blast cells, producing an additional anti-leukaemic effect to that generated by LAK cells (Price et al 1987). As yet we do not know whether these largely desirable effects of IL2 will translate into a reduction in the incidence of infection or relapse after autologous or TCD-BMT.

CLINICAL RESULTS AND INDICATIONS FOR ALLOGENEIC BMT IN LEUKAEMIA

In the treatment of AML in 1st remission several studies have reported an improved leukaemia free survival (LFS) for recipients of HLA identical BMT compared to conventional chemotherapy (Powles et al 1980, Applebaum et al 1984, Champlin et al 1985, Santos et al 1983, Zwaan & Jansen 1984). Of necessity these are never strictly randomised studies but this does not invalidate the observations. These studies fail to reach clinical significance for LFS because of the modest numbers that can be entered by single institutions and the confounding complications of allogeneic BMT. The largest single institution study is reported by the Seattle team (Clift et al 1987). In 231 patients (adults and children) with a median age of 25 years who have been followed for up to 10 years, the 5 year LFS is 46% and the relapse risk 25%. In this major centre there has been no improvement in outcome when transplants performed prior to 1982 are compared to those undertaken subsequently despite several changes to the management protocol. Increasing age had a profound effect on survival (p = 0.0001) most marked beyond the age of 20. Acute GvHD had a profound negative effect on survival but extensive cGvHD imparts the benefit of a decreased relapse risk (22% versus 8% for 100 day survivors) irrespective of the presence or not of prior aGvHD. A surprising observation from this series has been an increased risk of relapse associated with recipient CMV seropositivity (34% vs 12%). The use of CSA + MTX for GvHD prophylaxis was associated with a two fold increase in relapse risk compared with other combined methods despite a lack of impact on the onset of cGvHD. Adjusted for the effect of cGvHD the CSA + MTX combination led to a relative risk of relapse of 2.36. In these studies the single most important cause of death was interstitial pneumonitis (40 of 231 patients).

A multicentre study from the Childrens Cancer Study Group (Feig et al 1987) confirms this observation in a substantial group of younger patients. Of 67 children transplanted in the 1st CR of AML, 64 had sustained engraftment following various conditioning regimens. The 2 year actuarial LFS was 59% and the relapse risk was 16%. These patients received MTX as anti-GvHD prophylaxis and 44% had grade II or greater aGvHD. Relapses were seen exclusively in children conditioned with single dose TBI but this group also had a lower risk of aGvHD (37% vs 64% grade II or more) and GvHD increased transplant related mortality. The 4 year estimated LFS was 53% and the relapse risk was 22% (33% in those without significant aGvHD).

These data largely confirm the previous report for single institutions. The Seattle experience with children (Sanders et al 1985) suggested that younger children (<5 years) were at increased risk of relapse and the Minnesota studies (Bostrom et al 1985) that a high presenting WBC or a French/American/British (FAB) (Bennett et al 1976) type of M4 or 5 was also an adverse feature.

The range in LFS in AML with chemotherapy has ranged from 22–51% at 3–6 years in recent studies in adults (Rees et al 1986, Yates et al 1982, Wolft et al 1987) and 41–50% in children at 4–5 years (Weinstein et al 1987, Creutzig et al 1985). Although for LFS there is some overlap in the results compared with BMT, the failures after chemotherapy are almost exclusively due to leukaemia relapse and in this respect the results of BMT are indisputably superior (see Table 8.3).

Beyond first remission the treatment of AML by chemotherapy, providing the initial treatment has been 'adequate', is very disappointing. A little more than 50% will achieve a second remission but probably less than 5% will be cured (Weinstein et al 1983). Three approaches to the treatment of these patients are of interest and each is likely to produce their benefit through immunological mechanisms. Allogeneic BMT shows a relative (to first CR BMT) relapse risk of 1.55 for patients in second remission and 3.97 for those with resistant relapse or 1.61 for those transplanted in untreated relapse. The corresponding 5 year LFS was 28%, 21% and 30% in the large Seattle study (Clift et al 1987). Autologous BMT has shown promise in studies by the Johns Hopkins team. Of 22 patients (2 in 1st CR others in 2nd or further CR) conditioned with a high dose busulphan/cyclophosphamide regimen and receiving marrow purged with a cyclophosphamide derivative (4 hydroxyperoxycyclophosphamide 4-HC) 13 were alive, free of disease for between 2 and 207 weeks (Kaizer et al 1985, Santos & Colvin 1986). This result has been attributed to a combination of the conditioning regimen and marrow purging. We suggest that immune disregulation may in fact be playing a significant role (Reittie et al 1988a) and we are currently attempting to mimic (and boost) some of the immunological consequences of BMT, in particular the development of LAK cells active against residual leukaemia blasts. One way of achieving this is to treat patients in (2nd CR) with the cytokine interleukin 2 (Gottleib et al 1988).

The management of acute lymphoblastic leukaemia is more problematical. The prospects for cure in children are now excellent with 60% or more cured by chemotherapy (Riehm et al 1987). Some children can be identified as having a worse prognosis and these can reasonably be considered for BMT (Pui & Crist 1987, Weinstein et

Table 8.3 Recently reported LFS/relapse risk (RR) from single institutions or collaborative groups for HLA identical sibling BMT or chemotherapy in 1st CR of AML. *Key*: LFS, leukaemia free survival; RR, relapse risk.

'Institution'	No	Chemotherapy LFS %	RR %	Actuarial point years	No	BMT LFS %	RR%	Actuarial point years	Reference
CCSG (children)	—	—	—	—	64	59	16	5	Feig (1987)
MS-K (children)	—	—	—	—	24	66	0	5	Brochstein (1987)
Minnesota (children and some adults)	—	—	—	—	39	55	21	3	Bostrom (1985)
Boston (children) VAPA	45	50	(22/45)	4	—	—	—	—	Weinstein
80–035	45	40	(26/45)	4	—	—	—	—	(1983, 1987)
BFM (children)	151	41	48	5	—	—	—	—	Creutzig (1985)
Seattle (children)	—	—	—	—	38	64	20	8	Sanders (1985)
	—	—	—	—	23	46	25	5	Clift (1987)
Royal Marsden Hospital (all ages)	44	15	(37/44)	(3–11)	98	52	18/98	4.5	Helenglass (1987)
Seattle (adults)	43	20	30/43	5	33	49	(5/33)	5	Applebaum (1984)
Johns Hopkins	—	—	—	—	35	47	0	2.5	Santos (1987)
UK Joint Trial (children)	73	35	37	3.5	15	70	?	3	Marcus (1987)
(adults)		38	59	3.5	8	36	?	3	
Royal Free Hospital (adults, some children)	—	—	—	—	29	73	6	5	Prentice (1988)
EBMT (all ages)	—	—	—	—	578	50	20	4	Gratwohl (1988)
(T cell depleted)	—	—	—	—	127	—	27	4	Prentice (1988a)
IBMTR (all ages)	—	—	—	—	704	48	20	5	Gale (1987)
Nashville/Cleveland/ Washington HD-ARA-C	55	51	(19/55)	6	—	—	—	—	Wolff (1987)

al 1987). In adults the outlook with chemotherapy is generally considered to be poor. Most clinicians consider that the overall outcome in adults under the age of 50 (i.e. potential BMT recipients) would be a 30% LFS. There are two studies which suggest that this could be an underestimate. First, the German BFM group have reported that, of 170 adults up to 65 years of age with ALL, 78% achieved a CR with a median duration of remission of 20 months, and a 4 year LFS of 39%. In this study, patients less than 35 years old with c-ALL or T cell ALL with low initial WBC who achieved a CR within 4 weeks had a 61 and 58% chance respectively of remaining in CR at 3 years. These patients performed better than all others, who had a median survival of only 13 months (Hoelzer et al 1984). Similarly the Memorial Sloan-Kettering Hospital have reported excellent results with the L10/10M and L17/17M programmes, obtaining remission rates of 87% (Ph′ +ve cases excluded) between the age of 15 and 50 (Clarkson et al 1985). Those patients who had cyclophosphamide containing protocols had a 57% projected 5 year survival. The overall 5 year LFS was 51% for those under 25 and 31% for the older patients. It remains to be confirmed if these protocols reflect results which can be achieved by others using similar treatment.

Bone marrow transplantation in children with ALL is mainly confined to those beyond first remission. A few BMTs have been undertaken in children with very high risk presenting features constituting a significantly poorer prognosis group than adults transplanted in 1st CR and are reported in a current IBMTR study (Barrett et al 1988). These children had a LFS of 56% which is not different from the 64%

Table 8.4   ALL in 1st or 2nd CR.

'Institution'	CR status	n	Chemotherapy LFS%	RR%	Actuarial point (years)	n	BMT LFS%	RR%	Actuarial point (years)	Reference
Children:										
IBMTR	1st		—	—		56	56	27	5	Barrett (1988)
BFM 70	1st	119	54	—	15	—	—	—	—	Riehm (1987)
76/83	1st	1258	67	—	6–9	—	—	—	—	
Memorial S-K	2nd		—	—		31	64	13	5	Brochstein (1987)
Genova	2nd	19	18	82	4	17	48	42	4	Bacigalupo (1986)
Seattle	⩾2nd	21	0	?	4.5–8	24	8/24	?	4.5–8	Johnson (1983) Storb (1985)
Adults and some children:										
BFM	1st	126	44	70/136	4	—	—	—	—	Holzer (1984)
IBMTR										
High risk	1st	—	—	—	—	245	39	30	5	Barrett (1988)
	>1st	—	—	—	—	391	28	51	5	
IBMTR										
High risk	2nd	—	—	—	—	208	22	56	4	} Herzig (1987)
	1st	—	—	—	—	236	45	26	5	
Standard risk	2nd	—	—	—	—	97	36	49	4.5	
Memorial S-K	1st	123	46	57/123	4	—	—	—	—	Andreff (1987)
Minnesota*	⩾2nd	23	5		3	15	33	—	3	Woods (1983)
Johns Hopkins										
Adults & children	1st	—	—	—	—	15	45	(1/15)	2	}
	2nd	—	—	—	—	24	45	(1/24)	2.75	} Santos (1987)
	3rd	—	—	—	—	17	30	(6/17)	3.5	
EBMTR	1st	—	—	—	—	260	50	27	5	} Gratwohl (1988)
Adults & children	⩾2nd	—	—	—	—	360	53	50	5	}

* Mainly children.

at 5 years after BMT in 2nd CR reported from the Memorial Sloan-Kettering Cancer Center (MS-K) (Brochstein et al 1987). This comparison does not necessarily support withholding BMT until 2nd CR since the patients were selected because of their very high risk features in the IBMTR study. The MS-K results using hyperfractionated TBI show a 42% leukaemia free survival in children transplanted in 3rd CR and even in 4th CR or relapse when no alternative therapy exists this treatment is still justified as it produces LFS of 23%. The relapse risk for children transplanted in 2nd CR was only 13% in this study.

A significant benefit for BMT compared to chemotherapy has been shown in two single centre studies for children transplanted beyond 1st CR (Bacigalupo et al 1986, Storb 1985) although this issue is still not resolved especially for those that relapse more than 18 months after first remission (Butturini et al 1987).

The important issue of timing of BMT for adults with poor risk features appears to be resolved by the IBMTR analysis (Herzig et al 1987) which shows a clear benefit for BMT in 1st CR (see Table 8.4).

Interestingly both in adults and children T-ALL is emerging as a good prognostic group for BMT as has also been the case for adults treated by chemotherapy in both the BFM and Memorial Sloan-Kettering studies. The use of high doses of either (or both) cyclophosphamide or cytosine arabinoside in each setting might be relevant (Riehm et al 1987, Clarkson et al 1985).

Adults who relapse after chemotherapy have a less than 5% chance of cure with chemotherapy (Hoelzer & Gale 1987) whereas those who have a BMT in 2nd CR have a 22–36% chance of long term LFS (Herzig et al 1987). In this setting BMT is clearly beneficial and in the absence of a suitable sibling donor a search should be made for an HLA identical unrelated volunteer donor (see below).

The issue of chronic granulocytic leukaemia is dealt with comprehensively in Chapter 7 and Goldman (1987). Other than BMT only the biological response modifiers in the form of α or γ interferon offer even a glimmer of hope for curative treatment at the present time (Talpaz et al 1986). Thus, bone marrow transplantation is currently the best option and cure rates with conventional HLA identical transplantation are likely to be in excesss of 50% when BMT is undertaken in 1st chronic phase. For those who lack a suitable sibling the use of HLA identical unrelated donors offers hope, and our own recent results suggest that such an approach is entirely feasible in first CR with the more effective immunosuppressive approaches now available (see below). Although T cell depletion has been associated with an increased graft rejection rate (Hale et al 1988) and a very substantial increased risk of leukaemia relapse in this disease (Apperley et al 1986), we suspect that this is a function of the better preserved recipient immune function in these patients and anticipate that the new conditioning regimens will have a substantial impact upon both of these problems.

ALTERNATIVE DONORS

Until recently almost all marrow transplants were undertaken between major histocompatibility complex (MHC) identical siblings. Identity at the MHC was deemed essential to reduce the risk of lethal GvHD or graft rejection. The complexity and extreme polymorphism of the MHC means that such identity is only likely to be found between siblings, who have a 1 in 4 probability of inheriting the same chromosome 6 (on which the MHC is situated) from each parent. As family sizes are now small, most people with the potential to benefit from bone marrow transplant do not have a suitable sibling donor. Three approaches have been employed to overcome this problem.

Mismatched family members

Attempts have been made to overcome the risks of rejection and GvHD by increasing conditioning of the recipient and by T cell depleting donor marrow. In experimental models, haploidentical transplants using such approaches have been successful, with prolonged recipient survival (Wagemaker et al 1981). Unfortunately achieving similar success in man has proved more elusive. Probably the largest reported series comes from Wisconsin (Trigg et al 1985, Ash et al 1987) who report that intensive conditioning with cyclophosphamide, cytosine arabinoside and 1400 rads fractionated TBI coupled with modest T cell depletion (<2 logs) and cyclosporin A treatment post-transplant allows engraftment (1 of 28 rejected), and leads to a death rate from graft versus host disease of 17.8% (5 of 28). With a median follow-up of 7 months, 11 of the 28 patients (39%) are alive. Although these figures represent an improvement on results obtained without T cell depletion, they still fall some way below the success rate of matched BMT.

Our own experience (25 mismatched BMT) has been less successful. With the most intensive conditioning regimens (HD ara-C, cytoxan, TBI $\pm$ TLI but no post-transplant CSA immunosuppression) we have seen graft failure in 40% rising to 60% with our standard (cytoxan, TBI) conditioning regimen. This has been in the context of similar levels of T cell depletion to Wisconsin. Only recipients of one HLA antigen mismatched transplants have in general become long term disease-free survivors.

Using conventional BMT the Seattle team have had more encouraging results (Beatty et al 1985, Hansen et al 1987) particularly with one locus mismatched BMT (probability of survival 40% at 8 years) although there has been considerable morbidity and mortality attributable to GvHD. This complication shows close correlation with the degree of HLA Class I or II disparity.

Although newer methods of immunosuppressing the recipient may improve results, the major emphasis has now switched to the use of HLA identical unrelated volunteer BM donors.

Unrelated but MHC matched donors

The use of central 'clearing houses' for solid organ grafts has proved highly successful. The tissue types of patients requiring grafts are entered on a central database and as MHC typed organs become available they are distributed to the appropriate recipients. It therefore seemed rational to set up similar systems for BMT, in which volunteer donors would be MHC typed and then called to give marrow to a recipient when the need arose. While in principle this remains an attractive prospect, in practice the successful operation of the scheme has been limited by logistical and conceptual problems.

The fundamental difference between bone marrow transplantation and solid organ grafting lies in the degree of MHC matching required between the donor and recipient. Solid organs predominantly express antigens coded only by class I MHC loci (B, C and A) and, in practice, matching at just A and B is often adequate. In contrast bone marrow progenitor cells express and recognise antigens of the MHC class II loci and so must be matched for these structures as well. The class II region is highly complex: it consists of at least three well defined sub-regions (DP, DQ, DR) each of which code for the two peptides which form the α and β chain of class II molecules (Trowsdale et al 1985). Both α and β chains may be polymorphic and each locus may code for more than one α or more than one β chain. In practice, then, the chances of finding two unrelated individuals who are both class I and class II MHC identical are remote. As a corollary, successful matching can only occur if the donor database is correspondingly large. At present we lack sufficient typing sera or the financial resources to undertake a full analysis of all the individuals who would be necessary to provide a 'complete' database. This problem has led many people to dismiss the concept of the marrow donor panel, but such a view seems unnecessarily pessimistic. It is unlikely that total MHC identity between donor and recipient is necessary for successful transplantation, even though we do not yet know how great a degree of matching is important, nor which loci are the most relevant for success. In addition, it may not be necessary to use vast quantities of typing sera for MHC analysis. Instead it is possible to study restriction fragment polymorphisms in the MHC coding region of recipient and potential donor, selecting those individuals with the closest match (Bidwell et al 1987). Alternatively a combination of allele specific oligonucleotide probes with gene amplification strategies may allow rapid analysis of the class II region. The application of such techniques, however, will obviously require a more detailed knowledge of the relationship between DNA sequence and surface antigen structure than we at present possess. Finally, the existence of strong linkage disequilibrium between the different class II loci in any given racial group means that once individuals have been matched at one class II locus there is a higher than expected probability that they will match at other class II loci.

In the United Kingdom, the original Anthony Nolan unrelated donor panel has now been supplemented by donor databases set up at regional transfusion centres; equivalent donor panels are becoming established in North America. Initial experience with matched unrelated transplants using T cell depletion of donor marrow and monoclonal antibody conditioning of the recipient has shown a low risk of rejection and of GvHD. At this centre we have transplanted 8 patients with advanced haematological malignancy (mainly CGL) who were conditioned with cytoxan, TBI, total lymphoid irradiation (TLI), busulphan and the monoclonal antibody Campath 1G. All patients engrafted, 5 had no GvHD and 1, in whom there was class II disparity had severe GvHD (Prentice et al 1988a). Goldman et al (personal communication) using a similar conditioning regimen have reported essentially identical results. It is likely that the number of matched unrelated donor transplants will increase exponentially over the next few years.

Autologous bone marrow transplantation

In the absence of an HLA compatible donor, patients with acute leukaemia eligible for bone marrow transplant can still benefit from high dose chemo/radiotherapy if they are subsequently rescued by infusion of autologous bone marrow that has been previously collected and stored. This procedure lacks the problems of rejection and GvHD associated with allogeneic BMT but carries three other risks.

1. The absence of alloreactivity means that loss of the GvL effect might be anticipated, but our preliminary studies suggest that some benefit could be preserved by endogenously generated activated killer cells (Reittie et al 1988a).

2. The possibility of infusing a bone marrow incapable of reconstituting complete haemopoiesis. This could be a consequence of previous exposure to myelotoxic therapy or of the process of in vitro manipulation and cryopreservation. This risk seems more potential than real; infusion of as few as 5×10^7 nucleated cells/kg or 4×10^4 CFU-C/kg is sufficient to restore complete haemopoiesis (Spitzer et al 1980). Similarly in vitro manipulation of marrow and cryopreservation (in liquid nitrogen with dimethylsulphoxide as cryoprotectant) results in an acceptable level of loss of bone marrow progenitor cells (Linch et al 1982). Clinical data over the past few years have shown that the great majority of patients receiving ABMT have adequate haemopoietic recovery, although recipients of marrow harvested in second or subsequent remission may have greatly prolonged reconstitution times, particularly of platelets (Knight et al 1983).

3. Risk of infusing residual leukaemia cells. This represents a much more serious drawback to the use of autologous bone marrow transplantation. Depending on the detection method used there may be as many as 5% malignant cells in the bone marrow of patients with acute leukaemia in apparent complete remission. With an average of 2×10^8 nucleated cells/kg infused the 'remission' bone marrow could therefore contain more than 10^8 malignant cells. Whether these cells are responsible for the increased relapse rate of ABMT compared to allogeneic BMT is controversial,

but there is a natural reluctance to inject any malignant cell into a patient who has received therapy designed to eradicate disease in vivo. Techniques have therefore been developed to purge autologous marrow, obtained in nominal remission, of any contamination with malignant cells. Three approaches have been adopted.

Methods of purging

Biophysical purging is based on differences in cell density or size between malignant cells and haemopoietic progenitors, which allows separation on density gradients (Hagenbeek & Martins 1983). The techniques are complex and are not widely used. An extension of this technique is the use of counterflow elutriation which can be adequately employed with T cell purging for allografting, but is probably inadequate in this setting.

Pharmacological purging is based on possible differences in sensitivity to chemotherapeutic agents between leukaemic cells and haemopoietic progenitors. Two cyclophosphamide derivatives, 4 hydroxyperoxycyclophosphamide (4-HC) (Santos & Colvin 1986, Hagenbeek & Martins 1983) and INN mafosfamide (AstaZ-7557) (Douay et al 1984) are used most widely, but other agents such as etoposides, deoxycoformycin and photoreactive membrane intercalating dyes (e.g. merocyanin) have been considered (Santos & Colvin 1987). However, as the human pluripotent stem cell has not yet been identified, there is at present absolutely no evidence that these normal progenitor cells are any more resistant than leukaemia progenitor cells to the action of such pharmacological agents. An additional disadvantage of the pharmacological approach is that the drugs leave only 1–10% of the original CFU-C (Herve et al 1983), although marrow regeneration appears unimpaired at this level.

Immunological purging relies on the assumption that a discernible pattern of antigenic structures is detectable on all malignant cells but is absent on human haemopoietic stem cells. Monoclonal antibodies raised against these antigenic structures should therefore allow the neoplastic cells to be eliminated. Although the hunt for antigens unique to tumour cells continues, it is likely to remain futile. For the moment, therefore, it is acceptable to destroy non-malignant cells as well as the desired targets provided that all malignant cells are included but that all marrow stem cells are *not* (Nadler et al 1982, Lowenberg & Bauman 1984). At present these strictures limit immunological purging to lymphoid malignancy and to certain solid tumours (for example neuroblastoma). Immunological purging generally uses mixtures of monoclonal antibodies to remove unwanted malignant cells by complement mediated lysis (Hale et al 1983, Simonsson et al 1988), by attaching toxins, such as Ricin A chain to the antibodies (Thorpe et al 1982, Cassellas et al 1985), or by attaching magnetic microspheres to the antibodies and removing the target cells using magnetic fields (Dicke et al 1984, Treleaven & Kemshead 1985).

The use of peripheral blood stem cells (PBSC) harvested during the recovery phase after chemotherapy appeals to us as a relatively simple method of harvesting stem cells with an improved possibility of being clear of contaminating malignant cells. ABMT undertaken with this source of stem cells also results in accelerated engraftment (To et al 1987).

Benefits of purging
There are two questions that must be asked of any purging technique. Does it remove malignant cells and their clonogenic precursors and does it increase the probability of patient cure? Answers to these questions have not yet been obtained.

Are malignant cells removed? Although apparent complete removal of cells with malignant phenotype has proved possible — for example in lymphoid malignancy — our assessment of the extent of depletion is limited by the sensitivity of present techniques of detection of minimal residual disease. Where the malignancies have a clear cut phenotypic pattern (e.g. T cell leukaemia), detection of 1 cell in 5–50 000 may be possible, but this still means that a purged marrow could contain upwards of 10^4 malignant cells/kg of recipient weight: moreover, leukaemic clonogenic progenitors may have an entirely different phenotype from the 'mature' tumour (Griffin et al 1983). When the cells are phenotypically indistinguishable from normal cells (e.g. many myeloid leukaemia blasts), this type of quality control is impossible. The application of the polymerase chain reaction (PCR) technology may go some way to solving these problems since detection of abnormalities in DNA sequences unique to malignant clone may be possible down to very low levels of contaminating cells. More importantly, as sequence abnormalities may be detectable in cells phenotypically indistinguishable from normal progenitors as well as in malignant clonogenic cells, the restrictions of phenotype based detection systems will no longer apply.

Is patient survival improved? If purging removed all malignant cells then the results of autografting for leukaemia/lymphoma should match the results obtained in identical twin (syngeneic) BMT. These patients have a long term survival approaching 55% with a relapse risk of 25%. Overall, patients receiving unpurged autografts in remission have a long term survival approaching 40% with a relapse risk of 30%. This means that any beneficial effect of purging will only be seen when a large cohort of patients receiving purged and unpurged ABMT are compared. In addition, since so many other variables also affect the outcome of ABMT (for example radiation dose, time from diagnosis to transplant) it would be desirable for such comparative trials to be conducted in a randomised fashion with centre stratification. This ideal has not been achieved, but over the past 2 years studies have been established and the results are awaited.

Clinical outcome of purged and unpurged autologous marrow transplantation
Few studies have been published which included more than a minimal number of patients and in which the treatment of both patients and the autologous bone marrow was identical. The working party on ABMT of the European Bone Marrow Transplant Association has published the preliminary results of the first European survey of ABMT in acute leukaemia in first CR in which marrow was purged with mafosfamide (Gorin et al 1988 in preparation). In AML a significant ($p = 0.02$) advantage was shown for purging (n = 57) over no purge (n = 138) with a DFS at 4 years of 58% vs 32%. The French study group have published a similar review of 120 patients (Herve et al 1984). No patient transplanted in relapse achieved long term disease-free survival, but 25 of 37 patients transplanted in complete remission with purged marrow were disease-free at a median follow-up time of 7 months. Both studies showed satisfactory

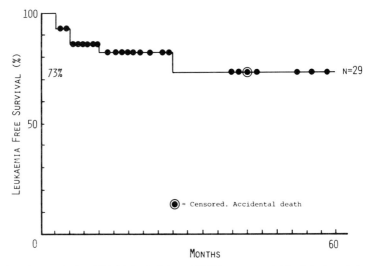

Fig. 8.1   T lymphocyte depleted HLA identical donor BMT in acute myeloblastic leukaemia in 1st CR using standard conditioning at The Royal Free Hospital, London.

haemopoietic recovery. Finally in a joint study between the Royal Free Hospital, University Hospital Uppsala, Sweden and the Royal Hospital for Sick Children, Glasgow, 54 patients with high risk ALL were treated with ABMT using marrow purged with selected MAbs. Disease free survival at 4 years was 64% for 21 patients transplanted in 1st CR (Simonsson et al 1988). The preliminary survival analysis for this group of patients is illustrated in Figure 8.2. From numerous studies in purged or unpurged ABMT two clear messages are evident.

1. Autologous bone marrow transplantation in complete remission with or without

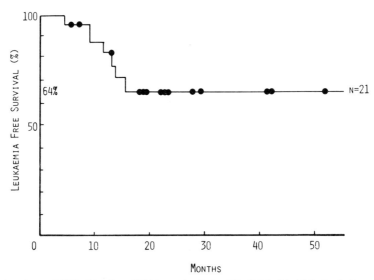

Fig. 8.2   Autologous BMT with selected MAb purging in 1st CR of high risk ALL. Preliminary analysis of Glasgow, Uppsala and Royal Free Hospital Collaborative Study, March 1988.

purging may increase the probability of disease-free survival over and above treatment with chemotherapy alone. It is also becoming clear that patients transplanted beyond first complete remission have a poor survival: they suffer from a higher relapse rate and a higher incidence of procedure related death than individuals grafted in first remission. As an extension of this observation:

2. Autologous bone marrow transplantation in relapse with or without bone marrow purging should be abandoned at present.

CONCLUSIONS

Recently reported results from centres or registries show that 47–73% of patients transplanted for AML in 1st CR are long term disease free survivors and the corresponding figures for ALL are 39–56%. Thus no clear progress has been documented over the past 10 years in the results of allogeneic BMT for acute leukaemia. We feel that this observation is misleading since advances have been made in several directions but their benefit is obscured by many outstanding problems. The major improvements have been in graft versus host disease prevention by T cell depletion and in antimicrobial support. The prevention of GvHD has been offset by complications such as graft rejection and an increased leukaemia relapse risk in CGL. We predict that recent advances in our understanding of the immuno-biology of leukaemia and marrow transplantation will result in clinical benefit in the near future. These will be in the areas of graft rejection and anti-leukaemic activity and will permit a rapid extension in the use of HLA matched unrelated donors.

Improvements in the safety of BMT along with a better ability to predict which groups with haematological malignancy have poor prognosis with conventional therapy will lead to a widening of the indications for BMT and allow a more clearly demonstrable benefit compared with chemotherapy alone.

Although autologous BMT clearly gives benefit over and above that seen with conventional therapy alone (especially in lymphoid malignancies) we see its role mainly as a method for achieving further tumour cytoreduction. Whilst we suspect a GvL benefit for ABMT (Reittie et al 1988a) we believe that ABMT by producing a state of 'minimal residual disease' will provide the ideal setting for the exploration of biological response modifiers including the interferons, tumour necrosis factor and interleukin 2.

Finally, with a better understanding of the function and interactions of the cytokines (especially IL2 and growth factors — Heslop et al 1988, Brandt et al 1988) we anticipate major improvements in the control of infection during the period of post-transplant immunoparesis.

REFERENCES

Andreeff M, Gaynor J, Chapman D, Little C, Gee T, Clarkson B D 1987 In: Büchner, Schellong, Hiddemann, Urbanitz, Ritter (eds) Hematology and Blood Transfusion 30: 111–124. Springer-Verlag, Berlin

Appelbaum F R, Dahlberg S, Thomas E D et al 1984 Annals of Internal Medicine 101: 581–588

Apperley J F, Jones L, Hale G et al 1986 Bone Marrow Transplantation 1: 53–68

Ash R C, Menitove J, Casper J et al 1987 Blood 70 (suppl 1): 289a

Atkinson K, Hansen J A, Storb R, Goehle S, Goldstein G, Thomas E D 1982 Blood 59: 1292

Ault K A, Antin J H, Ginsburg D et al 1985 Journal of Experimental Medicine 161: 1483–1502
Bacigalupo A, Frassoni F, Van Lint M T 1986 Cancer 58: 2307–2311
Baehner R L, Kennedy A, Sather H, Chard R L, Hammond D 1981 Medical Pediatric Oncology 9: 393–403
Barrett A J, Horowitz M M, Biggs J C et al 1988 Disease features and treatment modalities affecting relapse and survival after allogeneic bone marrow transplantation for acute lymphoblastic leukaemia (in preparation)
Baumgartner C, Morell A, Hirt A et al 1988 Blood 71: 1211–1217
Beatty P G, Clift R G, Mickelson E M et al 1985 New England Journal of Medicine 313: 765–771
Bell A J, Hamblin T J, Oscier D G 1987 Hematological Oncology 5: 45–55
Bennett J M, Catovsky D, Daniel M-T et al 1976 British Journal of Haematology 33: 451–458
Bidwell J L, Bidwell E A, Klouda P T, Goffin R V, Bradley B A, Brenner M K 1987 Bone Marrow Transplantation 1: 413–414
Borel J F, Feurer C, Magnee S, Stahelin H 1977 Actions 6: 468
Bortin M M 1987 Progress in Bone Marrow Transplantation 243–264
Bostrom B, Brunning R D, McGlave P et al 1985 Blood 65: 1191–1196
Brandt S J, Peters W P, Atwater S K et al 1988 New England Journal of Medicine 318: 869–876
Brenner M K, Wimperis J Z, Reittie J E et al 1987 British Journal of Haematology 64: 125–132
Brenner M K, Reittie J E, Grob J-P et al 1986b Transplantation 42: 257–261
Brochstein J A, Kernan N A, Groshen S et al 1987 New England Journal of Medicine 817: 1618–1624
Buckner C D, Appelbaum F R, Thomas E D 1981 In: Karow A M, Pegg D E (eds) Organ preservation for transplantation. Marcel Dekker, New York. p 355
Butturini A, Rivera G K, Bortin M M, Gale R P 1987 Lancet i: 429–432
Casellas P, Canat X, Fauser A A et al 1985 Blood 65: 289
Champlin R E, Ho W G, Gale R P et al 1985 Annals of Internal Medicine 102: 285–291
Clarkson B, Ellis S, Little C et al 1985 Seminars in Oncology 12(2): 160–179
Clift R A, Buckner C D, Thomas E D et al 1987 Bone Marrow Transplantation 2: 243–258
Cobbold S P, Martin G, Qin S, Waldmann H 1986 Nature 323: 164–166
Crawford D H, Mulholland N, Iliescu V, Powles R 1985 Experimental Hematology Suppl 17: 13, 71
Creutzig U, Ritter J, Riehm H et al 1985 Blood 65: 298–304
Cryz S J, Fürer E, Cross A S, Wegmann A, Germanier R, Sadoff J C 1987 Journal of Clinical Investigation 80: 51–56
Deeg H J, Doney K, Sullivan K M, Witherspoon R P, Appelbaum F R, Storb R 1987 Progress in Bone Marrow Transplantation 265–276
de Witte T, Hoogenhout J, de Pauw B et al 1986 Blood 67: 1302
Dicke K A, Van Bekkum D W 1978 Experimental Hematology 20: 126
Dicke K A, Van Hooft J, Van Bekkum D W 1968 Transplantation 6: 562–570
Dicke K A, Poynton C H, Reading C L 1984 In: Lowenberg B, Hagenbeeck J (eds) Minimal residual disease in acute leukemia. Martin Nijhoff, The Hague. p 209
Douay L, Gorin N C, Laport J-P, Lopez M, Najman A, Duhames G 1984 Investigational New Drugs 2: 187
Drexler H G, Brenner M K, Wimperis J Z, Signac S M, Hoffbrand A V, Janossy G, Prentice H G 1987 Clinical and Experimental Immunology 68: 662–668
Elfenbein G J, Bellis M M, Ravlin H M, Santos G W 1982 Experimental Hematology 19: 551
Favrot M, Janossy G, Tidman N et al 1983 Clinical and Experimental Immunology 54: 59–72
Feig S A, Nesbit M E, Buckley J et al 1987 Bone Marrow Transplantation 2: 365–374
Filipovich A H, Ramsay J A, Warkentin P I, McGlave P B, Goldstein G, Kersey J H 1982 Lancet 266: 1982
Filipovich A H, Vallera D, Youle R J et al 1984 Lancet i: 469–472
Filipovich A H, Ramsay N K C, Arthur D C, McGlave P, Kim T, Kersey J H 1985 Transplantation 39: 282
Fischer A, Griscelli C, Blanche S et al 1986 Lancet i: 1058–1061
Gale R P, Horowitz M M, Bortin M M 1987 Blood 70 No. 5 (suppl 1): 293a
Goldman J M 1987 Hematological Oncology 5: 265–279
Gorin N C 1984 In: Dicke K A, Spitzer G, Bander A R (eds) Autologous bone marrow transplantation. The University of Texas and MD Anderson Hospital and Tumor Institute, Houston p 17–22
Gorin N C et al 1988 in preparation
Gottlieb D J, Heslop H E, Prentice H G, Brenner M K 1988 British Journal of Haematology 69: 104
Gratwohl A, Zwaan F G, Hermans J, Lykleman A 1986 Bone Marrow Transplantation 1 (suppl 1): 177–181
Gratwohl A, Hermans J, Barrett A J et al 1988 Lancet i: 1379–1382
Griffin J D, Larcom P, Schlossman S F 1983 Blood 62: 1300
Grob J-P, Grundy J E, Prentice H G et al 1987 Lancet i: 774–776

Hagenbeek A, Martens A C M 1983 In: Gale R P (ed) Recent advances in bone marrow transplantation. Liss, New York, p 717

Hale G, Bright S, Chumbley G et al 1983 Blood 62: 873

Hale G, Cobbold S, Waldmann H 1988 Transplantation (in press)

Hansen J A, Beatty P G, Anasette C et al 1987 Progress in bone marrow transplantation. Fourth international symposium on bone marrow transplantation p 667–675

Hazlehurst G R, Brenner M K, Wimperis J Z, Knowles S M, Prentice H G 1986 Scandinavian Journal of Haematology 37: 1–3

Helenglass G, Lakhani A, Powles R et al 1987 Hematological Oncology 5: 245–254

Herve P, Tamayo E, Peters A 1983 British Journal of Haematology 53: 683

Herve P and the French study group on autologous bone marrow transplantation in acute leukemia 1984 In: Dicke K A, Spitzer G, Zander A R (eds) Autologous bone marrow transplantation in acute leukemia: a French review of 120 patients. Autologous Bone Marrow Transplantation, The University of Texas and MD Anderson Hospital and Tumor Institute, Houston, p 23

Herzig R H, Bortin M M, Barrett A J 1987 Lancet i: 786–788

Heslop H E, Price G M, Prentice H G et al 1988 Journal of Immunology 140: 3461–3467

Hoelzer D, Thiel E, Löffler H et al 1984 Blood 64: 38–47

Hoelzer D, Gale R P 1987 Seminars in Hematology 24: 27–39

Hows J, Beddoe K, Gordon-Smith E et al 1986 Blood 67: 177–181

Janossy G, Prentice H G, Grob J-P et al 1986 Clinical and Experimental Immunology 63: 577–586

Johnson F L, Thomas E D, Clark B S, Chard R L, Hartmann J R, Storb R 1981 New England Journal of Medicine 305: 846–851

Kaizer H, Stuart R K, Brookmeyer R et al 1985 Blood 65: 1504–1510

Kashahara T, Djeu J Y, Dougherty S F, Oppenheim J J 1983 Journal of Immunology 131: 2329

Keever C A, Welte K, Small T et al 1987 Blood 70: 1893–1903

Knight W A, Roodman G D, Clark G M 1983 Proceedings of the American Association Cancer Research 14: 163 (Abstract)

Kohler G, Milstein C 1975 Nature 256: 495–497

Leger O, Brenner M K, Drexler H G, Reittie J E, Secker-Walker L, Prentice H G 1987 British Journal of Haematology 67: 273–279

Linch D C, Knott L J, Patterson K G, Cowan D A, Harper P G 1982 Journal of Clinical Pathology 35: 186

Lindholm A, Zucker W, Ringden O, Lonnqvist B 1986 Bone Marrow Transplantation 1: 1–372

Lopez C, Kirkpatrick D, Livnat S et al 1980 Proceedings of the National Academy of Sciences USA. 79: 2663

Lowenberg B, Bauman J 1984 In: Lowenberg B, Hagenbeek J (eds) Minimal residual disease in acute leukemia. Martin Nijhoff, The Hague. p 197

Lum L G 1987 Blood 69: 369–380

Lum L G, Seigneuret M C, Storb R F et al 1981 Blood 58: 431

Lopez C, Kirkpatrick D, Livnat S et al 1980 Lancet ii: 1025

Malkovsky M, Brenner M K, Hunt R et al 1986 Cellular Immunology 103: 476–481

Marcus R E, Catovsky D, Prentice H G et al 1987 In: Büchner, Schellong, Hiddemann, Urbanitz, Ritter (eds) Haematology and Blood Transfusion 30: 346–351. Springer-Verlag, Berlin

Martin P J, Hansen J A, Buckner C D et al 1985 Blood 66: 664–672

Mitsuyasu R T, Champlin R E, Ho W G et al 1986 Annals of Internal Medicine 105: 20–26

Nadler L M, Ritz J, Griffin J D et al 1982 Progress in Haematology 12: 187

O'Reilly R J, Colling N H, Brochstein J et al 1986 In: Hagenbeek, Löwenerg (eds) Minimal residual disease in acute leukemia. p 337

Pahwa S G, Pahwa R N, Friedrich W et al 1982 Proceedings of the National Academy of Science USA 79: 2663

Patterson J, Prentice H G, Brenner M K et al 1986 British Journal of Haematology 63: 221–230

Perreault V, Pelletier M, Landry D, Gyger M 1984 Blood 63: 807–811

Pollard C M, Powles R L, Millar J L 1986 Lancet (Letter) ii: 1343

Powles R L, Barrett A J, Clink H M, Kay H E M, Sloane J, McElwain T J 1978 Lancet ii: 1327–1331

Powles R L, Clink H M, Spence D et al 1980a Lancet i: 327

Powles R L, Morgenstern G, Clink H M et al 1980b Lancet i: 1047

Prentice H G, Ganeshaguru K, Bradstock K F et al 1980c Lancet i: 170

Prentice H G, Blacklock H A, Janossy G et al 1982 Lancet i: 700–704

Prentice H G, Blacklock H A, Janossy G et al 1984 Lancet i: 472–476

Prentice H G, Zwaan F E, Hermans J 1988a Bone marrow transplantation (in press)

Prentice H G, Burnett A K, Brenner M K et al 1988b T cell depletion for acute leukaemia in first remission — a 5 year follow up report (in preparation)

Prentice H G, Goldman J, Waldmann H et al 1988c Immunological conditioning for unrelated donor transplants (in preparation)

Price G, Brenner M K, Prentice H G, Hoffbrand A V, Newland A C 1987 British Journal of Cancer 55: 287–290

Pui C-H, Crist W M 1987 Blood Reviews 1: 25–33

Rees J K H, Gray R G, Swirsky D, Hayhoe F G J 1986 Lancet ii: 1236–1241

Reisner Y, Kapoor N, O'Reilly R J, Good R A 1980 Lancet ii: 20–27

Reisner Y, Kapoor N, Kirkpatrick D et al 1981 Lancet ii: 327–331

Reittie J E, Leger O, Gottlieb D et al 1988a Analysis of endogenously generated activated killer cells after autologous and allogeneic bone marrow transplantation (submitted)

Reittie J E, Poulter L W, Prentice H G et al 1988b Transplantation 45: 1084–1090

Riehm H, Feickert H-J, Schrappe M, Henze G, Schellong G 1987 In: Büchner, Schellong, Hiddemann, Urbanitz, Ritter (eds) Haematology and Blood Transfusion 30: 139–158. Springer-Verlag, Berlin

Ringden O, Lonnqvist B, Sundberg B 1987 Lancet (Letter) ii: 105–106

Ringden O, Backman L, Tollemar J, Lonnqvist B 1988 Journal of Cellular Biochemistry Suppl 12c: 94

Ritz J, Sallan S E, Bast R C Jr et al 1982 Lancet ii: 60

Rodt H, Kolb H J, Netzel B et al 1981 Transplantation Proceedings 13: 257–261

Rooney C M, Wimperis J Z, Brenner M K, Patterson J, Hoffbrand A V, Prentice H G 1986 British Journal of Haematology 62: 413–420

Sallan S E, Bast R C, Lipton J M, Ritz J 1984 In: Lowenberg B, Hagenbeek J (eds) Minimal residual disease in acute leukemia. Martin Nijhoff, The Hague p 255

Saltzman R L, Quirk M R, Jordan M C 1988 Journal of Clinical Investigation 81: 75–81

Sanders J E, Thomas E D, Buckner C D et al 1985 Blood 66: 460–462

Santos G W, Colvin O M 1986 In: Goldstone A H (ed) Clinics in Haematology 15(1): 67–83

Santos G W, Tutschka P J, Brookmeyer R et al 1983 New England Journal of Medicine 309: 1347–1353

Santos G W, Yeater A M, Saral R 1987 In: Büchner, Schellong, Hiddemann, Urbanitz, Ritter (eds) Haematology and blood transfusion 30: 226–232. Springer-Verlag, Berlin

Saxon A, Mitsuyasu R, Stevens R, Champlin R E, Kimata H, Gale R P 1986 Journal of Clinical Investigation 78: 959

Scala G, Allavena P, Djeu J Y, Kasahara T, Ortaldo J R 1984 Nature 309: 57

Simonsson B, Burnett A K, Prentice H G et al 1988 Autologous bone marrow transplantation with monoclonal antibody purged marrow for high risk acute lymphoblastic leukaemia (submitted)

Singer C R J, Tansey P H, Burnett A K 1983 Clinical and Experimental Immunology 51: 455

Spitzer G, Verma D S, Fisher R et al 1980 Blood 55: 317

Stepan D E, Bartholomew R M, LeBien T W 1984 Blood 53: 1120

Stiff P J, Wustrow T, DeRisi M et al 1982 Blood 60: (1), 17a

Storb R 1985 Experimental Hematology (suppl 17) 13: 6–8

Storb R, Epstein R B, Graham T C et al 1970 Transplantation 9: 240–246

Storb R, Deeg H J, Whitehead J et al 1985 Blood 5 (suppl 1): 66

Sullivan K M, Deeg H J, Sanders J, Shulman H, Storb R, Thomas E D 1985 Blood 65 (suppl 1): 262a

Talpaz M, Kantarijian H M, McCredie K, Trujillo J M, Keating M J, Gutterman J U 1986 New England Journal of Medicine 314: 1065–1069

Thomas E D 1986 Cold Spring Harbor Symposia on Quantitative Biology, Volume L1

Thomas E D, Storb R, Clift R A et al 1975 New England Journal of Medicine 292: 832–843, 895–902

Thorpe P E, Mason D W, Brown A N F et al 1982 Nature 297: 594

To L B, Dyson P G, Banford A L et al 1987 Bone Marrow Transplantation 2: 103

Treleaven J G, Kemshead J T 1985 Hematology & Oncology 3: 65–75

Trigg M E, Billing R, Sondell P M et al 1985 Cancer Treatment Reports 69: 377

Trowsdale J, Young J A T, Kelly A P et al 1985 Immunological Review 85: 5

Uphoff D E 1958 Proceedings of the Society of Experimental and Biological Medicine 99: 651–653

Vyakarnam A, Brenner M K, Reittie J E, Lachmann P J 1985 European Journal of Immunology 15: 606

Wagemaker G, Vriesendorp H M, Van Bekkum D W 1981 Transplantation Proceedings 13: 875

Weiden P L, Flournoy N, Thomas E D 1978 New England Journal of Medicine 300: 1068–1073

Weinstein H, Grier H, Gelber R et al 1987 In: Büchner, Schellong, Hiddemann, Urbanitz, Ritter (eds) Haematology and Blood Transfusion 30: 88–92. Springer-Verlag, Berlin

Weinstein H J, Mayer R J, Rosenthal D S, Coral F S, Camitta B M, Gelber R D 1983 Blood 62: 315–319

Welte K, Ciobanu N, Moore M A S, Gulati S, O'Reilly R J, Mertelsmann R 1984 Blood 64: 380

Welte K, Keever C A, Levick J et al 1987 Blood 70: 1595–1603

Wimperis J Z, Brenner M K, Prentice H G et al 1986 Lancet i: 339–343

Wimperis J Z, Brenner M K, Drexler H G, Campana D, Hoffbrand A V, Prentice H G 1987a Clinical and Experimental Immunology 69: 601–608

Wimperis J Z, Brenner M K, Prentice H G, Thompson E J, Hoffbrand A V 1987b Journal of Immunology 138: 2445–2450
Witherspoon R P, Storb R, Ochs H P et al 1981 Blood 58: 360
Witherspoon R P, Lum L G, Storb R, Thomas E D 1982 Blood 59: 844
Witherspoon R P, Matthews D, Storb R et al 1984a Transplantation 37: 145
Witherspoon R P, Lum L G, Storb R 1984b Seminars in Haematology 21: 2–10
Wolff S N, Herzig R H, Phillips G L 1987 Seminars in Oncology 14 (2) suppl 1: 12–17
Woods W G, Nesbit M E, Ramsay N K C et al 1983 Blood 61: 1182–1189
Yates J, Glidewell O, Wiernik P et al 1982 Blood 60: 454–462
Zander A R, Vellekoop L, Spitzer G et al 1981 Cancer Treatment Reports 65: 377
Zwaan F E, Jansen J 1984 Seminars in Hematology 21: 35–42

9. Chronic lymphocytic leukemia and related diseases

K. A. Foon   R. P. Gale

Chronic lymphocytic leukemia (CLL) is a hematologic neoplasm characterized by proliferation and accumulation of relatively mature-appearing lymphocytes. In most cases a single clone of B lymphocytes undergoes malignant transformation; a small proportion of cases involve T lymphocytes. CLL is the commonest leukemia in the United States and Europe, accounting for approximately 30% of all cases, but is extremely rare in the Orient. A familial tendency has been suggested, as well as concordance in several identical twins, but no pattern of inheritance has been reported (Conley et al 1980). Even in cases of concordance in twins, the molecular events are distinct, suggesting different transforming events (Brok-Simoni et al 1987). CLL typically occurs in persons over 50 years (median age, 60 years), but occasionally it develops in young adults or even children; it affects males more than females at a ratio of 2:1.

Recently, there have been important advances in our understanding of CLL. The complex immunology, cell physiology, and biochemistry associated with CLL have become more fully appreciated. Various chromosomal abnormalities, a suggested viral etiology, and major molecular discoveries have also been reported. We review recent developments in the biology and treatment of CLL.

Immune features

In most instances, CLL develops from the malignant transformation of an immature B lymphocyte; a small proportion of cases (less than 5%) involve T lymphocytes. When CLL occurs in B lymphocytes, the disease is clonal. Clonality is suggested by the expression of a single immunoglobulin light chain, either kappa (κ) or lambda (λ), on the cell surface membrane (Aisenberg & Bloch 1976a). More sophisticated techniques have confirmed clonality by showing unique immunoglobulin-idiotype specificities, a single pattern of glucose-6-phosphate dehydrogenase activity, clonal chromosomal abnormalities, or immunoglobulin gene rearrangements (Hamblin et al 1980, Fialkow et al 1978, Korsmeyer 1985). Patients with T cell CLL may also have clonal chromosomal abnormalities and likely will have clonal rearrangements of T cell antigen receptor genes as reported for other T cell malignancies (Minden et al 1985).

CLL typically involves small, relatively mature-appearing cells with round, compact nuclei and clumped chromatin without distinct nucleoli (Fig. 9.1 Top). These cells are similar to those observed in malignant lymphoma, small lymphocytic (Fig. 9.1 Bottom) by the working formulation (Non-Hodgkins Lymphoma Project 1982) or diffuse well-differentiated lymphocytic lymphoma by the Rappaport classification. The B lymphocytes characteristic of CLL display a relatively small amount of surface immunoglobulin, cytoplasmic immunoglobulin can also be identified, and distinct differences at the molecular level between cytoplasmic, surface, and secretory

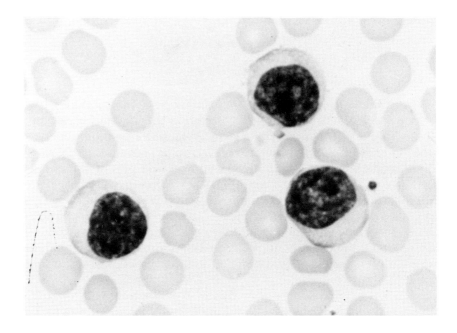

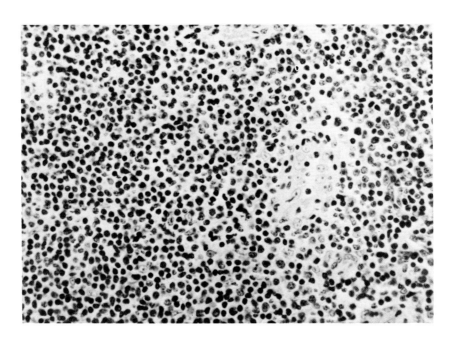

Fig. 9.1   (Top) Chronic lymphocytic leukemia (Wright's stain; original magnification, ×800). (Bottom) Malignant lymphoma, small lymphocytic (hematoxylin and eosin; original magnification, ×65).

immunoglobulin have been reported (Rubartelli et al 1983).

Immunoglobulin isotype analysis indicate that most cells display a single heavy chain class, typically (μ). Some cells display both μ and δ. Less commonly, gamma, alpha, or no heavy chain determinant is found. CLL cells display either κ or λ light chains but never both. Some data suggest that heavy chain switching can occur in B-CLL consistent with increasing maturity of the malignant cell (Ligler et al 1983). Other studies suggest that CLL cells contain only μ, or μ and δ, and that γ is extrinsic and not synthesized by the leukemia cells (Stevenson et al 1981). One characteristic feature of CLL cells is the excess production of free light chains. Whether this production represents an abnormality of the malignant cell or is typical of all B cells at this level of development is unknown. Using high-resolution electrophoresis/immuno-fixation, circulating monoclonal IgM paraproteins can be identified in 25–50% or more of patients (Deegan et al 1984). In some instances oligoclonal immunoglobulin is detected in patients with CLL; rarely, patients may have biclonal M-components. Recently, Cooper and coworkers (Cooper et al 1985) have shown that a small proportion of plasma cells from patients with B-CLL express the same idiotype as the malignant cells, indicating that the concept that the cells are 'frozen' at a specific level of maturation is not correct.

Other surface features of CLL cells are listed in Table 9.1. The cells have receptors

Table 9.1   Surface features of chronic lymphocytic leukemia cells

Present
Low intensity immunoglobulin staining on the cell surface membrane
Heavy chain, usually μ or μ and δ
Light chain κ or λ
Mouse erythrocyte receptors
Complement receptors (CR2 > CR1)
Ia antigens
Fc-receptor for IgG
B cell-associated antigens CD19, CD20, CD21, CD24 and others
T cell-associated antigen CD5 and TQ1

Absent
T-cell antigens (other than those listed above)
CD10 (CALLA) antigen
Sheep erythrocyte receptor
Terminal deoxynucleotidyl transferase

for mouse erythrocytes, a marker of immature B lymphocytes, as well as receptors for the Fc fragment of IgG and for complement. There is a relative increase of C'3d receptors (CR2) over C'3b receptors (CR1) typical of immature B cells. CLL cells show several antigens, including D-related human leukocyte antigens (HLA-DR or Ia) and human B cell antigens such as BA-1 or CD24, B1 or CD20, B2 or CD21, and B4 or CD19 (Foon & Todd 1986). CLL cells do not express the common acute lymphoblastic leukemia antigen (CALLA or CD10). A recently described antigen termed cCLLa, molecular weight 69 kilodaltons, has been reported to be expressed on the surface membrane of all patients cells with B cell CLL and hairy cell leukemia (Agee et al 1986). This antigen was not reported on normal lymphocytes or any other B cell or T cell malignancies. In contrast, FMC-7, an antigen common to hairy cell leukemia and prolymphocytic leukemia, is uncommon on CLL cells (Brooks et al 1981). One unanticipated finding was that CLL cells display a 65–69 kilodalton glycoprotein antigen (CD5) identified by the anti-Leu-1, T101, and anti-T1 monoclonal antibodies that was previously thought to be restricted to T lymphocytes (Foon & Todd 1986). The precise meaning of this anomalous expression of a T cell antigen is unclear. Recent studies report a normal B cell counterpart in human tonsil lymph nodes that expresses this surface antigen and may be the normal cell counterpart of CLL cells (Caligaris-Cappio et al 1982). Terminal deoxynucleotidyl transferase is not present in CLL cells.

Cell differentiation

The malignant B lymphocyte that is the usual target of transformation in CLL is an intermediate cell with some but not all morphologic features of mature B cells. The lymphocyte appears to be 'frozen' in its normal differentiation scheme and does not normally progress to the final stages of B cell development. Incubation of CLL cells in vitro with tumor promotors such as phorbol esters or B cell mitogens induces the cells to differentiate into an activated cell similar to prolymphocytic leukemia (PL) cells (Totterman et al 1980, Robert et al 1983) or mature-appearing plasma cells (Fu et al 1978). Under these conditions, the cells may begin to actively secrete immunoglobulin. Mitogen-induced switching from cell surface IgM to secreted IgG has also been reported (Juliusson et al 1983). These changes are associated with development of the endoplasmic reticulum and other morphologic features typical of mature plasma cells. Immunoglobulin secretion is preceded by a rapid increase in mRNA coding for the secretory form of IgM (Cossman et al 1984). This preferential transcription of secretory rather than membrane mRNA is similar to that seen in plasma cells. Under certain circumstances, cells resembling hairy cells with filamental projections develop when typical CLL cells are treated with phorbol ester (Caligaris-Cappio et al 1985) and in a synergistic fashion with phorbol ester and calcium ionophore (Drexler et al 1987). This finding is consistent with recent data suggesting that hairy cell leukemia cells have immunologic surface markers consistent with a more mature B cell than CLL cells, and in fact have some features of 'pre-plasma cells' (Anderson et al 1985). These data suggest that the malignant B cells typical of CLL are not irreversibly frozen at an immature level of B cell development but can be driven to mature end cells (plasma cell) under appropriate in vitro conditions. An alternative view is that the malignant cell in B-CLL represents a rare B cell phenotype rather than a cell frozen at one step of maturation.

Other chronic lymphocytic leukemias

Our current classification of the chronic lymphoid leukemias is shown in Table 9.2. Although a detailed analysis is beyond the scope of this chapter, certain morphologic and clinical features deserve discussion.

In contrast to the cell that appears morphologically mature, typical of B-derived CLL, B-derived PL is characterized by larger, less mature-appearing cells with condensed nuclear chromatin and prominent nucleoli (Galton et al 1974). Expression of surface immunoglobulin is increased and mouse-rosette formation is decreased, as compared with CLL cells. PL cells typically have cytogenetic abnormalities, particularly those involving chromosome 14. In contrast, abnormalities of chromosome 12 are present in 50% of cases of B-CLL, abnormalities of chromosome 14 are not as common (Brito-Bapapulle et al 1987). FMC-7 antigen is typically found on PL

Table 9.2 Clinical and laboratory features of the chronic leukemias. *Key:* $T_{H/I}$, helper/inducer phenotype; $T_{C/S}$, T cytotoxic/suppressor phenotype; HTLV, human T cell leukemia/lymphoma virus.

	Median age at diagnosis (years)	Male/female	Leukocyte count ($\times 10^9/l$)	Lymph nodes (%)	Spleen (%)	Skin (%)	Other
B lymphocytes							
Chronic lymphocytic leukemia	60	2/1	10–200	50	50	5	
Prolymphocytic leukemia	65	4/1	100 to >500	25	>90	5	—
Waldenstrom's macroglobulinemia	50	1/1	Normal to 50	30	30	<5	Elevated IgM
Leukemic phase of poorly differentiated lymphoma (follicular or diffuse)	50	2/1	Normal to >100	90	75	5	—
Hairy cell leukemia	50	5/1	<1–100	30	>75	<5	Pancytopenia
T lymphocytes							
Chronic lymphocytic leukemia	60	M > F	>20–200	50	50	10	—
Adult T cell leukemia/lymphoma	40	M > F	Normal to >150	90	>50	>50	$T_{H/I}$, HTVL-1, hypercalcemia, lytic bone lesions
Prolymphocytic leukemia	60	M > F	100 to >500	25	>90	<10	—
T gamma-chronic lymphoproliferative disease	50	2/1	Normal to >30	10	30	<10	$T_{C/S}$, granulocytopenia
Cutaneous T cell lymphoma	50	M > F	Normal to >150	>50	10	100	$T_{H/I}$
Hairy cell leukemia	0–60	M > F	Lowered	30	>75	—	HTLV-2

cells but not on B-CLL cells (Brooks et al 1981). Conversely, CD5 reactivity is far greater on CLL cells than PL cells. It is generally agreed that the blastic morphology is a marker of cellular activation (Robert et al 1983). Several clinical and laboratory features are also distinctive of B-PL including extreme leukocytosis ($>100 \times 10^9$) and prominent splenomegaly, without substantial lymphadenopathy. A small but significant proportion of otherwise typical cases of CLL undergo transformation to a 'prolymphocytoid' leukemia (Enno et al 1979).

The relationship between PL and CLL is complex (Table 9.3). At the extremes

Table 9.3 Relationship between CLL, CLL/PL and PL. *Key:* M-RFC, mouse-rosette forming cells; IGIR, G, germline; R, rearranged.

	CLL	CLL/PL	PL
Age	60	60	70
WBC($\times 10^9$/l)	10–200	10–200	>100–>500
%PL	<10%	10–55%	>55%
↑ spleen	+ +	+ + +	+ + + +
↑ lymph nodes	+ +	+ + + +	+ + + +
M-RFC	>50%	>50%	<30%
CD5	>50%	>50%	<50%
FMC-7	<20%	<20%	>50%
SmIg	+/−	+/− to + +	+ + + +
Chromosomes	+12 (50%)	+12	14q+ (100%)

are classic CLL and classic PL. The prolymphocytoid variant of CLL has some features of both diseases. Clinically, there is a spectrum of increasing aggressiveness more like PL. While the cells morphologically appear 'activated' and look like classic PL cells, they share most phenotypic features with CLL cells (Melo et al 1987).

In Waldenström's macroglobulinemia the malignant lymphocytes have plasmacytoid features (Krajny & Pruzanski 1976), often with abundant basophilic cytoplasm. The periodic-acid-Schiff reaction is frequently positive, indicating the presence of polysaccharide; occasionally, this occurs in globules leading to the term 'grape cells.' The cells typically have both surface and cytoplasmic IgM, and secrete substantial IgM into the serum resulting in a monoclonal peak on protein electrophoresis. An increase in relative serum viscosity is found in about two thirds of patients; only half of these have symptoms associated with hyperviscosity. Waldenström's macroglobulinemia has a peak incidence in the sixth and seventh decades, and is frequently an indolent disease with prolonged survival. With disease progression, lymphadenopathy, splenomegaly, and hepatomegaly become prominent and the clinical pattern resembles a lymphoma. In contrast to multiple myeloma, bone lesions are infrequent.

A fourth type of chronic B-derived leukemia is sometimes referred to as 'lymphosarcoma cell leukemia' (Isaacs 1937). This condition usually represents the leukemic phase of a follicular or diffuse small cleaved-cell lymphoma, but can rarely represent the leukemic phase of large-cell lymphomas (histiocytic) or Burkitt's lymphoma. The typical cells from follicular or diffuse lymphomas are often pleomorphic with small, prominent nucleoli (nuclear clefting), and a finer chromatin pattern than typical CLL cells. This disorder typically presents as a lymphoma rather than as leukemia, but up to one half of patients have bone marrow involvement at diagnosis. Some patients present with bone marrow and peripheral blood involvement without lymph node involvement, which is difficult to distinguish from CLL. In the absence of a lymph node biopsy, the diagnosis should be made by morphologic features as well as immunologic features associated with poorly differentiated lymphomas, such as lack of mouse erythrocyte rosetting, normal capping, and bright surface membrane immunoglobulin fluorescence (Aisenberg 1976b). Most cases of poorly differentiated lymphoma do not express the CD5 antigen identified by the T101, anti-Leu-1 and equivalent antibodies, whereas almost all cases of CLL react with these antibodies (Foon & Todd 1986). Furthermore, most cases of follicular lymphomas express the common acute lymphoblastic leukemia antigen, whereas CLL cells do not (Ritz et al 1981).

The term 'lymphosarcoma cell leukemia' is best avoided. Lymphoma with bone marrow and peripheral blood involvement should indicate the histiologic subtype followed by a notation of hematologic involvement. If there is no lymph node involvement, the morphologic and immunologic features of poorly differentiated lymphoma cells described above should distinguish them from CLL cells. The distinction between poorly differentiated lymphoma cells and prolymphocytic leukemia cells is less clear; immunologic features are similar, and proper identification rests on morphologic and clinical parameters such as the extremely high leukocyte count and the extensive splenomegaly without lymph node enlargement that is typical of prolymphocytic leukemia.

Hairy cell leukemia is a fifth form of B lymphocyte-derived chronic leukemia. The disease is so-termed because 'hairy' cytoplasmic projections are sometimes visible under light, phase, or electronmicroscopy (Bouroncle 1958, Golomb et al 1978). The cells are of moderate size, with eccentric, oval nuclei; spongy chromatin; and variably prominent nucleoli. Monoclonal surface immunoglobulin is found in most cases and the cells often react with B cell-specific monoclonal antibodies (Foon & Todd 1986). The cells may be phagocytic and usually contain tartrate-resistant isoenzyme 5 of acid phosphatase (Yam et al 1971). Hairy cell leukemia has a marked male predominance with pancytopenia and prominent splenomegaly. Although most patients are leukopenic, some have a leukocytosis with a high percentage of hairy cells.

The chronic T lymphocyte leukemias are also shown in Table 9.2. These disorders parallel to a large extent the leukemias of the B lymphocyte axis. Six interrelated syndromes characterized by proliferation of T lymphocytes have been reported. Although there is some overlap in morphologic features, we feel it is useful to distinguish these syndromes at present. These disorders are T-CLL, adult T cell leukemia/lymphoma (ATL), T-PL, chronic T-gamma-lymphoproliferative disease, cutaneous T cell lymphoma (Sézary syndrome/mycosis fungoides), and T-hairy cell leukemia.

The leukemic cells in T-CLL are morphologically indistinguishable from the B cell form of the disease. T-CLL accounts for less than 5% of cases of CLL. The only distinctive clinical feature is an increased frequency of skin involvement. ATL is more aggressive than CLL and occurs in slightly younger individuals of median age 50 years. It is included in the chronic leukemias because of the mature appearance of the cells which are described as small pleomorphic with convoluted nuclei (Uchiyama et al 1977, Bunn et al 1983). In contrast to B-derived CLL, skin involvement in ATL occurs in up to two thirds of cases; splenomegaly and hepatomegaly occur in

50%. 35% of patients have lytic bone lesions associated with hypercalcemia. Leukocytes are typically greater than $50 \times 10^9/l$. In most instances the T helper subset is involved and human T cell leukemia/lymphoma virus-1 (HTLV-1) has been isolated from several cases. Serum from almost all patients contains antibodies to HTLV-1. Two forms of ATL have been identified, an endemic form in Japan, the Carribean and the southwest United States and non-endemic forms. These are relatively rare disorders, less than 500 cases have been reported worldwide. The T-derived variant of PL is morphologically identical to B cell PL, but is more often associated with lymphadenopathy than the B cell variant (Catousky et al 1973).

A new disorder termed chronic T-gamma-lymphoproliferative disease or natural killer cell leukemia has recently been reported (Reynolds & Foon 1984, Newland et al 1984). The distinguishing morphologic feature is the presence of abundant cytoplasm usually containing azurophilic granules. These cells have been termed large granular lymphocytes. Clinical features include relatively low levels of circulating leukocytes and granulocytopenia; recurrent infections are common, whereas lymphadenopathy and skin involvement are typically absent.

A fifth type of T cell chronic leukemia typically occurs in patients with prominent cutaneous involvement and is referred to as cutaneous T cell lymphoma or Sézary syndrome/mycosis fungoides (Lutzner et al 1975). The cells are typically large with cerebriform nuclei, coarse chromatin, and inconspicuous nucleoli. Cutaneous T cell lymphoma occurs in younger persons more often than does typical CLL. Mycosis fungoides refers to the cutaneous form of this desease, which may be present for several years before the development of clinically evident systemic involvement. When both skin and systemic involvement occur, the disease is referred to as the Sézary syndrome.

The final form of T cell chronic leukemia is the T cell equivalent of B hairy cell leukemia (Saxon et al 1978). Morphologic, clinical, and laboratory features are similar to the B cell form, but the T cell form is extremely rare. Immune studies are used to distinguish the two forms. Recently, a second retrovirus, human T cell leukemia/lymphoma virus-II, has been isolated from cases of T derived hairy cell leukemia (Kalyanaraman et al 1982).

Lymphoproliferative disorders and normal lymphopoiesis

A proposed scheme of B lymphoid development is shown in Figure 9.2. This scheme is based primarily on detailed studies of malignant B cells. Stem cells committed to B lymphocyte development are the earliest detectable precursors. Although some investigators have developed putative assays for B lymphoid stem cells, none is uniformly accepted and morphologic identification of these cells has not been accomplished. These cells probably express surface Ia antigens and nuclear terminal deoxynucleotidyl transferase. It seems likely that the most primitive non-T acute lymphoblastic leukemia cells reflect this phenotype.

At a relatively early stage of development, the cells display surface antigens typical of B lymphocytes beginning with the CD19 antigen and followed by CD20, CD24, and CD21 (Nadler et al 1984). The (CLLA) CD10 antigen is also expressed early in B-cell differentiation and can be induced in early B cells by incubation with phorbol esters (Nadler et al 1982). On a molecular level, the earliest detectable commitment to B cell development is the rearrangement of heavy chain immunoglobulin genes followed by rearrangement of light chain genes proceeding from mu to kappa

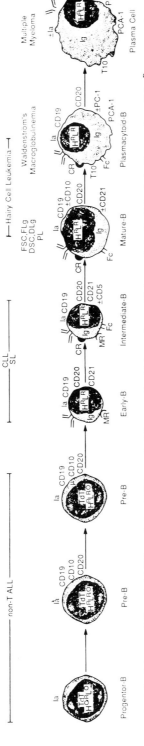

Fig. 9.2 Scheme of B lymphoid differentiation. TdT, terminal deoxynucleotidyl transferase; H, heavy chain; L, light chain; ^{R}, rearranged allele; MR, mouse rosette receptor; CR, complement receptor; Fc,Fc receptor for IgG; ALL, acute lymphoblastic leukemia; CLL, chronic lymphocytic leukemia; SL, malignant lymphoma, small lymphocytic; FSC, malignant lymphoma, follicular small cleaved cell; FLg, malignant lymphoma, follicular large cell; DSC, malignant lymphoma, diffuse small cleaved cell; DLg, malignant lymphoma, diffuse large cell; PL, prolymphocytic leukemia.

to lambda (Korsmeyer 1985). If these gene rearrangements are unproductive, the cell cannot develop along the normal B cell axis.

The next identifiable level of B cell differentiation involves expression of the rearranged immunoglobulin heavy chain genes in the form of an intracytoplasmic mu chain; kappa or lambda light chain expression is not detected, although productive light chain gene rearrangements may have already occurred. Cells at this stage are commonly referred to as pre-B cells and their malignant counterpart is the pre-B acute lymphoblastic leukemia cell (Foon & Todd 1986).

After successful immunoglobulin gene rearrangement, the cells begin to show surface membrane immunoglobulin, usually IgM with or without IgD. These immature B cells have receptors for mouse erythroytes. These are the likely normal counterpart to CLL cells and malignant lymphoma, small lymphocytic cells (Non-Hodgkin's Lymphoma Project 1982). As the cells continue to mature, surface IgM increases and the cells lose receptors for mouse erythrocytes and acquire the ability to synthesize and secrete immunoglobulin after antigen stimulation. The shift from intracytopasmic to membrane and finally to secreted forms of IgM is accomplished by differential mRNA splicing. On a cellular level the process of B cell differentiation is characterized by differences between lymphoma cells, PL cells, hairy cell leukemia, and Waldenström's macroglobulinemia cells. Mature B cells are further capable of switching from μ, or μ and δ, to γ α, or ε class immunoglobulin synthesis. Most data indicate that heavy chain switching occurs via genomic immunoglobulin-gene rearrangements.

In the final stages of B lymphocyte development, the cell is irreversibly committed to becoming a plasma cell. Surface markers typical of immature lymphocytes are lost as are surface immunoglobulin and B cell antigens including Ia. Interestingly, new surface antigens such as the PC-1 and PCA-1 antigens may be expressed (Foon & Todd 1986). The predominant feature of the plasma cell is the ability to synthesize and secrete large amounts of immunoglobulin of a specific isotype. The malignant counterpart to this cell is the myeloma cell. A parallel, albeit less detailed, scheme of the relationship between T cell chronic leukemias and normal T cell development has also been suggested (Foon & Todd 1986).

IMMUNE ASPECTS OF CHRONIC LYMPHOCYTIC LEUKEMIA

Immune function of chronic lymphocytic leukemia cells

Several investigators have studied the immune function of CLL cells. As indicated, low levels of surface Ig and absence of Ig capping suggest abnormalities of surface membrane motility. Despite the fact that CLL cells have Ia antigens, they show limited or no stimulatory activity in autologous and allogeneic mixed lymphocyte culture (Halper et al 1979). Other cell activities are also abnormal, including in vitro response to B-cell mitogens such as pokeweed mitogen, lipopolysaccharide, and Epstein-Barr virus, and decreased activity in antibody-dependent cellular cytotoxicity (Smith et al 1972). CLL cells have a decreased proliferative response to B cell growth factor which is likely secondary to the impaired expression of cell surface receptors for B cell growth factors (Perri 1986). Cytochalasin B appears to be a potent mitogen for CLL cells (Larson & Yachnin 1983). Culture techniques that permit the in vitro growth in semisolid agar of colonies of malignant B cells derived from patients with

CLL have been reported (Perri & Kay 1982). These techniques may help analyze details of immune function in CLL.

Immune function of the T lymphocytes and natural killer cells

A significant increase in the absolute number of circulating T lymphocytes has been reported in untreated patients with CLL, and levels of T cells have been found to fluctuate during the course of the disease (Kay et al 1979). In general, patients with CLL show a marked inversion of the normal T-helper cell (CD4) to T suppressor cell (CD8) ratio in the peripheral blood (Kay 1981, Platsoucas et al 1982). There are increases in the percentage and absolute number of T suppressor cells; in some studies these correlated with the degree of hypogammaglobulinemia commonly seen with CLL. Additional T cell surface marker abnormalities include a decreased proportion of T cells reactive with the pan-T anti-CD3 antibody and the presence of circulating cells simultaneously expressing helper-associated and suppressor-associated antigens, a characteristic that is normally present on some thymocytes but not circulating T lymphocytes (Kay 1981). These abnormalities of T cell subsets may correlate with disease stage or therapy or both (Kay et al 1982).

Functional studies of T cells from patients with CLL indicate that mitogenic responses to plant lectins, such as phytohemagglutinin, are usually but not always normal (Han et al 1981). In contrast, reactivity to autologous or allogeneic B cells is impaired (Han et al 1982). The T progenitor cells, assayed by colony growth in semisolid agar, have been reported to be decreased in some (Foa et al 1980) but not all studies (Fernandez et al 1984). Spontaneous and antibody-dependent cytotoxicity are reduced, suggesting an abnormality in the large granular lymphocyte (natural killer cell) population (Platsoucas et al 1980). Reduced reactivity with the anti-Leu-11 antibody and additional antibodies that recognize normal natural killer activity have also been reported (Foa et al 1986). In another study, the emergence of a population of granular lymphocytes with natural killer cell markers (Leu-7 and M1) in addition to the helper antigen (CD4) was reported which may provide for an alternative explanation for the multiple functional T cell defects described in CLL patients (Velardi et al 1985).

Recently, functional studies of T helper and T suppressor cells in patients with CLL have been reported (Kay 1981, Kay et al 1982, Lauria et al 1983). Many of these data are contradictory and difficult to critically interpret. Most but not all studies suggest decreased T helper function; increased T suppressor function has been more difficult to convincingly establish. It is probable that patients with CLL are heterogeneous with regard to these abnormalities. Furthermore, disease stage and treatment are likely to be important determinants. Splenectomy and splenic irradiation have been reported to correct some T cell abnormalities, and some of the natural killer cell abnormalities can be corrected by in vitro or in vivo exposure of cells to either interferon or synthetic thymic hormones (Hokland & Ellegaard 1981, Lauria et al 1984).

The precise origin of these T cell abnormalities in CLL is unknown, and it is uncertain whether they are a cause or an effect of the disease. The T cells in CLL are probably not a product of the malignant clone, as indicated by the lack of chromosome abnormalities and by heterozygosity for glucose-6-phosphate dehydrogenase. It should be noted, however, that these studies have been performed on individuals with B-CLL or relatively brief duration; long lived T cells may have been tested that preceded the onset of leukemia. Therefore, this does not necessarily exclude involvement of a very immature stem cell with both T and B cell differentiation potential. Clonal rearrangement of the T cell β receptor has been reported in the malignant B cells in about 10% of cases of B-CLL suggesting its origin in a very immature B cell (O'Connor et al 1985, Norton et al 1988). It is also possible that abnormalities of additional cell populations such as macrophages may be responsible for some of the immune abnormalities typical of CLL. Finally, B cells may function abnormally in CLL by achieving independence from T cell regulation.

Hypogammaglobulinemia
Hypogammaglobulinemia occurs in approximately 50% of patients with CLL depending on the value used as the lower limit of normal. Infections, particularly with encapsulated microorganisms, are a frequent cause of morbidity and mortality (Cohn & Uhr 1964). The pathogenesis of hypogammaglobulinemia is poorly understood. The decreased immunoglobulin levels are probably the result of impaired B cell function. Several studies have reported decreased in vitro immunoglobulin synthesis in response to polyclonal mitogens or antigens (Fernandez et al 1983). Regulatory abnormalities of T cells may also be important in inducing hypogammaglobulinemia, including the reversal in T helper/T suppressor ratios. The hypogammaglobulinemia characteristic of CLL is likely to be the result of several interrelated factors.

Autoimmunity in chronic lymphocytic leukemia
Patients with CLL may develop features of autoimmunity. For example, autoimmune hemolytic anemia occurs in 10–25% of patients at some time during the course of the disease. These are often IgG antibodies and sometimes have specificity for the Rh blood group system, specifically the C antigen, although they are not always definable. Interestingly, these antibodies are not produced by the malignant B cell clone. Some patients develop either idiopathic thrombocytopenic purpura or neutropenia related to autoantibodies to platelets or neutrophils, respectively (Bergsagel 1967). Rarely, patients develop a syndrome resembling pure red cell aplasia; this is most commonly associated with T- rather then B-CLL (Mangan et al 1982). Why patients should develop these autoimmune disorders with such high frequency in CLL, particularly in the face of diminished B-cell function, is unknown. One interesting hypothesis is that in some cases previous radiation therapy and alkylating agents may 'trigger' autoimmune complication in some of these patients (Lewis et al 1966). Other theories relate autoimmune phenomena to the imbalance of T cell subsets characteristic in these patients (described above). Apparently this propensity to develop autoantibodies is not random but restricted to the hematopoietic system because there is no increased frequency of other autoantibodies such as antinuclear antibodies (Hamblin et al 1986). However, there is an increased risk of autoimmune diseases in relatives of patients with CLL (Conley et al 1980). It has recently been reported (Kipps et al 1986) that B cells from most patients with B-CLL are restricted to the V_kIIIb light chain sub-subtype. This sub-subtype also occurs in increased frequency in rheumatoid antibodies (anti-Ig antibodies) which occur in patients with rheumatoid arthritis. mRNAs from several patients with V_kIIIb positive CLL have been analyzed. These data show considerable sequence homology suggesting that κ light chains are derived from a limited number of conserved germline V_k genes.

Transformation

The phenotypic expression of CLL is usually stable over months to years. Rarely, the disease evolves into an acute phase. Several forms of transformation have been reported including development of a diffuse lymphoma (Richter Syndrome), 'prolymphocytoid' transformation, an acute (or blast) crisis, or progression into multiple myeloma.

In 1928, Richter (1928) reported the development of a lymphoma of large pleomorphic cells in a patient with typical CLL. Subsequently, more than 300 cases have been reported; the projected incidence is 3–15% of the total cases of CLL (Long & Aisenberg 1975). This syndrome has been variously termed Richter syndrome, reticulum cell sarcoma, or diffuse histocytic lymphoma. Some data, albeit limited, suggest that CLL and Richter syndrome can arise from a single transformed clone of B lymphocytes (Bertoli et al 1987). Transformation to a diffuse large-cell lymphoma is characterized by a rapidly evolving terminal illness with increasing tumor mass. In some cases, however, the cells display different heavy or light chains, as well as different rearrangements of heavy chain genes suggesting distinct B cell malignancies (Van Dongen et al 1984). This high frequency of independent large cell lymphomas in B-CLL is similar to that observed in other immune deficiency states such as severe combined immune deficiency, Wiskott-Aldrich syndrome and transplant recipients receiving immune suppression treatment.

We previously discussed PL as a distinct clinical entity with B and T cell variants. A small but significant proportion of patients with CLL will develop cells with morphologic features of prolymphocytes (Enno et al 1979). Usually, transformation to 'prolymphocytoid' leukemia occurs gradually over several years and is associated with increasing anemia, thrombocytopenia, lymphadenopathy, splenomegaly, and resistance to treatment. The blood usually contains two distinct populations, typical CLL cells and the immature-appearing 'prolymphocytoid' cells. The latter express the same immunoglobulin isotype as the CLL cells; unlike de-novo PL cells, these cells express little immunoglobulin on the surface membranes. This prolymphocytoid transformation of typical B-CLL should be distinguished from patients with CLL/PL from the time of diagnosis.

The third type of transformation in CLL is the development of acute (blast) crisis (Brouet et al 1973). Acute transformation occurs in less than 1% of patients with CLL. This contrasts with the invariant progression to acute transformation which occurs in patients with chronic myelogenous leukemia. In acute transformation of CLL, the cells are immature lymphoblasts with fine chromatin and prominent nuclei and in most cases have the L-2 structure usually found in adults with acute lymphoblastic leukemia (Bennett et al 1976). Patients with acute transformation of CLL have clinical and laboratory features of acute lymphoblastic leukemia in adults. Treatment with antileukemic chemotherapy is usually ineffective, perhaps as a result if the advanced age of the patients.

The final and rarest form of transformation involves differentiation into multiple myeloma. In most cases, the heavy and light chains of the myeloma cells have been reported to be identical to the CLL cells (Brouet et al 1985). Two separate clones were identified with anti-idiotype antibodies in a limited number of cases, suggesting the simultaneous occurrence of two unrelated diseases (Brouet et al 1985). In another case where a patient developed multiple myeloma 10 years after the diagnosis of

CLL was made, idiotypic determinants were shared by the myeloma IgG and IgA and the CLL cells (Fernand et al 1985).

Transformation of one morphologic subtype of lymphoma to another is not uncommon. Similarly, disease evolution in CLL is probably commoner than is generally appreciated. Although we have discussed transformation in the context of four distinct entities — diffuse histiocytic lymphoma (Richter's syndrome), 'prolymphocytoid' transformation, acute transformation, and multiple myeloma — it is reasonable to consider these as entities along a spectrum of B lymphoid differentiation.

Chromosomes

Detailed cytogenetic studies of chromosomes from patients with acute leukemia and chronic myelogenous leukemia indicate a high incidence of clonal chromosome abnormalities. It has been considerably more difficult to study chromosome abnormalities in cells from patients with CLL due to difficulty in obtaining sufficient metaphases for analysis. Recently, several investigators have reported clonal chromosome abnormalities using B cell mitogens such as pokeweed mitogen, lipopolysaccharide, protein A, or Epstein-Barr virus. Based on the most recent studies, these abnormalities have

Table 9.4   Common chromosome abnormalities reported in patients with B cell chronic lymphocytic leukemia

Chromosome abnormality	Comments
+12	Commonest; may also be seen in Waldenström's macroglobulinemia, hairy cell leukemia, and prolymphocytic leukemia
14q+	Found in B and T cell chronic lymphocytic leukemia
del(14q)	
t(11q;14q)	
inv(14q)	
del(3)(p13)	Prolymphocytic leukemia

been reported in 50% of patients (Table 9.4) (Han et al 1984c, d, Juliusson et al 1985, Pittman & Catovsky 1984).

Most abnormalities involve chromosome 12 and 14. Trisomy 12 is the commonest abnormality, although in one study the 14q+ marker was more frequently identified (Pittman & Catovsky 1984). Han and coworkers (Han et al 1984c) reported that trisomy 12 was usually the only abnormality in patients with early disease, whereas trisomy 12 in combination with other chromosome changes is more frequent in advanced disease (Han et al 1984c). Abnormalities were found in 20% of patients with stage 0, 33% of those with stage 1–2, and 75% of those with stage 3–4. The % of abnormal metaphases are correlated with the cytogenetic abnormality, 30% of those with +12, 60% of those with +12 and additional abnormalities, and 30% of those with abnormalities other than +12. These data suggest that trisomy 12 may be the earliest karyotypic change, and other chromosomal abnormalities result from clonal evolution, de-differentiation, or treatment. Interestingly, patients who had a normal karyotype did not develop karyotypic abnormalities with disease progression. In contrast, those with an abnormal karyotype and progression continued to exhibit an abnormal karyotype. In their study, survival for patients with trisomy 12 as the sole abnormality was not different from patients with normal karyotypes, whereas patients with additional abnormalities had poorer survival (Han et al 1984c). Response rates to therapy were also correlated with karyotype; 90% in those with a normal karyotype and 30% in those with an abnormal karyotype. This translated into a difference in 5 year survival of 70% versus 30%. Patients with abnormal karyotypes were also more likely to enter into a Richter syndrome.

In contrast, Juliusson and coworkers (Juliusson et al 1985) reported that patients with trisomy 12 required therapy earlier than patients with normal karyotypes. One possible explanation for these disparate results is that in the latter study there was a greater percentage of patients with more advanced disease with trisomy 12 as the sole abnormality, suggesting they were studying a different patient population. Both studies agreed, however, that patients with complex karyotype abnormalities had a poorer prognosis. A high incidence of trisomy 12 or 12q+ in patients with the closely related (or identical) disorder, malignant lymphoma, small lymphocytic cell has also been reported (Yunis et al 1982). Using a recently developed cytogenetic method that allows simultaneous analysis of cell morphology, immunologic phenotype and karyotype in the same mitotic cell, Knuutila and coworkers demonstrated that trisomy 12 in B cell CLL occurs in the neoplastic B cells but not in the T cells (Knuutila et al 1986). They propose that this provides an explanation for the common finding of mitoses with normal karyotypes in patients with CLL. These patients, therefore, had CLL for relatively brief periods. It is possible, therefore, albeit unlikely, that T cell involvement might not have been detected since most of these cells would have been produced prior to the onset of CLL.

Abnormalities of chromosome 14 are also common with 14q+ (breakpoint q32) the predominant finding (Pittman & Catovsky 1984). Interestingly, patients with T cell CLL more frequently have chromosome 14 abnormalities with breaks involving band q11 often associated with breaks at q32 (Zech et al 1984). Abnormalities of chromosome 14 are particularly common in patients with PL. Similar findings have been reported in patients with other types of T-cell leukemia/lymphomas, and in patients with ataxia telangiectasia which is a rare hereditary disorder characterized by cutaneous and cerebellum telangiectasia and immune deficiency. The latter have an increased risk of developing T cell CLL. Of interest is the recent mapping of the gene encoding the alpha-chain of the T cell receptor to chromosome 14 (Croce et al 1985). A number of cases of t(11;14)(q13;q32) have been reported and are discussed in the section on oncogenes.

Although the importance of these chromosomal abnormalities is unknown, it is interesting that most of the chromosomes involved in CLL contain either immunoglobulin genes such as 14(heavy chain), 2 (κ light chain), or 22(λ light chain) or cellular homologues of viral transforming genes (oncogenes) such as 8 (c-myc,c-mos), 12 (c-ras-Kirsten), or 11 (c-ras-Harvey). Mutation of Kirsten-ras, however, has recently been reported to be absent in B-CLL (Browett et al 1988).

Oncogenes

CLL shows some features similar to Burkitt's lymphoma, and because similar chromosomes can be involved in these disorders or their murine counterparts, it will be important to study CLL cells for evidence of oncogene rearrangements or abnormal immunoglobulin gene expression. Recently, two cell lines derived from patients with PL with a t(11;14) (q13;q32) translocation have been studied in detail (Tsujimoto et al 1984). The break on chromosome 14 occurs in the J region of the IgH locus.

The rearrangement on chromosome 11 involves a postulated oncogene designated B cell lymphoma/leukemia 1 (bcl-1) that appears involved in the transformation of human B cells with the t(11;14) translocation including a cell line from diffuse histiocytic lymphoma. No known human homologue of a retroviral transforming oncogene has been mapped to the long arm of chromosome 11. Interestingly, a high proportion of cases of B cell lymphoma, a related disorder, carry a t(14;18) translocation (Yunis et al 1987). In these cases, the abnormality on chromosome 18 seems to involve another putative oncogene B-cell lymphoma-2 or bcl-2. The mechanism of rearrangement between the IgH locus and bcl-2 appears to involve the aforementioned recombination normally implicated in immunoglobulin gene rearrangement.

Viruses and leukemia

The RNA tumor viruses (retroviruses) are a common cause of lymphoid leukemias in animals. There has been considerable effort to detect a viral origin for leukemias in man. In 1980, a type C retrovirus identified as the cause of an unusual form of T-cell leukemia in Japan termed adult T cell leukemia/lymphoma (ATL) (Gallo et al 1983). This virus does not contain conventional retroviral oncogenes, but recent data suggest that one of the viral genes encodes a trans-acting protein capable of stimulating other cellular genes (Sordoski et al 1984).

This type of leukemia is now known not to be restricted to Japan but occurs in the southeastern United States, the Carribean, and elsewhere. Recently, it has become apparent that there is a chronic form of ATL; in some instances this resembles T-CLL. Investigation of the leukemia cells show clonal integration of HTLV-1. Chronic ATL is typically manifest by cutaneous lesions with minimal involvement of spleen or lymph nodes. Other related disorders which have been variously associated with HTLV-1 include persistent T lymphocytosis (Kinoshita et al 1985) and chronic T helper cell leukemia (Pandolfi et al 1985). Recently antibodies to HTLV-1 were reported in 6 of 17 patients from Jamaica with B-CLL; there was, however, no integration of provirus in these cases suggesting that HTLV-1 was not the etiologic agent.

A second related retrovirus HTLV-2 has also been identified. This has been reported in cases of T-PL and T cell hairy cell leukemia (Kalyanaraman et al 1982).

A preliminary report described isolation of retroviral-like particles and reverse transcriptase activity in cultured cells of patients with B derived CLL (Garver et al 1984). A monoclonal antibody was developed to the viral particles that cross-reacted with human T cell leukemia/lymphoma virus-I. Additionally, antibody to the 19 000-dalton core protein of human T cell leukemia/lymphoma virus-I reacted with this putative 'chronic lymphocytic leukemia virus.' Confirmation of this finding is lacking despite several years since the initial report.

The possible role of DNA viruses such as Epstein Barr Virus (EBV) or cytomegalovirus (CMV) in CLL is unknown. Direct involvement of EBV seems unlikely. B-CLL cells can be infected by EBV, as indicated by expression of Epstein Barr nuclear antigen (EBNA), but this does not lead to immortalization (Rickinson et al 1982). Recently, one EBV infected cell line was shown to produce tumors in nude mice (Lee et al 1986). However, a more likely role for EBV might be in causing a polyclonal expansion of B cells; a similar role has been discussed in the context of Burkitt lymphoma. It is sometimes referred to as 'hit and run'. Finally in one unusual case, complete regression of CLL was reported in a patient who developed severe disseminated Herpes zoster infection (Rozman, personal communication).

Animal models and a model of CLL

The unusual phenotype of B cells typical of B-CLL has been studied in a number of animal models: CBA/N mice carrying the X-linked immunodeficiency (Xid) genetic mutation and a series of Ly1 cell tumor models (BCL1, CH lymphomas, and the NFS-5 pre-B). CBA/N Xid mice (Scher 1982) lack a mature set of normal B lymphocytes (as defined by the Lyb-5 antigen) and are unable to respond to thymus-independent antigens. It is believed by some investigators that the lack of this mature B cell population leads to a reduced autoantibody production. There are several murine B cell tumors that express the Ly1 antigen (Davidson et al 1984) which is homologous to the human CD5 antigen which is found on CLL cells. Analogous to the human CD5 antigen on a minor population of B cells, Ly1-B-cell subpopulation can be identified in certain strains of mice; 1–2% and 5–10% of splenocytes in Balb/c and NZB mice (Hayakawa et al 1983). Ly1-B-cells secrete IgM antibodies, primarily to self-antigens. They are long-lived appearing early in ontogeny. Interestingly, secondary in vitro antibody responses of these cells are V_H restricted. We previously discussed the V_KIIIb restriction of B-CLL cells.

Three typical tumors of Ly1-B cells have been described: BCL_1, and CH lymphomas and NFS-5 pre-B tumor. BCL_1 which is syngeneic to Balb/c mice, has a striking clinical resemblance to PL whereas morphologic and immune features are more similar to CLL. CH lymphomas of B10H mice (Haughton et al 1986) are of interest because the antibodies of the malignant clone react with erythrocytes and the main autoimmune syndrome accompanying CLL is autoimmune hemolytic anemia. In addition, the 27 independently derived known CH tumors exhibit idiotypic cross-reactivity suggesting their origin from a restricted family of germline genes (Pennel et al 1985). The NFS-5 pre-B tumor expresses SmIg on the surface membrane in addition to Ly1 similar to CLL.

A model of B-CLL is proposed in Figure 9.3. This model attempts to consider

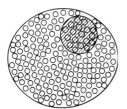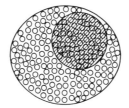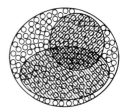

Fig. 9.3 Pathogenesis of B cell chronic lymphocytic leukemia. In the left panel and middle panel there exists an expanding population of a subset of B lymphocytes within the universe of B lymphocytes. In the right panel there is transformation of a single target cell and clonal expansion of this malignant cell which is representative of the B-CLL population.

several factors including the high incidence of polyclonal or oligoclonal autoantibodies, particularly to cellular structural proteins and to hematopoietic cells, and the monoclonal nature of the malignant cells. The initial abnormality in B-CLL might be a polyclonal expansion of the subclass of B cells involved in autoimmune responses. For example, this would encompass B-CLL of the λ VIIIa isotype subclass as well as anti-RhD reactive clones. The origin of this initial polyclonal expansion is unclear but might be intrinsic or extrinsic. A parallel can be drawn to Burkitt lymphoma where both malaria and EBV infection probably result in a polyclonal B cell expansion. It is possible that this B cell expansion might reflect an intrinsic or acquired abnormality of T cells. For example, viral infection of T cells could impair the normal production of B cells. In some instances, a rare transforming event, such as a chromosomal trisomy or translocation, occurs within one B cell in the expanded population leading to the clonal B cell proliferation typical of B-CLL. Similar mechanisms have been proposed for other human malignancies.

Prognostic factors and staging

One of the major problems in the clinical management of CLL is to determine the optimal therapeutic strategy for each patient. The clinical course of chronic lymphocytic leukemia is highly variable; many patients are older (median age, 60 years), have only an elevated lymphocytes or asymptomatic lymphadenopathy or splenomegaly, and have other complicating medical disorders. These patients may require no specific treatment and are unlikely to die as a result of their leukemia. In contrast, occasional patients with CLL may present with lymphoma-like symptoms or features of bone marrow failure, including severe anemia and thrombocytopenia. These patients may have a rapid, progressive course with median survival of less than 2 years in some series. Most patients fall into an intermediate group who do reasonably well for several years without therapy but eventually require specific treatment. Rarely, spontaneous remissions have even been observed in patients with well documented CLL (Han et al 1986).

Ideally, one would like to be able to identify potential prognostic factors in CLL so as to design optimal therapeutic strategies. In 1975, Rai and coworkers (1975) proposed a five-stage staging system for CLL in which patients were categorized on the basis of lymphocytes, lymphadenopathy, splenomegaly, hepatomegaly, anemia (<11 g/dl) and thrombocytopenia ($<100 \times 10^9$/l). Patients with lymphocytosis (stage 0) and those with associated lymphadenopathy (stage I) had a median survival of greater than 10 years and greater than 8 years, respectively. Patients with more advanced disease with hepatosplenomegaly (stage II), anemia (stage III), or thrombocytopenia (stage IV), had progressively shorter median survival of less than 7 years, 2–5 years, and less than 2 years, respectively. Basically, the Rai classification divides patients into low-risk (0), intermediate-risk (I, II), and high-risk (III, IV) groups. These groups constitute approximately 25%, 50%, and 25% of patients, respectively.

Although this staging system is useful, it has limitations. One problem is that the intermediate group is heterogeneous with respect to prognosis. Survival of some patients is comparable to that of the low-risk group, whereas survival in others is comparable to high-risk patients. Other limitations of the Rai classification are that the impact of isolated organomegaly is not considered, and immune versus nonimmune anemia and thrombocytopenia are not distinguished. Several staging systems have been developed in an attempt to address these limitations.

In 1981, Binet and coworkers (Binet et al 1981) proposed a new system in which patients are divided into stages A, B, and C. Patients with anemia (<10 g/dL) or thrombocytopenia ($<100 \times 10^9$/L) were designated as stage C. These 20% of patients were found to have the worst prognosis, with median survival of 3 years or less.

Survival of the remaining 80% of patients was found to depend on the number of lymph node sites clinically involved. Five potential sites of involvement were identified: cervical, axillary, or inguinal lymph nodes (unilateral or bilateral), spleen, and liver. Patients with two sites or less of involvement were considered stage A (median survival 7 years or greater), and those with three or more sites were considered stage B (median survival, 5 years or less).

In the International Workshop of Chronic Lymphocytic Leukemia it was suggested that the Binet staging be integrated with the Rai system, such that patients with stage A would be classified as A (0) (lymphocytosis only), A (I) (lymphadenopathy, A (II) (hepatosplenomegaly), and so forth. This has proven to be cumbersome, and most investigators use either the Rai or the Binet system. Presently there are two points of ongoing debate: (1) whether stage A should be distinguished from stage 0 and (2) whether the cut-off point for anemia should be 10 or 11 g/dl. The first issue is being studied by several groups and likely to be resolved shortly. The decision regarding anemia is arbitrary since this is certainly a continuous variable; a 10.5 g/dl compromise may be reasonable.

The Binet staging system resolves some problems associated with the Rai classification, but fails to resolve the heterogeneity of stage B or stage II patients. Although as a group, median survival of these patients is intermediate between low- and high-risk patients; individual patients tend to segregate with either the low- or higher-risk group. Other investigators have attempted to address this problem by analyzing the effect of lymphocyte count in intermediate-risk patients (Rozman et al 1982, Baccarani et al 1982). Patients whose lymphocyte count was $40 \times 10^9/l$ or less had improved survival similar to low-risk patients, whereas patients with higher lymphocyte counts did not fare as well. In addition, a significant correlation between bone marrow pattern and survival has also been reported in some (Rozman et al 1984b) but not all studies (Han et al 1984a). Patients with nodular or interstitial patterns of bone marrow involvement had longer survival than patients with diffuse involvement. Lymphocyte doubling time may also be an important prognostic factor.

A second problem with current staging systems is their inability to distinguish between persons with low-stage disease, who are stable for many years and require no therapy, and the small but important cohort who develop progressive disease and require treatment. Both groups are considered A in the Binet staging. An interesting group of 20 patients with Rai stage 0 disease have been reported (Han et al 1984b) who had normal karyotypes and stable disease for 6.5–24 years. This form of CLL has been termed 'benign monoclonal lymphocytosis.' These data suggest that chromosome studies may be important in further subclassifying patients with low-stage disease. Clearly, chromosome studies may prove to have an important role in prognosis of patients in all disease stages (discussed below).

Immunoglobulin isotype has been correlated with clinical stage and prognosis; patients with surface IgM had more advanced disease than those with IgG (Ligler et al 1983). In a different study, it was reported that patients in Binet stage A who had only mu-type surface immunoglobulin had a significantly poorer prognosis that those with mu and delta (Baldini et al 1985). Other factors reported to predict the prognosis of patients with low stage CLL include cell size, serum immunoglobulin levels, response to mitogens, glucocorticoid receptor levels, proliferative index, changes in surface glycoprotein patterns, elevated levels of serum lactate dehydrogenose activity, serum deoxythymidine kinase levels, and increased levels of beta$_2$-microglobulin. Recently the density of the CD5 antigen on lymphocytes from stage A patients was reported to correlate with disease progression (Caggiano et al 1986). All of these data are controversial and need to be verified in prospective clinical trials.

THERAPY

Response criteria
One major problem in evaluating therapeutic trials in CLL is the lack of uniform response criteria. Complete remission is typically defined as normalization of leukocytes, hemoglobin, and platelets, a normal bone marrow; and resolution of enlarged lymph nodes, spleen, and liver. These criteria describe a complete clinical response and are probably useful and reproducible. Some investigators include normalization of depressed serum immunoglobulins, normal levels of mouse rosette-forming cells, and the presence of a polyclonal B cell population in the bone marrow as determined by a normal ratio of kappa to lambda light chains. A more sensitive indicator of complete remission is the absence of cells in the peripheral blood and bone marrow that express the idiotype of the leukemic B cells. However, this indicator would require developing anti-idiotype antibodies for individual patients with CLL cells, which is impractical and cannot be done in most patients. Another approach, which will likely prove to be the most sensitive and practical, is to study DNA from 'remission' cells for a clonal rearrangement of heavy- or light-chain immunoglobulin genes corresponding to the initial malignant clone.

Partial response is widely defined as a greater than 50–75% decrease in peripheral blood lymphocytes, a 50% decrease in enlarged lymph nodes and spleen, hemoglobin greater than $11\,g/dl$, and platelets greater than $100 \times 10^9/l$; or improvement of these values by 50–70% of their deviation from normal. In the following studies, in which responses and survivals are evaluated, comparisions between studies are inherently flawed by a lack of uniform response criteria.

Systemic complications requiring therapy
Patients with CLL commonly develop hypogammaglobulinemia, which may be severe. The etiology is complex and is probably related both to intrinsic and extrinsic abnormalities of B and T lymphocyte function and these patients also respond abnormally to immunization. Intramuscular immunoglobulin therapy has been evaluated; no benefit was seen, but most investigators consider the dose and schedule inadequate to achieve clinically meaningful elevations in systemic immunoglobulin levels. The recent availability of intravenous immunoglobulin has led to prospective randomized trials. Preliminary analysis of these data suggest that intravenous immunoglobulin can prevent or modify bacterial or viral infections or both. Intravenous gammaglobulin is also being investigated for treatment of immune thrombocytopenia and anemia that develop in patients with CLL (Besa 1984).

Immune-mediated hemolytic anemia, thrombocytopenia, and neutropenia are generally treated with prednisone. Patients who fail to respond may require splenectomy. Chemotherapy may be required to control the underlying disease. Patients with CLL may, in rare instances, develop a hyperviscosity syndrome and require plasmapheresis, corticosteroids, or chemotherapy. Patients with CLL may develop a hypermetabolic state and hyperuricemia, particularly after therapy; these conditions are usually treated with hydration and allopurinol.

TREATMENT OF CHRONIC LYMPHOCYTIC LEUKEMIA

One unresolved question in the treatment of CLL is when to initiate therapy. There are no data to suggest that therapeutic intervention in patients with elevated leukocyte counts and lymphadenopathy prolongs survival. Two recent trials in patients with low stage disease (stages I and II or A) with chlorambucil alone or with prednisone showed no advantage in survival over no treatment (Shapiro et al 1984). The Medical Research Council is also prospectively evaluating this problem. Treatment remains an important issue as recent data suggest that survival of untreated patients with early disease is significantly shorter than age-matched normals (Rozman et al 1984a). When limited lymph node enlargement causes symptoms, local or systemic therapy may be initiated. Most physicians initiate systemic therapy for patients with organomegaly or cytopenias. Three classes of therapeutic agents are commonly used, radiation therapy, alkylating agents, and corticosteroids.

Radiation therapy

External radiation was the first therapy used to treat CLL (Osgood 1961), but it was abandoned in the mid-1940s when radiophosphorus (^{32}P) became available. In the late 1960s interest was revived in the use of whole body radiation in patients with advanced disease. These patients received a dose of 0.5–1 Gy/d, 3–5 times per week, to a total dose of 10–40 Gy; greater than 80% response rates and improved survival in complete responders were reported (Johnson 1976). In other similar trials, response rates for total body irradiation were reported; however, severe hematologic toxicity paralleled the response rate, and response was not better than that achieved with chlorambucil and prednisone (Rubin et al 1981). Despite these limitations, total body radiation may have a role in the therapy of patients unresponsive to chemotherapy.

Local radiation has been used to treat lymph nodes compromising vital organ function and for relief of painful bone lesions. Splenic radiation has also been used to treat painful splenomegaly, progressive lymphocytosis, anemia, and thrombocytopenia (Byhardt et al 1975). Complete remission after splenic radiation in a subgroup of patients who present with primarily splenomegaly has been reported (Han et al 1967). Thymic radiation was reported to be of benefit in one study (Richards et al 1978), but no beneficial effect and severe toxicity was reported by others (Sawitsky et al 1976). Extracorporeal blood radiation has been used in patients with advanced disease but has not shown superiority over conventional radiation therapy or chemotherapy (Chanana et al 1976); trials in patients with limited disease have not been reported. Radiophosphorus is no longer used to treat CLL.

Single-agent chemotherapy

The first chemotherapeutic drugs used to treat CLL were urethane, nitrogen mustard, and triethylenemelamine (Bigley 1963, Huguley 1974, 1977). Chlorambucil was introduced in 1952 and has remained the most popular drug (Table 9.5). Chlorambucil is an aromatic derivative of nitrogen mustard absorbed orally. The standard dose

Table 9.5   Response to chemotherapy in chronic lymphocytic leukemia

Drugs	Partial remission (%)	Complete remission (%)	Total remissions (%)
Chlorambucil, daily	36	9	45
Chlorambucil, biweekly	50	10	60
Cyclophosphamide			40
Busulfan			30
Fludarabine monophosphate	35	4	39
Deoxycoformycin	12	2	25
Corticosteroids			5–50
Chlorambucil daily + prednisone	67	13	80
	21	17	38
Chlorambucil biweekly + prednisone	25	52	77
	51	8	59
Chlorambucil monthly + prednisone	40	10	50
Cyclophosphamide + vincristine + prednisone	11	33	44
	28	44	72
	25	52	77
	29	2	31
Cyclophosphamide + vincristine + carmustine + melphalan + prednisone	44	17	61

of chlorambucil is 0.1–0.2 mg/kg body weight/d. The dose is reduced once the disease is under control or if toxicity supervenes. A response rate of 60% is common, with 10–20% complete remissions. Often several months are required to obtain a complete response. Some investigators suggest that patients be pretreated with corticosteroids before receiving chlorambucil. Chlorambucil may also be given as a pulse of 0.4–0.6 mg/kg given once every 2–4 weeks. Responses are comparable to those achieved with a daily dose and with less hematologic toxicity (Knospe et al 1974).

Cyclophosphamide is probably as effective as chlorambucil (Huguley 1977) and can be given intravenously as well as orally. Cyclophosphamide may be useful in patients unresponsive to chlorambucil; cross-resistance is unusual. The usual dose is 2–3 mg/kg/d or 20 mg/kg every 2–3 weeks. Busulfan also has activity in CLL (Livingston & Carter 1970a) but is less effective than chlorambucil and cyclophosphamide and may worsen thrombocytopenia.

Corticosteroids have been used to control leukocytes and to treat immune mediated hemolytic anemia and thrombocytopenia (Ezdinli et al 1969, Livingston & Carter 1970b). The usual dose of prednisone is 30–60 mg/m^2 body surface area/d. Corticosteroids can rapidly decrease lymphadenopathy and hepatosplenomegaly; this may be accompanied by a striking lymphocytosis thought to be related to lymphocyte redistribution. Complete remissions are rarely induced with corticosteroids, which should not be used alone to treat CLL except in the presence of autoimmune hemolytic anemia and thrombocytopenia, or in advanced disease unresponsive to other therapies. Patients with extensive disease are frequently treated with corticosteroids before initiating cytotoxic chemotherapy; typically, this treatment consists of prednisone 20–60 mg/d for 1–3 weeks. Dramatic improvement in anemia or thrombocytopenia may suggest an immune component.

Fludarabine monophosphate, the 2-fluoro, 5′ phosphate derivative of 9-β-D-arabino-furano-syladenine has activity in patients with advanced CLL. Ten of 26 evaluable patients achieved clinical improvement with one complete responder (Grever et al

1986). A 25% response rate has been reported for patients treated with 2′-deoxycofor-mycin, an adenosine deaminase inhibitor (Grever 1987).

Combination chemotherapy

The precise role of multidrug chemotherapy in CLL is controversial. Prednisone alone was compared to prednisone plus daily chlorambucil and to prednisone plus monthly chlorambucil in 96 patients with stage III or IV disease (Table 9.5) (Sawitsky et al 1977). Response rates were 11% for prednisone alone, 37% for daily chlorambucil and prednisone, and 47% for monthly chlorambucil and prednisone. Responders lived longer than non-responders in each treatment group but there was no substantial difference in median survival among the three groups. In another study, 24 patients were randomly assigned to receive daily low-dose chlorambucil with or without predni-sone (Han et al 1973). A response rate of 80% was reported with 20% complete remission for patients receiving chlorambucil plus prednisone versus 45% response rate and 9% complete remission for those receiving chlorambucil alone (p = 0.05).

These studies suggest that there may be a small therapeutic advantage to the combi-nation of chlorambucil with prednisone over chlorambucil as a single agent, but a prospective randomized trial has not been reported. Intermittent rather than daily treatment with chlorambucil may be less toxic, is more convenient, and is probably more effective than daily therapy.

Combination chemotherapy with cyclophosphamide, vincristine, and prednisone has been used in patients with advanced disease. In one study, 36 patients received these drugs (Liepmen & Votaw 1978); overall response rate was 72% with 44% com-plete remissions. Eight of 13 previously treated patients responded with partial or complete remissions. In another study of 18 previously treated patients, the response rate was 44% (Oken & Kaplan 1979). Patients achieving complete or partial response had a mean survival of 38 months; nonresponding patients survived only 5 months. In one study, 71 previously untreated patients with advanced CLL were randomized to receive either chlorambucil and prednisone or a combination of cyclophosphamide, vincristine, and prednisone (Montserrat et al 1985). No differences in response or survival were reported between these two groups. In another study, 124 patients were randomized to receive either chlorambucil and prednisone or cyclophosphamide, vincristine, and prednisone. Complete remission rate and survival were the same for both groups (Bennett et al 1987). In another large study, patients receiving CVP were more frequently downstaged than those receiving chlorambucil and prednisone, although there was no difference in survival between the 2 groups (French Cooperative Group 1986). At present, it is reasonable to treat patients unresponsive to chlorambucil (with or without prednisone) with the combination of cyclophosphamide, vincristine, and prednisone.

Therapy with more intensive regimens containing doxorubicin has also been evalu-ated in patients with CLL. Seventy patients with advanced disease were randomized between cyclophosphamide, vincristine and prednisone and the same drugs with the addition of 25 mg/m² of doxorubicin on the first day of each course (French Coopera-tive Group 1986, Cooperative Group on CLL 1986). There were 21 deaths in the former group and 14 deaths in the group receiving doxorubicin (p = 0.003). Median survival for patients treated with doxorubicin is >4 years versus <2 years in controls. These investigators concluded that the addition of low-dose doxorubicin to cyclophosphamide, vincristine and prednisone was beneficial.

Sixty-three patients with stage II, III, or IV disease were treated on the M2 protocol consisting of vincristine, cyclophosphamide, carmustine, melphalan, and prednisone; the overall response rate was 62% (18% complete remission and 44% partial remission) (Kempin et al 1982). Median survival of complete responders was 76 months, significantly larger than partial responders (40 months) and nonresponders (14 months). Previous therapy was found to be the only significant negative prognostic variable with respect to response; median duration of survival for patients who received no previous therapy was 47 months, as opposed to 15 months for previously treated patients.

Several innovative studies are currently in progress. In one study, the efficacy of combination chemotherapy with cyclophosphamide, and prednisone with and without total body radiation (10–20 Gy), is being examined in patients with advanced disease (Kempin et al 1983). Although it is too early to determine whether it improves responses, total body radiation in this study has no substantial toxicity. Another recent study reported responses in 10 of 20 patients with advanced CLL treated with dexamethasone, high-dose cytarabine and cisplatin (Valesquez et al 1986). Recently five young patients with CLL were treated by high-dose chemotherapy and radiation followed by bone marrow transplantation. Results are too preliminary for critical analysis (Michallet et al 1986).

One major concern in the use of multiagent chemotherapy in patients with CLL is the risk of developing acute myelogenous leukemia linked to therapy. An increased risk of acute leukemia after chemotherapy with an alkylating agent is well documented (Reiner et al 1977). This risk is particularly true with alkylating agents such as melphalan, chlorambucil, and nitrosoureas, and is probably substantial.

In summary, patients with low stage disease (0, 1 or A) have not been shown to benefit from treatment. The initial therapy for patients with CLL who require treatment is usually chlorambucil or cyclophosphamide with or without prednisone given in a pulse therapy every 2–4 weeks. Combination therapy with other chemotherapeutic agents should be reserved for patients with more advanced disease. Patients with intermediate stage disease (1, 2 or B) have comparable response rates to chlorambucil and prednisone compared to CVP. Patients with advanced disease (3, 4 or C) have shown favorable responses to CHOP over CVP in one large study (French Cooperative Group 1986, Cooperative Group on CLL 1986). Although similar survival results to CHOP using CVP were reported in another large study when the drugs were given more often and for a longer duration (Bennett et al 1987).

Maintenance therapy

Another unanswered question in the therapy of CLL is whether maintenance chemotherapy is useful in patients who respond to initial chemotherapy. In one study, responding patients were randomized to six additional courses of chlorambucil and prednisone or to four courses of cycle-active cyclophosphamide and cytarabine (Keller et al 1983). Cycle-active therapy showed no benefit and was more toxic. Maintenance chemotherapy is ineffective in related disorders such as Hodgkin's disease, lymphomas, and multiple myeloma. Currently, there is little evidence of a role for maintenance chemotherapy in CLL once a response has been obtained. It should be emphasized, however, that in one large study (Bennett et al 1987) prolonged treatment of up to 18 months may have had a major influence on prolonging survival of primarily Rai stage III and IV patients to 4.2 years as compared to 19 months in earlier trials where therapy was usually stopped at 6–9 months.

Splenectomy

There is no curative role for splenectomy in CLL. Splenectomy has been used in patients with hemolytic anemia, thrombocytopenia (either steroid-dependent or unresponsive to steroids), pancytopenia, and painful splenomegaly. Splenectomy has been reported to lead to a sustained improvement in previously depressed hematologic parameters in patients with splenomegaly (Merl et al 1983). Patients with massive splenomegaly were most likely to benefit. Some patients with immune cytopenias unresponsive to corticosteroids may also respond to splenectomy. Except for these unusual circumstances, splenectomy is not beneficial for patients with CLL.

Intensive leukapheresis

There has been recent interest in the treatment of CLL by intensive leukapheresis using blood cell separators. Leukapheresis is sometimes considered for patients with bone marrow failure unable to tolerate chemotherapy. Although substantial elevations in hemoglobin and platelets and a reduction in organomegaly have been reported, this finding is not consistent. One recent review suggested that leukapheresis was safe and effective and should be considered as an interim therapy in patients refractory to chemotherapy and in those with chemotherapy-induced anemia and thrombocytopenia (Marti et al 1983). Routine use of leukapheresis is probably not justified but selected patients may benefit.

Monoclonal antibodies

Several investigators have studied the response of both B and T cell CLL and other chronic lymphoid leukemias to monoclonal antibodies. Patients with typical B-derived CLL received T101 monoclonal antibody (anti-CD5) reactive with normal and malignant T lymphocytes and B-CLL cells (Foon & Todd 1986). This led to transient reductions in circulating leukemia cells, without an effect on the bone marrow or involved lymph nodes or other organs. This therapy resulted in some intravascular cell injury, but destruction in the spleen, liver, and lungs was probably more important. Patients with T cell CLL may also respond. Patients with cutaneous T cell lymphoma treated with T101 or a similar antibody (anti-Leu-1) have had only transient improvement in skin lesions and lymphadenopathy (Foon & Todd 1986). Side effects of monoclonal antibody therapy are usually minor; however, respiratory distress after the rapid infusion has been reported as have transient elevations of creatinine and liver enzymes.

Several problems with monoclonal antibody therapy must be addressed. First, treatment with some antibodies such as T101 result in modulation of the antigen off of the cell surface membrane. Loss of antigen expression prevents antibody from binding to the tumor cells. A portion of the T101 antigen antibody complex is rapidly pinocytosed into the cytoplasm (Schroff et al 1984); this might be advantageous when drugs or toxins are linked to the antibody to enhance its cytotoxicity. Early trials using T101 antibody conjugated to the A-chain of ricin have not demonstrated a beneficial clinical effect in patients with CLL (Laurent et al 1986). Another potential problem is circulating free antigen, which could prevent the antibody from reaching the tumor cells. Furthermore, murine antibodies may stimulate production of human anti-mouse antibodies and lead to antibody neutralization. This problem may be overcome by treatment with high initial doses of antibody (greater than 500 mg) or by simultaneous treatment with immunosuppressive drugs to induce tolerance in the host. Another problem is heterogeneity of antigen expression on tumor cells that would require therapy with more than one antibody. Clearly, monoclonal antibody therapy for leukemia and lymphoma is in its earliest stages.

One interesting therapeutic approach with monoclonal antibodies is the use of anti-idiotype monoclonal antibody reactive with the idiotype of the immunoglobulin on malignant B cells. Such an antibody is tumor-specific for only a single patient's tumor cells. One patient with B cell lymphoma in an accelerated phase, no longer responsive to conventional therapies, was treated with an IgG_{2b} antiidiotype monoclonal antibody (Miller et al 1982). After 8 intravenous infusions, the patient entered a complete remission sustained for over 3 years. Results were less impressive in 7 other patients with lymphoma treated with this approach; two failed to respond, one had a minimal response, and four responded for 1–6 months (Meeker et al 1985). Interestingly, 1 patient with prolymphocytic leukemia with high circulating leukemia cell counts had a transient reduction of circulating and bone marrow leukemia cells. We developed several monoclonal antiidiotype antibodies to cells from patients with leukemia and lymphoma (Giardina et al 1985). The first patient treated had Rai stage IV CLL. No benefit was seen to sequential antiidiotype monoclonal antibody therapy with IgG_{2b} and IgG_1 antibody. This patient's therapy was limited because of circulating idiotype immunoglobulin that blocked the binding of the antiidiotype antibody to the leukemia cells. We were unable to sufficiently reduce the circulating idiotype with extensive plasmapheresis.

Although antiidiotype antibody therapy remains an interesting area of investigation, its applicability is limited by specificity for a single patient, and by circulating antibody in the serum in many patients. The recent observation that some tumors are biclonal and would require more than one antibody for successful therapy also suggests limitations (Sklar et al 1984). An additional problem is that the idiotype may be unstable due to somatic mutation within the immunoglobulin variable region genes (Raffeld et al 1985).

Interferon

Crude α-interferon preparations were reported to be active in patients with advanced CLL (Gutterman et al 1980). In a phase 2 trial of recombinant leukocyte α-interferon in 19 patients with advanced disease only two brief partial responses were reported (Foon et al 1985). Five patients had disease progression while receiving recombinant leukocyte α-interferon. In contrast, a recent preliminary study reported responses in 10 successive patients with untreated early stage disease treated with low-dose (2×10^6 units/m^2/3 times per week) recombinant α-interferon (Rozman et al 1988). Recombinant γ-interferon is currently being studied in phase II trials for patients with CLL; results will be forthcoming shortly. Interferon has been shown to induce cell differentiation in vitro from most patients with CLL (Ostlund et al 1986). Interestingly, some patients' cells (3 of 29) also proliferated in vitro when exposed to interferon which might explain the rapid disease progression seen in patients.

These findings contrast responses in patients with chemotherapy-refractory low-grade and histologic intermediate-grade non-Hodgkin's lymphoma and cutaneous

T cell lymphoma (Roth & Foon 1986). Over 50% of these patients have had good partial responses and some complete responses.

Hairy cell leukemia is highly responsive to α-interferon. Excellent responses were reported in 7 patients with hairy cell leukemia (3 complete and 4 partial responses) treated with crude α-interferon (Quesada et al 1984). Similar data have been reported by a number of investigators using recombinant α-interferon (Roth & Foon 1986). Response rates have been comparable with recombinant preparations after 3 times a week or daily with dosages ranging from $3–6 \times 10^6$ units intramuscularly or subcutaneously. Although the initial reports suggested that complete responses were frequent, this has not been confirmed (of 158 responses reported, only 22 were complete). More important, however, is that virtually all of the patients with responses demonstrated normalization of peripheral blood cell counts. Many of these patients had no prior therapy including splenectomy. For responding patients the disease has not been reported to become refractory to α-interferon; many patients have been followed for more than 3 years. In some studies interferon has been discontinued after approximately 1 year of therapy. Less then half of the patients relapse within 6–12 months and most can be reinduced into remission with interferon. In addition, improvement in natural killer activity and immunologic surface markers parallels the hematologic recovery. The mechanism of action of interferon in HCL and CLL is uncertain. Cordingley et al (1988) have shown that tumor necrosis factor acts as a growth factor in CLL and HCL and this is antagonised by interferon. These observations may be relevant.

Pentostatin (2'-Deoxycoformycin)
Pentostatin is an adenosine deaminase inhibitor. The administration of pentostatin in low doses every 2 weeks produced complete and partial responses in approximately 25% of patients with refractory CLL (Grever 1987). Pentostatin has remarkable activity in hairy cell leukemia. Over half of the patients treated enter complete remissions and virtually all of the remaining patients enter a partial remission (Spiers 1987). This treatment has been effective in previously untreated patients, those with prior splenectomy or those who had failed interferon. Pentostatin is continued only until a response and then it is discontinued. It is too early to draw firm conclusions but thus far very few patients have relapsed. Pentostatin may prove to be superior to interferon as the period of treatment is shorter, the incidence of complete remission is greater and it has been effective in patients who have failed interferon. Currently a prospective randomized trial of pentostatin and α-interferon is underway to address this question.

CONCLUSION

With the availability of monoclonal antibodies to differentiation antigens on lymphocytes, and molecular probes for immunoglobulin and T cell receptor genes, our understanding of the development of normal B and T lymphocytes has progressed rapidly. We can now more precisely define the level of development of the malignant cell involved in CLL. Clonal chromosomal abnormalities have been identified in CLL cells and may even help to determine the prognosis of the disease. Other prognostic factors and staging systems have been identified. Although none of these staging systems is ideal, they are useful in predicting the course of the disease. In early stages of CLL, patients are generally not treated. When chemotherapy is required, chlorambucil, with or without prednisone, is frequently useful. Most data suggest that treatment with prednisone and chlorambucil every 2–4 weeks is less toxic and as effective as daily chlorambucil. Whole body radiation and combination chemotherapy are usually reserved for patients who relapse after receiving alkylating agents with or without prednisone and those with advanced disease. None of these combinations is clearly superior to chlorambucil and prednisone for initial therapy. It is hoped that newer biological therapies such as γ-interferon and monoclonal antibodies, perhaps conjugated to drugs, toxins, or isotopes, will prove useful in the treatment of CLL. New chemotherapy reagents and new combinations of drugs, possibly including biological agents, may improve the therapy of this disease.

REFERENCES

Agee J F, Garver F A, Faguet G B 1986 Blood 68: 62–68
Aisenberg A C, Bloch K J 1976a N Engl J Med 287: 272–27
Aisenberg A C, Wilkes B 1976b Blood 48: 707–715
Anderson K C, Boyd A W, Fisher D C, Leslie D 65: 620, 1985
Baccarani M, Cabol M, Gobbi M, Lauria F, Tura S 1982 Blood 59: 1191–1196
Baldini L, Mozzana R, Cortelezzi A et al 1985 Blood 65: 340–344
Bennett J M, Catovsky D, Daniel M T et al 1976 Br J Haematol 33: 451–458
Bennett J M, Raphael B, Moore D F, Silber R, Oken M M, Rubin P 1987 In: Chronic lymphocytic leukemia: recent progress and future directions. Liss, New York
Bergsagel D E 1967 Can Med Assoc J 96: 1615–1620
Bertoli L F, Kubagawa H, Borzillo G P et al 1987 Blood 70: 45–50
Besa E C 1984 AM J Med 76 (suppl 3a): 209–218
Bigley R H 1963 Cancer Chemother Rep 30: 27–43
Binet J L, Catovsky D, Chandra P et al 1981 Br J Haematol 48: 365–367
Bouroncle B A 1958 Blood 13: 609–630
Brito-Babapulle V, Pittman S, Melo J V, Pomfret M, Catovsky D 1987 Hematol Path 1: 27–33
Brok-Simoni F, Rechavi G, Katzir N, Ben-Bassat I 1987 Lancet 1: 329–330
Brooks D A, Beckman G R, Bradley J et al 1981 Journal of Immunology 126: 1373
Brouet J C, Preud'Homme J L, Seligmann M, Bernard J 1973 Br Med J 4: 23–24
Brouet J C, Fernand J P, Laurent G et al 1985 Br J Haematol 59: 55–66
Browett P J, Ganeshaguru K, Hoffbrand A V, Norton J D 1988 Leukemia Research 12: 25–31
Bunn P A J R, Schechter G P, Jaffe E et al 1983 N Engl J Med 309: 257–264
Byhardt R W, Brace K C, Wiernik P H 1975 Cancer 35: 1621–1625
Caggiano V, Paglieroni T 1986 Blood 68 (suppl 1): 196a
Caligaris-Cappio F, Gobbi M, Bofill M, Janossy G 1982 J Exp Med 155: 623–628
Caligaris-Cappio F, Pizzolo G, Chilosi M et al 1985 Blood 66: 1035–1042
Carey R W, McGinnis A, Jacobson B M, Carvalho A 1976 Arch Intern Med 136: 62–66
Catovsky D, Galletto J, Okos A, Galton D A G, Wiltshaw E, Stathopoulos G 1973 Lancet 2: 232–234
Chanana A D, Cronkite E P, Rai K R 1976 Int J Radiat Oncol Biol Phys 1: 539–548
Conley C L, Misiti J, Laster A J 1980 Medicine 5: 323–333
Cooper M D, Bertoli L F, Borzillo G V, Burrows P D, Kubagawa H 1985 In: Gale R P, Golde D W (eds) Leukemia: recent advances in biology and treatment. Liss, New York, p 453–466
Cooperative Group on CLL of the Societe Francaise d'Hematologie 1986 Blood (Abstract) 86 (suppl 1): 219a
Cohn L, Uhr J W 1964 J Clin Invest 43: 2241–2248
Cordingley F T, Hoffbrand A V, Heslop H E et al 1988 Lancet i: 969–971
Cossman J, Neclers L M, Braziel R M, Trepel J B, Korsmeyer S J, Bakhshi A 1984 J Clin Invest 73: 587–592
Croce C M, Isobe M, Polumbo A et al 1985 Science 227: 1044–1047
Davidson W F, Fredrickson T N, Rudikoff E K et al 1984 J Immunol 133: 744–753
Deegan M J, Abraham J P, Sawdy K M, Van Slyck E J 1984 Blood 64: 1207–1211
Drexler H G, Brenner M K, Coustan-Smith E, Wickremasinghe R G, Hoffbrand A V 1987 Blood 70: 1536–1542
Enno A, Catovsky D, O'Brien M, Cherchi M, Kumaran T O, Galton D A G 1979 Br J Haematol 41: 9–18
Ezdinli E Z, Stutzman L, Aungst C W, Firat D 1969 Cancer 23: 900–909
Fernand J P, Herait J P, Brouet J C 1985 Blood 66: 291–293

Fernandez L A, MacSween J M, Langley G R 1983 Blood 62: 767–774
Fernandez L A, MacSween J M, Langley R 1984 Br J Haematol 57: 97–104
Fialkow P J, Najfeld V, Reddy A, Singer J, Sternmann L 1978 Lancet 2: 444–446
Foa R, Catovsky D, Lauria F, Dalton D A G 1980 Br J Haematol 46: 623–625
Foa R, Fierro M T, Lusso P et al 1986 Br J Haematol 62: 151–154
Foon K A, Bottino G C, Abrams P G et al 1985 Am J Med 78: 216–20
Foon K A, Todd R F III 1986 Blood 68: 1–31
French Cooperative Group on Chronic Lymphocytic Leukemia 1986 Lancet 1: 1346–1349
Fu S M, Chiorazzi N, Kunkel H G, Halper J P, Harris S I 1978 J Exp Med 148: 1570–1578
Gallo R C, Kalyanaraman V S, Sarngadharan M G et al 1983 Cancer Res 43: 3892–3899
Galton D A G, Goldman J M, Wiltshaw E, Catovsky D, Henry K, Goldenberg G J 1974 Br J Haematol 27: 7–23
Garver F A, Kiefer C R, Moscoso H, Testino A, Beezhold D H, Kestler D P 1984 Blood 64 (suppl 1): 202a
Giardina S L, Schroff R W, Woodhouse C S et al 1985 J Immunol 135: 653–658
Golomb H M, Catovsky D, Golde D W 1978 Ann Intern Med 89: 677–683
Grever M R, Coltman C A, Files J C et al 1986 Blood 68 (suppl 1): 223a
Grever M 1987 In: Gale R P, Rai K (eds) Chronic lymphocytic leukemia: recent progress and future directions. Liss, New York. p 399–409
Gutterman J U, Blumenschein G, Alexanian R et al 1980 Ann Intern Med 93: 399–406
Halper J P, Fu S M, Gottlieb A B, Winchester R J, Kunkel H G 1979 J Exp Med 64: 1141–1148
Hamblin T J, Abdul-Ahad A K, Gordon J, Stevenson F K, Stevenson G T 1980 Br J Cancer 42: 495–502
Hamblin T J, Oscier D G, Young B J 1986 J Clin Pathol 39: 713–716
Han T, Ezdinli E Z, Sokal J E 1967 Cancer 20: 243–253
Han T, Ezdinli E Z, Shimaoka K S, Desai D V 1973 Cancer 31: 502–508
Han T, Ozer H, Henderson E S et al 1981 Blood 58: 1182–1189
Han T, Bloom M L, Dadey B et al 1982 Blood 60: 1075–1081
Han T, Barcos M, Enrigh L et al 1984a J Clin Oncol 2: 562–570
Han T, Ozer H, Gavigan M et al 1984b Blood 64: 244–252
Han T, Ozer H, Sadamori N et al 1984c N Engl J Med 310: 288–292
Han T, Sadamori N, Ozer H et al 1984d J Clin Oncol 2: 1121–1132
Han T, Gomez G A, Henderson E S 1986 Blood 68 (suppl 1): 199a
Hayakawa K, Hardy R R, Parks D R et al 1983 J Exp Med 157: 202–218
Haughton G, Arnold L W, Bishop G A et al 1986 Immunol Rev 93: 35–52
Hokland V P, Ellegaard J 1981 Leuk Res 5: 349–355
Huguley C M J R 1974 Cancer Chemother Rep 16: 241–244
Huguley C M J R 1977 Cancer Treat Rev 4: 261–273
Isaacs R 1937 Ann Intern Med 11: 657–662
Johnson R E 1976 Cancer 37: 2691–2696
Juliusson G, Robert K-H, Hammerström L, Smith C I E, Biberfeld G, Gahrton G 1983 Scand J Immunol 17: 51–59
Juliusson G, Robert K-H, Ost A et al 1985 Blood 65: 134–141
Kalyanaraman V S, Sarngadharan M G, Robert-Guroff M, Miyoshi I, Golde D, Gallo R C 1982 Science 218: 561–563
Kay N E, Johnson J D, Stanek R, Douglas S D 1979 Blood 54: 540–544
Kay N E 1981 Blood 57: 418–420
Kay N E, Howe R B, Douglas S D 1982 Leuk Res 6: 345–348
Keller J W, Knopse W H, Bartolucci A A, Huguley C M, Johnson K, Raney M 1983 Blood 62 (suppl 1): 204a
Kempin S, Lee B J III, Kosiner B et al 1982 Blood 60: 1110–1121
Kempin S, Kurland E, Koziner B et al 1983 Blood 62 (suppl 1): 204
Kinoshita K, Amagasaki P, Ikedas et al 1985 Blood 66: 120–127
Kipps T J, Fong S, Goldfien R D et al 1986 Blood 68 (suppl 1): 248a
Knospe W H, Loeb V J R, Huguley C M J R 1974 Cancer 33: 555–562
Knuutila S, Elonen E, Teerenhovi L et al 1986 N Engl J Med 314: 865–869
Korsmeyer S J 1985 In: Waldman T A (moderator) Ann Intern Med 102: 497–510
Krajny M, Pruzanski W 1976 Can Med Assoc J 114: 899–905
Larson R A, Yachnin S 1983 J Clin Invest 72: 1268–1276
Laurent G, Pris J, Farcet J-P et al 1986 Blood 67: 1680–1686
Lauria F, Foa R, Mantovani B, Fierro M T, Catovsky D, Tura S 1983 Br J Haematol 54: 277–284
Lauria F, Raspadore D, Tura D 1984 Blood 64: 667–671
Lee C L Y, Uniyal S, Fernandez L A, Lee S H S, Ghose T 1986 Cancer Res 46: 2497–2501

Lewis F B, Schwartz R S, Dameshek W 1966 Clin Exp Immunol 1: 3–11
Liepman M, Votaw M L 1978 Cancer 41: 1664–1169
Ligler F S, Kettman J R, Smith R G, Frenkel E P 1983 Blood 62: 256–263
Livingston R B, Carter S K (eds) 1970a Single agents in cancer chemotherapy. IFI/Plenum Data, New York. p 112–129
Livingston R B, Carter S K (eds) 1970b Single agents in cancer chemotherapy. IFI/Plenum Data, New York. p 337–358
Long J C, Aisenberg A C 1975 Am J Clin Pathol 63: 786–795
Lutzner M, Edelson R, Schein P, Green I, Kirkpatrick C, Ahmed A 1975 Ann Intern Med 83: 534–552
Mangan K F, Chikkappa G, Farley P C 1982 J Clin Invest 70: 1148–1156
Marti G E, Folks T, Longo D L, Klein H 1983 J Clin Apheresis 1: 243–248
Meeker T C, Lowder J N, Maloney D G et al 1985 Blood 65: 1349–1363
Melo J V, Catovsky P, Gregory C M, Galton D A G 1987 Br J Haematol 65 (in press)
Merl S A, Theodorakis M E, Goldberg J, Gottlieb A J 1983 Am J Hematol 15: 253–259
Michallet M. Corrant B, Chabanon C, Hollard D 1986 Blood 68 (suppl 1): 277a
Miller R A, Maloney D G, Warnke R, Levy R 1982 N Engl J Med 306: 517–522
Minden M D, Toyonaga B, Ha K et al 1985 Proc Natl Acad Sci USA 82: 1224–1227
Montserrat E, Alcala A, Parody R et al 1985 Cancer 56: 2369–2375
Nadler L M, Ritz J, Bates M P et al 1982 J Clin Invest 70: 433–442
Nadler L M, Korsmeyer S J, Anderson K C et al 1984 J Clin Invest 74: 332–340
Newland A C, Catovsky D, Linch D et al 1984 Br J Haematol 58: 433–436
The Non-Hodgkin's Lymphoma Pathologic Classification Project 1982 Cancer 49: 2112–2135
Norton J D, Pattinson J, Hoffbrand A V, Jani H, Yaxley J C, Leber B F 1988 Blood 71: 178–185
O'Connor N T J, Wainscoat T S, Weatherall D J et al 1985 Lancet 1: 1295–1297
Oken M M, Kaplan M E 1979 Cancer Treat Rep 63: 441–447
Osgood E E 1961 Nucl Med 6: 421–432
Ostlund L, Einhorn S, Robert K-H, Juliusson G, Biberfeld P 1986 Blood 67: 152–159
Pandolfi F, Monzari V, Derossi J et al 1985 Lancet 2: 633–636
Pennel C A, Arnold L W, Lutz P M et al 1985 Proc Natl Acad Sci USA 82: 3799–3803
Perri R T, Kay M E 1982 Blood 59: 247–249
Perri R T 1986 Blood 67: 943–948
Pittman S, Catovsky D 1984 Br J Haematol 58: 649–60
Platsoucas C D, Fernandes G, Gupta S L et al 1980 Immunol 125: 1216–1223
Quesada J R, Reuben J R, Manning J T, Hersh E M 1984 N Engl J Med 310: 15–18
Platsoucas C D, Galiniski M, Kempin S, Reich L, Clarkson B, Good R A 1982 J Immunol 129: 2305–2312
Raffeld M, Neckers L, Longo D L, Cossman J 1985 N Engl J Med 312: 1653–1658
Rai K R, Swaitsky A, Cronkite E P, Chanana A, Levy R N, Pasternak B S 1975 Blood 46: 219–234
Reiner R R, Hoover R, Fraumeni J F, Jr Young R C 1977 N Engl J Med 197: 177–181
Reynolds C W, Foon K A 1984 Blood 64:1146–1158
Richards F J R, Spurr C L, Ferree C, Blake D D, Raben M 1978 Am J Med 64: 947–954
Richter M N 1928 Am J Pathol 4: 295–292
Rickinson A B, Finerty S, Epstein M A 1982 Clin Exp Immunol 50: 347–354
Ritz J, Nadler L M, Bhan A K et al 1981 Blood 58: 648
Robert K-H, Juliusson G, Biberfeld P 1983 Scand J Immunol 17: 397–401
Roth M S, Foon K A 1986 Am J Med 67: 152–159
Rozman C, Montserrat E, Feliu E et al 1982 Blood 59: 1001–1005
Rozman C, Montserrat E, Fernandes J M R et al 1984a Sangre (Barc) 29: 156–163
Rozman C, Montserrat E, Rodrigues-Fernandez J M et al 1984b Blood 64: 642–648
Rozman C, Montserrat E, Viñolas N et al 1988 Blood 71: 1295–1298
Rubartelli A, Sitia R, Zicca A, Grossi C E, Ferrarini M 1983 Blood 62:495–504
Rubin P, Bennett J M, Begg C, Bozdech M J, Silber R 1981 Int J Radiat Oncol Biol Phys 7: 1623–1632
Sawitsky A, Rai K R, Aral I et al 1976 Am J Med 61: 892–896
Sawitsky A, Rai K R, Glidewell O, Silver R T 1977 Blood 50: 1049–1059
Saxon A, Stevens R H, Golde T W 1978 Ann Intern Med 88: 323–326
Scher I 1982 Adv Immunol 33 1–71
Schroff R W, Farell M M, Klein R A, Oldham R K, Foon K A 1984 J Immunol 133: 1641–1648
Shapiro L, Shustic C, Anderson K, Sawitsky A 1984 Proc Am Soc Clin Oncol 3: 191
Sklar J, Cleary M L, Thielemans K, Gralow J, Warnke R, Levy R 1984 N Engl J Med 311: 20–27
Smith J L, Cowling D C, Barker C R 1972 Lancet 1: 229–233
Sordoski J G, Rosen C A, Haseltine W A 1984 Science 225: 381–385
Spiers A S D 1987 Blood Reviews 1: 106–110

Stevenson F K, Hamblin T J, Stevenson G T 1981 J Exp Med 154: 1965–1969
Tötterman T H, Nilsson K, Sunström C 1980 Nature 288: 176–178
Tsujimoto Y, Yunis J, Onorato-Showe L, Erikson J, Nowell P C, Croce C M 1984 Science 224: 1403–1406
Uchiyama T, Yodo J, Sagawa K, Takatsuki K, Uchino H 1977 Blood 15: 481–492
Valesquez W S, McLaughlin P, Swan F, Kantarjian J, Cabanillas F, Barlogie B 1986 Blood 68 (suppl 1): 234a
Van Dongen J J, Hooijkaas H, Michiels J J et al 1984 Blood 64: 571–575
Velardi A, Prchal J T, Prasthofer E F, Grossi C E 1985 Blood 65: 149–155
Yam L T, Li C Y, Lam K W 1971 N Engl J Med 284: 357–360
Yunis J J, Oken M M, Kaplan M, Ensrud K M, Howe R R, Theologides A 1982 N Engl J Med 307: 1231–1236
Yunis J J, Frizzera G, Oken M M, McKenna J, Theologides A, Arnesen M 1987 N Engl J Med 316: 79
Zech L, Gahrton G, Hammerström L et al 1984 Nature 308: 858–860

10. The management of Hodgkin's disease and the non-Hodgkin's lymphomas

D. C. Linch   B. Vaughan-Hudson

INTRODUCTION

The major advances in the management of the malignant lymphomas have been the development of radical radiotherapy in the 1940s and combination chemotherapy regimes in the mid-1960s and early 1970s. Progress since then has been slow. There is increasing awareness of the importance of a variety of prognostic factors in patients with lymphoma and the consequent need for patient stratification both for the assignment of appropriate treatment and for the evaluation of treatment results. Such stratification, intended to maximise therapeutic efficacy while minimising treatment related toxicity, necessarily leads to smaller treatment groups, and few single centres have sufficient patients for adequate randomised trials. The problems of patient selection may be large, especially in secondary and tertiary referral centres where the initial selection is not made by the trial investigators. Multi-centre groups have the patient numbers but adherence to protocols may be less strict and several authors have pointed out the importance of delivering in full the drug dosages prescribed in the trial protocols at the appropriate times (Longo et al 1986, Carde et al 1983). In evaluating therapeutic options it is therefore necessary to analyse results from both single centres and multi-centre groups. Encouraging preliminary results in small studies from the former are frequently not upheld in larger randomised trials by the latter and the reasons for these discrepancies are not usually clear.

This article attempts to survey the current management of both Hodgkin's disease and the non-Hodgkin's lymphomas in adults. It is not an exhaustive review. Alternative strategies not discussed may be as valid as those that are and emphasis is given to the more recent developments which are in general less well tried and more contentious.

HODGKIN'S DISEASE

Patient stratification

Staging
The Ann Arbor staging system has been the major means of stratification in Hodgkin's disease (Carbone et al 1971) (Table 10.1). In patients with clinically localised disease the staging process has traditionally included a staging laparotomy (pathological staging = PS). In patients with clinical stage (CS) I and II supradiaphragmatic disease 25–30% of patients are advanced to PS III or IV on the findings of laparotomy (Jelliffe & Vaughan Hudson 1987). Despite these findings, the role of a staging laparotomy has been questioned and it has been abandoned by some (Table 10.2). This is not a reflection of improved imaging techniques for intraabdominal disease. CT scanning will detect retroperitoneal nodes but is probably not better than well performed lymphangiography (Blackledge et al 1980, Castellino et al 1984). CT scanning is not a sensitive

Table 10.1   Ann Arbor staging system (+modifications) for Hodgkin's disease

Stage I	Involvement of a single lymph node region or a single extralymphatic organ or site (IE)	I I	(above thyroid notch) (below thyroid notch)
Stage II	Involvement of two or more lymph node regions on the same side of the diaphragm or an extralymphatic organ or site with nodes on the same side of the diaphragm (IIE)	II$_n$	where n = number of node regions involved
Stage III	Involvement of lymph node regions on both sides of the diaphragm This may be accompanied by localised involvement of an extralymphatic organ or site (IIIE) or spleen (IIIS) or both (IIISE)	IIIA$_1$ IIIA$_2$	indicates involvement of spleen, splenic coeliac or porta hepatitis nodes only within the abdomen indicates involvement of paraaortic iliac or mesenteric nodes
Stage IV	Diffuse or disseminated of one or more extralymphatic organs or tissues		

Each stage is divided into A or B categories, B being defined as the presence of systemic symptoms (pruritus excluded)

Table 10.2   Arguments for and against staging laparotomy

For	Against
1. Identifies intra-abdominal disease in 25–30% of CSI and II	1. Early morbidity and mortality
2. Optimal recognition of patients curable by radiotherapy alone	2. Late fulminant infections following splenectomy
3. Spleen removed (smaller radiation field)	3. Staging laparotomy fails to detect intra-abdominal disease in 30% of cases when it is present
	4. Effective chemotherapy salvage is possible after radiotherapy relapses
	5. Increased use of chemotherapy as primary treatment
	6. Recognition of other prognostic variables identifying patients requiring primary chemotherapy

means of detecting hepatic or splenic involvement. Ultrasound investigation of the liver and spleen is also insensitive and gives a high rate of false positives and false negatives (Glees et al 1977). Magnetic resonance imaging may be an advance on previous scanning techniques in some situations but it is still to be fully evaluated in intraabdominal Hodgkin's disease.

The reasons for which some centres have abandoned the staging laparotomy are multiple. The procedure is of course unpleasant and has a significant early and late morbidity. The procedure associated mortality is low but not negligible (approximately 0.5%). Within the BNLI series there have been 6 deaths from fulminant infections in splenectomised patients in remission at the time of death. The procedure is also not as sensitive as was originally hoped. In the British National Lymphoma Investigation (BNLI) studies, 610 patients with CS I and IIA disease underwent a staging laparotomy. Intraabdominal disease was detected in 130 patients (21%), but a further

61 patients (10%) relapsed in the abdomen, indicative of occult intraabdominal disease not detected at laparotomy. More importantly it has become apparent that for many patients, effective salvage with chemotherapy is possible after radiotherapy relapse (Canellos et al 1972, Timothy et al 1979). Furthermore primary chemotherapy is used increasingly in those patients with the highest chance of intraabdominal disease (see below). The use of radiotherapy in patients with localised disease who have been only clinically staged will result in a higher relapse rate but in two small studies no survival advantage attributable to the improved staging associated with laparotomy was detected (Haybittle et al 1985, Reddy et al 1986). This would suggest that treating clinically occult lower half disease at presentation is no more successful than waiting until it is manifest clinically. This does not mean that a staging laparotomy has no role. The long term toxicity of radiotherapy followed by chemotherapy may be greater than that of chemotherapy alone with particular reference to the development of secondary solid tumours within the irradiation field. The higher relapse rate following radiotherapy in clinically staged patients also causes significant psychological trauma. Which patients might be selected for laparotomy staging ultimately becomes a matter of philosophy. In patients with CS I and IIA (upper half) disease of mixed cellularity subtype the risk of intraabdominal disease is nearly 50% (Table 10.3). This could

Table 10.3 Influence of histological subtype on risk of intra-abdominal disease in 599 patients with CS I and IIA (upper half) Hodgkin's disease (BNLI)

Histological subtype	No. of patients	Intra-abdominal disease detected at laparotomy (%)	Initial intra-abdominal relapse (%)	Total intra-abdominal disease (%)
Lymphocyte predominant	37	0	5	5
Nodular sclerosis				
Grade I	366	24	14	38
Grade II	109	15	8	23
Mixed cellularity	87	29	19	48

be interpreted as an indication for a staging laparotomy by some or as an indication for primary chemotherapy, and thus no staging laparotomy, by others. In patients with CS IIB upper half disease the incidence of intraabdominal disease is in the order of 70% and many centres use chemotherapy as initial therapy.

Perhaps the strongest argument for a staging laparotomy is in the young man with localised disease with poor prognostic features who has no family and does not wish to risk the infertility associated with some forms of chemotherapy, unless absolutely essential to his survival.

The value of other staging procedures also continues to be debated. Bilateral bone marrow biopsies are positive in 9–15% of patients at diagnosis (Bartl et al 1982) but this information is of very limited value in determining treatment strategy in individual patients. An analysis of 613 staging bone marrow trephines (unilateral biopsies in most cases) by Macintyre et al (1987) revealed infiltration in 40 cases (6.5%). Thirty-six of these patients were stage III or IV by other criteria and only 4 patients were advanced from localised disease to advanced disease as a result of the biopsy. Two of these patients had hepatosplenomegaly, and all had a raised alkaline phosphatase, but further investigations were not performed because of the positive marrow result. Bone marrow biopsy thus altered management in less than 1% of cases and may not have done so in any.

Histological classification
The Rye classification (Lukes et al 1966) divides Hodgkin's disease into four categories: lymphocyte predominant, nodular sclerosis, mixed cellularity and lymphocyte depleted. This classification has limited prognostic significance by virtue of the fact that the large majority of patients have nodular sclerotic disease. Bennett et al (1985) have therefore divided this subtype into grade 1 and grade 2 where grade 2 indicates easily recognised areas of lymphocyte depletion or numerous pleomorphic Hodgkin's cells. This revised classification has considerable prognostic value (Fig. 10.1) which

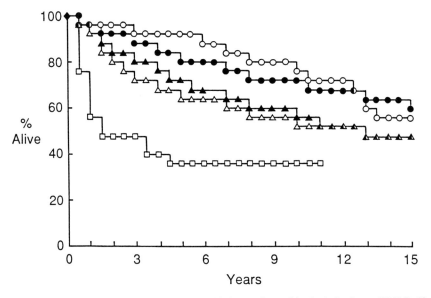

Fig. 10.1   Overall survival in Hodgkin's disease divided according to histological subtype (BNLI). *Key:* ○ LP, 149; ● NSI, 1255; △ NSII, 671; ▲ MC, 482; □ LD, 41; LP, lymphocyte predominant; NSI, nodular sclerosis: low grade; NSII, nodular sclerosis: high grade; MC, mixed cellularity; LD, lymphocyte depleted.

has been confirmed by others (Jairam et al 1987). Lymphocyte predominant and nodular sclerosis grade 1 have a good prognosis whereas nodular sclerosis grade 2 and mixed cellularity have a considerably worse prognosis. The prognosis of lymphocyte depleted Hodgkin's disease is particularly poor. Although the histological subtype and stage are related at presentation the histology is an independent prognostic factor with regard to survival (Table 10.4). It should be noted that in stage IA and IIA disease treated by radiotherapy alone there is no significant difference in the CR rate between the histological types with nearly all patients achieving CR. The difference in survival reflects the difference in relapse rate and response to second line chemotherapy. In stage IIIB and IV, all initially treated by chemotherapy, the histological subtype influences the complete remission rate as well as the 5-year survival.

A cell marker profile of Hodgkin's cells has been determined in recent years using monoclonal antibodies. The malignant cells typically react positively with antibodies

Table 10.4 Influence of stage and histological subtypes on survival in 2062 patients with Hodgkin's disease* entered into BNLI studies from 1970 to 1986

Stage**	Symptoms	Histological grade†	% of patients	CR rate on initial therapy (%)	Actuarial 5-year survival (%)
I	A	I	13	99	92
		II	7	98	83
	B	I	<0.5	67	100
		II	0.5	80	79
II	A	I	13	96	94
		II	8	90	77
	B	I	3	74	78
		II	4	55	70
III	A	I	11	85	80
		II	6	70	71
	B	I	6	69	77
		II	7	60	55
IV	A	I	3	62	74
		II	2	44	56
	B	I	5	61	64
		II	9	43	64

* All adult patients are included with no upper age limit. The 5-year survival figures include intercurrent deaths.
** Includes both clinically and pathologically staged patients.
† Grade I, lymphocyte predominant and Grade 1 nodular sclerosis; Grade II, grade 2 nodular sclerosis, mixed cellularity and lymphocyte depleted.

to class II MHC antigens, the IL-2 receptor (CD 25) and the CD 30 (Ki1) and CD 15 (e.g. leu M1) antigens (Sloane 1987). Such immunophenotype analysis may be of value in the differential diagnosis of Hodgkin's disease but has not to date been of value in subclassifying the disease.

Other prognostic factors

Numerous centres have now identified independent prognostic factors by univariate and multivariate analysis. Particular attention has been paid to patients with localised disease as it is in this group that such information has been most likely to influence treatment, helping to define the need for a staging laparotomy or for primary chemotherapy. The prognostic factors determined by any one centre will depend on the population of patients studied and the therapy used, but there is considerable agreement as to the relevant factors (Table 10.5). Prognostic indexes have been constructed to give appropriate weighting to the various factors and using this the BNLI have defined three prognostic categories (Fig. 10.2) (Haybittle et al 1985). Similarly others have divided CS I and II patients into different categories and have recommended chemotherapy for the worst prognostic category. The prognostic factors for relapse are not necessarily identical to those for overall survival. Age makes little difference to the relapse rate but a large difference to the overall survival (Vaughan Hudson et al 1983, Selby & McElwain 1987). In the BNLI series of localised disease the 5-year survival rate in patients aged 16–39 years, 40–59 years and 60–77 years is 91%, 83% and 68%, with the mortality from Hodgkin's disease being 7%, 10% and 20% respectively. The significance of mediastinal involvement as an independent prognostic factor is not clear. It is generally (but not universally) accepted however that patients with large mediastinal masses do have a higher relapse rate and many centres use chemotherapy as well as radiotherapy in such circumstances. Poor prognostic

Table 10.5   Identification of poor prognostic factors in localised Hodgkin's disease (CS I and II) by multivariate analysis

	EORTC (n = 1139, Tubiana et al 1985)	BNLI (n = 743, Haybittle et al 1985)	Royal Marsden (n = 294, Horwich et al 1986)	Princess Margaret Hospital, Toronto (n = 252, Sutcliffe et al 1985)
Survival:				
Age	⩾40 years	Progressive	⩾60 years	⩾50 years
Sex	Male	Male		
Histology	MC or LD	NSII, MC or LD		MC or LD
Symptoms	A + ESR ⩾50 B + ESR ⩾30			
ESR		ESR >40		
Number of sites	Stage IIn ⩾ 3		Stage II	Stage II
Mediastinal involvement		Positive		
Relapse free survival:				
Age	⩾40			⩾50
Sex	Male			
Histology		NSII, MC or LD		MC or LD
Symptoms	A + ESR ⩾ 30 B + ESR ⩾ 50			
ESR		⩾40		
Number of sites	Stage IIn ⩾ 3	Stage II	Stage II	Stage II
Mediastinal involvement				

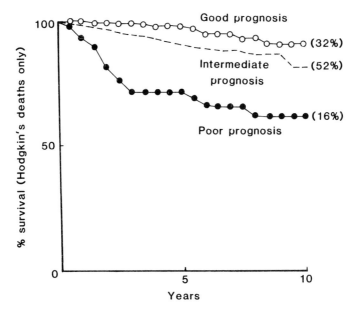

Fig. 10.2   Actuarial survival in CSI and IIA Hodgkin's disease divided according to prognostic index (BNLI).

factors predicting relapse after radiotherapy do so in part by predicting occult intra-abdominal disease but the predictive value for this is not precise. Thus in the EORTC H6 trial although the incidence of a positive laparotomy is twice as high in the unfavour-able group of patients, the incidence in the favourable group is still 18% (Tubiana et al 1985). Brada and colleagues from the Royal Marsden Hospital evaluated different prognostic factors predicting for a positive laparotomy. The factors were different from those predicting for relapse free survival with age and sex independently prognos-tic, as well as the size and bulk of nodes in CSI disease (Brada et al 1986). Three categories of risk were identified with risk of occult intraabdominal disease being >50%, 15–50% and <15% in the high, intermediate and low risk groups. Women in general had a lower risk of a positive laparotomy and the greatest risk was in men under 20 years of age. Prognostic factors thus vary, not only with the patient population and the treatment used but also with the event to be analysed. Determi-nation of risk of intraabdominal disease is important for those committed to staging laparotomy in most patients but is of limited interest to those who have abandoned the procedure on other criteria.

Prognostic factors may also be defined in advanced disease. In the BNLI series of patients, the main factors indicating a poor prognosis in univariate analyses are low presentation albumin level (strongly associated with low haemoglobin and high ESR), age, aggressive histology, and 'B' symptoms. It should be noted that in advanced disease the prognosis is poorer in older patients because of a lower response to treatment as well as intercurrent deaths. Prognostic factors in advanced disease may become increasingly important in selecting patients for more intensive first and second line chemotherapy.

Treatment

Role of radiotherapy

Radiotherapy is undoubtedly the treatment of choice in selected patients with localised Hodgkin's disease. The selection of appropriate patients and the choice of radiation field will depend on the attitude of the physician or centre. In general terms, the use of limited radiation fields results in higher relapse rates but ultimately similar survival due to effective second line therapy. Glatstein (1984) has suggested that a radiotherapy failure rate in excess of 35% is unacceptable but this figure is of course debatable.

In the small number of patients with CS IA disease above the thyroid notch involved field radiotherapy produces excellent results, with CR rates approaching 100% and 5-year disease-free survivals (DFS) of the order of 90% (Russell et al 1984, Sutcliffe et al 1985). Neither staging laparotomy nor more extensive therapy would appear justified in this situation.

In other cases of upper half CS I and II treated by mantle fields the relapse rate is well in excess of 40% the majority of relapses being below the diaphragm. In pathologically staged patients (PS I and II upper half) the relapse rate appears to be less (Table 10.6). Extended field irradiation to include infradiaphragmatic fields (paraaortics or inverted Y) results in a lower relapse rate, particularly in patients who have not been pathologically staged. The use of a mantle field alone in CS I and II disease may seem totally inadequate from this data but the relapse rate is

Table 10.6   Relapse rates following irradiation in localised Hodgkin's disease

Treatment by mantle field			Treatment by mantle and infradiaphragmatic irradiation		
Reference	No. of patients	Relapse rate	Reference	No. of patients	Relapse rate
Clinical stage I and II:					
Rubin et al (1974)	83	64% (5 y)	Rubin et al (1974)	50*	28% (5 y)
Tubiana et al (1975)	52**	58% (5 y)	Tubiana et al (1981)	156	33% (5 y)
Liew et al (1983)	64	52% (5 y)			
Sutcliffe et al (1985)	130	37% (10 y)	Sutcliffe et al (1985)	51**	30% (10 y)
Pathological stage I and II:					
Liew et al (1983)	66	33% (5 y)	Tubiana et al (1981)	106	19% (5 y)
			Hoppe et al (1982)	109**	23% (10 y)
Anderson et al (1984)	55	31% (5 y)	Nissen & Nordentoft (1982)	128	32% (9 y)
BNLI	203†	38% (10 y)	Willet et al (1987)	122††	25% (5 y)

* 32 of these patients received a laparotomy but results are not taken into account in this analysis.
** Includes some patients with lower half disease.
† I and IIA nodular sclerosis only.
†† I and IIA. 14 patients clinically staged only.

reduced if patients with B symptoms or high risk prognostic factors are excluded from this treatment approach, and it must be emphasised that the more conservative initial treatment does not appear to prejudice ultimate survival. Indeed some centres elect to give involved field irradiation only, even in clinically staged patients. This increases the relapse rate further (Glatstein 1977, Jelliffe 1979, Hagemeister 1982) but has less toxicity and again does not mitigate against survival.

A further factor requiring consideration when using radiotherapy is the influence of bulky mediastinal disease. Several centres have reported a high risk of intrathoracic relapse in patients with bulky mediastinal disease (>0.33 the widest thoracic diameter) and advocated treatment with chemotherapy as well as irradiation (Hagemeister et al 1982, Liew et al 1984) although this has been deemed to be unnecessary except in the most enormous masses (>0.5 × the thoracic diameter) by members of the EORTC (Cosset et al 1984).

Localised infradiaphragmatic disease is relatively uncommon. In CS I (approximately 10% of cases) the results of radiotherapy are excellent. In CS II disease, especially if the paraaortic nodes are involved there is a high incidence of splenic involvement or more advanced disease (Barrett et al 1981, Sutcliffe et al 1985) and many authorities would recommend chemotherapy in this situation if a staging laparotomy is not performed.

The reported results of radiation therapy alone (total nodal irradiation) in CS IIIA disease are poor with relapse occurring in at least half the patients (Peckham et al 1975, Prosnitz et al 1978, Hellman & Mauch 1982). The results in PS IIIA are also poor for DFS (Prosnitz et al 1978, Hellman & Mauch 1982). It thus seems appropriate to use chemotherapy as first line treatment in IIIA disease. Several authors have however emphasised that high abdominal disease ($IIIA_1$) which is usually only detected at staging laparotomy has a better prognosis than $IIIA_2$ disease and radiotherapy may be appropriate in these cases (Prosnitz et al 1978, Hellman & Mauch 1982) though the relapse rate still exceeds 40%.

Role of chemotherapy

Chemotherapy as first line treatment has largely been used on its own in advanced disease or as an adjuvant to radiotherapy in localised disease. Its use in advanced disease is discussed first as this is the scenario in which it has been developed.

Combination chemotherapy is the only effective therapy in stage IIIB and IV disease and is probably also the treatment of choice in CS IIB and IIIA disease. The MOPP regime was introduced by De Vita and others in the 1960s and the long term follow up of 188 patients was published in 1986 (Longo et al 1986). 84% of patients obtained complete remission and 66% of these patients have remained disease free for more than 10 years. The overall survival is 48% with 19% of patients dying of intercurrent illness free of Hodgkin's disease. Numerous other studies report CR rates between 60% and 80% (Table 10.7). The reasons for the variability of the results is not clear, although there is a tendency for multi-centre groups to report less satisfactory results.

Table 10.7 Selected results of combination chemotherapy in advanced Hodgkin's disease

Type of regime	Regime	Centre	Reference	Stage	No. of patients	CR rate	Overall survival
MOPP	MOPP	NCI	Longo et al (1986)	95% III & IV	188	84%	65% (5 y) 51% (10 y) 48% (15 y)
	MOPP	BNLI		ALL III & IV	461	63%	64% (5 y) 50% (10 y)
	MOPP	ECOG	Bakemeier et al (1984)	93% III & IV	146	73%	61% (5 y)
	MOPP	Milan	Bonadonna et al (1986)	IIB & III	114	81%	68% (7 y)
	MOPP			IV	43	74%	64% (8 y)
MOPP variants	MVPP	St Barth- olomews, London	Sutcliffe et al (1978)	IIIB & IV	49	76%	65% (5 y)
	Ch1VPP	Royal Marsden, London	Dady et al (1982)	80% III & IV	59	73%	66% (5 y)
	LOPP	BNLI	Hancock (1986)	III & IV	136	59%	68% (5 y)
	Bleo-MOPP	SWOG	Jones et al (1983)	No details	125	67%	71% (3 y)
	BCVPP	ECOG	Bakemeier et al (1984)	I & II recurrents + III & IV	147	76%	67% (5 y)
	MOP-BAP	SWOG	Jones et al (1983)	III & IV	166	77%	77% (3 y)
Non cross-resistant regimes	ABVD + RT	Milan	Santoro et al (1987)	IIB & III	109	92%	77% (7 y)
	SCAB	NCI	Diggs et al (1981)	IIIB & IV	20	75%	77% (3 y)
Sequential	MOPP/ABVD	Milan	Bonadonna et al (1986)	IV	45	89%	84% (8 y)
	LOPP/EVAP	BNLI		80% III & IV	151	72%	84% (3 y)
	MOPP/ CAVmp/RT	EORTC	Wagener et al (1983)	III & IV	47	87%	86% (3 y)
	MOPP-CABS	NCI	Young et al (1985)	No details	43	85%	80%* (4 y)
	MOPP/ ABVD/RT	Memorial Kettering	Straus et al (1984)	68% III & IV	34	78%	85% (4 y)
	CAD-MOPP/ ABVD/RT	Memorial Kettering	Straus et al (1984)	59% III & IV	37	82%	90% (4 y)
Hybrids	MOPP/ABV	Vancouver	Klimo & Connors (1985)	75% III & IV	52	88%	90%* (4 y)
	MA/MA + RT	Milan	Bonadonna et al (1985)	Bulky I & IIA, IIB, III & IV	40	93%	—

* Median follow up only 27 months.

This may be a reflection of the fact that centres participating in multi-centre trials see a less selected group of patients or that smaller centres are less capable of looking after their patients. This latter possibility is highly contentious and is without firm evidence. It is of interest that in the BNLI series in which the CR rate was only 62.5% the 10 year overall survival of 50% is not dissimilar from the NCI results.

The early MOPP studies indicated that maintenance therapy was unnecessary and this has been subsequently confirmed (Bakemeier et al 1984, Nissen et al 1979). It is now common practice to give chemotherapy until CR, then 2–4 further cycles, and then stop.

Numerous MOPP variant regimens have been devised. In general they replace mustine with an alternative alkylating agent such as a nitrosourea, chlorambucil or cyclophosphamide, and replace vincristine with vinblastine. The use of an alternative alkylating agent results in less nausea and vomiting and less alopecia and the use of vinblastine causes less neurotoxicity. The efficacy of these less toxic variants has been shown to be the same as MOPP in single centre studies and large randomised clinical trials (Bakemeier et al 1984, Hancock 1986).

The addition of bleomycin to MOPP or to a MOPP variant has been tested by several groups. Overall there is little evidence that this leads to an improved survival.

A more drastic departure from MOPP was the use of four completely different and hopefully non cross-resistant drugs (ABVD). This regime was compared with MOPP in three trials (Santoro et al 1987) all of which also employed radiotherapy. ABVD was shown to be at least as good as MOPP for initial therapy. ABVD has the advantage of being less sterilising than MOPP, and may produce fewer leukaemias (Bonadonna 1985). ABVD does however produce severe nausea and vomiting, and several multi-drug regimens containing adriamycin but not DTIC have been developed. These are probably as efficacious as MOPP although direct comparisons have not been made.

The major problem with such regimens is the development of chemotherapy resistance, and the Goldie–Coldman somatic mutation hypothesis (Goldie & Coldman 1984) predicts that the early introduction of multiple agents would reduce this problem and so increase the response rate and durability of those responses. The Milan group piloted the use of alternating cycles of MOPP and ABVD and updated the results in 1986 (Bonadonna et al 1986). In this study the CR rate and freedom from progression were significantly better in those patients receiving alternating chemotherapy compared to MOPP. The overall survival was also better with alternating MOPP/ABVD than MOPP although this did not achieve statistical significance. It should also be noted that half the MOPP patients ultimately received ABVD. Numerous other studies of alternating therapy are in progress or have been reported in preliminary form (Table 10.7). The NCI study comparing MOPP with alternating MOPP/CABS has not yet shown an advantage for the alternating regime (Young et al 1985). In a large prospective randomised trial by the BNLI comparing LOPP with alternating LOPP/EVAP, the complete remission rate and disease free survival are significantly better with the alternating therapy although this has not as yet been converted to overall survival.

A further extension of this approach has been the development of hybrid regimens in which 7 or 8 of the most active drugs are introduced into each cycle given monthly. Klimo & Connors (1985) using a MOPP/ABV hybrid reported that 46 of 52 previously untreated and evaluable patients (88%) achieved CR with an actuarial overall survival at 4 years of 90% and actuarial freedom from relapse in the complete responders of 93% at 41 months. The Milan group have also reported encouraging results with a MOPP/ABVD hybrid regime (Bonadonna et al 1985). A further possible advantage of hybrid regimes is that they may enable the period of therapy to be considerably reduced (Klimo & Connors 1985).

Combined modality

As discussed above (Table 10.6) the relapse rate following radiotherapy for apparently localised Hodgkin's disease is considerable even when patients are carefully selected and extended radiation fields are used. For this reason chemotherapy is often added to the radiation schedule, the rationale being that chemotherapy will reduce the volume of a large tumour mass and allow a smaller and safer radiation field to be used (e.g. in the mediastinum), that it will produce further tumour kill in the irradiated area (non cross-resistant) and that it will eliminate occult disease outside of the radiation field. The majority of studies indicate that combined modality treatment results in a significantly better disease free survival than radiotherapy alone (Table 10.8). The

Table 10.8   Randomised trials of radiotherapy versus combined modality treatment

Centre	Reference	Stage	No. of patients	Treatment	Relapse-free survival	Overall survival
Stanford	Hoppe et al (1982)	PS I & II	109	TLI	77% (10 y)	84% (10 y)
			121	RT + CHEMO*	84% (10 y)	84% (10 y)
		PS I & II	14	TLI	45% (10 y)	84% (10 y)
		Bulky mediastinum (subgroup of above)	27	RT + CHEMO*	77% (10 y)	74% (10 y)
Finsen Institute	Nissen & Nordentoft (1982)	PS I & II	128	TNI	67% (7 y)	92% (7 y)
			133	Mantle + MOPP	92% (7 y)	92% (7 y)
Manchester	Anderson et al (1984)	PS I & II	55	Mantle	69% (7 y)	94% (7 y)
			59	Mantle + MVPP	93% (7 y)	91% (7 y)
EORTC	Tubiana et al (1984)	CS I & II	46	TLI	78% (3.5 y)	86% (3.5 y)
			20	EF (pelvis excluded)	58% (3.5 y)	89% (3.5 y)
			55	EF + MOPP	89% (3.5 y)	92% (3.5 y)
New York	Dutcher & Wiernik (1985)	PS I & II	29	EF	66% (14 y)	78% (14 y)
			17	EF + MOPP	94% (14 y)	100% (14 y)
		PS IIIA	12	EF	42% (14 y)	58% (14 y)
			16	EF + MOPP	95% (14 y)	79% (14 y)

*RT was either IF, EF or TLI. Chemo was predominantly MOPP.

overall survival is not significantly different however, because of the efficacy of chemotherapy given after relapse from radiotherapy. There is limited data on chemotherapy alone in localised Hodgkin's disease. In a report by Pavlovsky and colleagues (1987) 131 CS I and II patients were treated by CVPP chemotherapy alone, 88% obtained a CR, with a disease free survival at 6 years of 61% and overall survival of 79%. This compares with a CR rate of 94%, disease free survival of 72% and overall survival of 92% in 136 patients randomised to radiotherapy + CVPP. Although the DFS was significantly better with combined modality treatment the survival was not significantly better.

A retrospective analysis of PS III patients treated in Boston by radiotherapy alone or by combined modality showed a significantly improved actuarial survival for combined modality treatment (Mauch et al 1985) but the results may again not be better than chemotherapy alone. In a retrospective analysis from the Royal Marsden Hospital of PS III and CS III patients combined modality treatment gave better survival than radiotherapy or chemotherapy alone but this did not achieve statistical significance when corrected for age (Brada et al 1987).

The studies shown in Table 10.8 all use 6 courses of MOPP. This regime causes infertility, may be leukaemogenic and can exacerbate radiation tissue damage. This strategy would not therefore appear to be advisable except in those cases with the very highest risk of relapse such as those with B symptoms or large mediastinal masses. Two developments may alter this situation. Firstly, several reports suggest that it may only be necessary to give two or three cycles of chemotherapy in the adjuvant setting, resulting in a lesser risk of chemotherapy side effects (Ferme et al 1984, Zittoun et al 1985). Secondly, the use of ABVD regimes rather than MOPP further reduces the risks of infertility and leukemogenesis. It is possible that in poor prognosis localised disease combined modality treatment using two courses of ABVD or equivalent could result in less ultimate toxicity than either radiotherapy or full dose chemotherapy given as initial treatment.

In advanced disease treated by chemotherapy, the majority of relapses occur at sites of previous bulk disease (Young et al 1978). It might be expected that adjuvant radiotherapy to such sites after chemotherapy would improve the complete remission rate disease free and perhaps overall survival. The dosage of radiotherapy required in the adjuvant setting might be less than the 35–40 Gy required for radical therapy. Several centres use such strategies and have reported good results (Bonadonna et al 1985, Strauss et al 1984, Wagener et al 1983), but randomised controlled trials are required to resolve this important issue.

Salvage therapy

CHEMOTHERAPY

Salvage therapy is the optimistic term used for the treatment of patients after chemotherapy failure, and it is in this setting that many of the newer drug regimes have been developed. Following chemotherapy failure the long term prognosis is poor as illustrated by the survival curve for patients failing 'MOPP-type' chemotherapy in the BNLI (Fig. 10.3). It must be noted however that the attrition rate is slow, and a significant proportion of patients are alive at 5 years as a result of many different salvage strategies. MOPP (or similar regimes) may be effective in inducing a CR even in MOPP relapses especially when there has been a prolonged first remission. Thus in selected patients the second CR rate may be very high. For those patients failing to achieve a CR on MOPP type treatment or relapsing quickly, then alternative 'non cross-resistant' regimes are required. In 54 MOPP resistant or early relapsed cases Santoro et al (1982) reported a complete remission rate of 59% with ABVD, but similar excellent results have not been obtained in other centres (Case et al 1977, Harker et al 1984). The response to ABVD is better in those who obtained a previous CR on MOPP than in those who did not, and in those who have only nodal disease and no symptoms at the time of relapse. Patients who have been heavily pretreated will also fare less well. These factors may account for some of the differences between

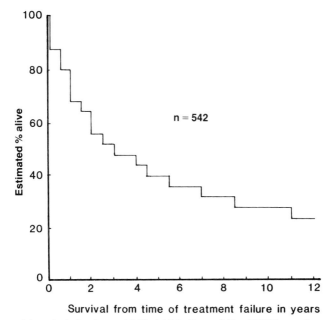

Fig. 10.3 Actuarial survival of patients with Hodgkin's disease failing MOPP type chemotherapy (all ages) (BNLI).

centres. Even in the best series, however, the long term disease free survival with ABVD is poor. Other second line non cross-resistant regimes nearly all contain adriamycin. Other drugs used include bleomycin, the nitrosoureas, VP16, VP26, cis-platinum, predmustine and hexamethylmelanine. There is little evidence to suggest that the results with many of these numerous regimes differ significantly from ABVD.

It should be noted that in patients with purely nodal relapses following chemotherapy alone, effective salvage and even long term survival can be achieved in some cases with radiotherapy (Fox et al 1987, Mauch et al 1987, Roach et al 1987).

Combinations of the various drugs listed above are also used to formulate third line regimes, the composition of the regime depending on what was used for first and second or initial alternating/hybrid therapy. Results with third line therapy are generally poor although some patients with chronic relapsing disease may have good partial responses on repeated occasions.

AUTOLOGOUS BONE MARROW TRANSPLANTATION

The use of very intensive chemo/radiotherapy with haematological rescue by bone marrow transplantation represents an alternative salvage strategy. Numerous pilot studies have now been reported using high dose chemo/radiotherapy and autologous bone marrow transplantation. The Bloomsbury transplant group have reported results of 50 adult patients who are evaluable post ABMT (Goldstone et al 1987a). The median age was 27 years. All patients were in relapse of disease following chemotherapy (two modalities of chemotherapy or alternating therapy) and over 50% had also received radiotherapy. The high dose therapy used in 39 of these patients was the BEAM regime (BCNU 300 mg/m^2 day 1, VP16 100–200 mg/m^2 days 2–5, cytosine arabinoside 100–200 mg/m^2 days 2–5 and melphalan 140 mg/m^2 day 6). Five patients died from sepsis during the aplastic phase and a further patient (aged 59 years) died of acute cardiac failure whilst in CR 8 months after the procedure and is regarded as a treatment related death. The treatment related mortality is thus high (12%), although it must be noted that many of these patients had been heavily pretreated. Nineteen patients entered CR post ABMT (38%). A further 2 patients defined as PR because of residual mediastinal masses have had no further treatment and have had no progression of their disease for 18 and 25 months. Three further patients obtaining a partial remission on the ABMT procedure have obtained a CR with subsequent radiotherapy. Of these 25 patients (50%) with a good response to treatment, 20 have freedom from progression with a median follow up of 19 months. This data is in broad agreement with results from other centres (Table 10.9). The majority

Table 10.9 Results of high dose chemo/radiotherapy and autologous bone marrow transplantation as salvage therapy in Hodgkin's disease

Centre	Reference	No. of patients	CR rate (%)	Overall survival
Lyon	Philip et al (1986)	17	41	18% approx (2 y)
Vancouver	O'Reilly et al (1987)	20	80★	—
New York	Ahmed et al (1987)	30	47	—
Bloomsbury	Goldstone et al (1987a)	50	50★★	50% (2 y)
Nebraska/M D Anderson	Jagannath et al (1988)	62	52†	41% (3 y)
EBMTG	Goldstone et al (1987b)	117††	56	42% (2 y)

★ Patients heavily treated to minimal disease state prior to autograft procedure.
★★ Includes 4 patients who went into CR after post transplant radiotherapy.
† Includes 5 patients who went into CR after post transplant radiotherapy.
†† Includes some patients reported by Goldstone et al and Philip et al.

of patients have received high dose chemotherapy rather than total body irradiation (TBI) because of the pulmonary complications associated with TBI after mantle radiotherapy (Phillips et al 1984). The results are in general encouraging but the precise role of such treatment, if any, has not been defined. If the procedure related morbidity is to be reduced, such intensive treatments must be given early in the course of the disease and this requires stratification to define the poor prognostic groups. Although the ultimate survival of patients failing MOPP type regimes is poor the rate of attrition is slow (Fig. 10.3). We have arbitrarily deemed that a patient to be eligible for an autograft procedure should have an expected 2 year survival <65% and a 5 year survival of <35%. Using these criteria we have identified 4 situations in which autografting is applicable (Table 10.10) (Gribben et al 1987b). This analysis based on presenting features is imperfect and more precise stratification must also take into account the prognostic factors that are present at the time of relapse.

Conclusions

In localised Hodgkin's disease the recent greater awareness of prognostic factors, the use of extensive radiation fields and the use of chemotherapy in the initial treatment programme have all enabled an improved relapse free survival to be obtained. Improved overall survival has not been demonstrated, however, and some centres continue to use very conservative treatment approaches even in clinically staged

Table 10.10 Possible indications for intensive therapy and autologous bone marrow transplantation in Hodgkin's disease defined by presentation criteria

---

Treated initially with chemotherapy
1. Failure to obtain CR on MOPP type therapy if:
    a. High grade histology (NS II, MC, LD)
    b. Low grade histology and ESR ⩾60
2. Treatment failure after two treatment modalities
3. Treatment failure after alternating or hybrid regimes

Treated initially with radiotherapy (Stage II)
4. Criteria as in 1 and 2 above ignoring the initial radiotherapy

---

patients. The overall survival in younger patients is good whatever the approach, and further improvements will be difficult to demonstrate.

The treatment of advanced Hodgkin's disease remains difficult with many patients still dying of their disease. Recent developments using more intensive chemo/radiotherapy as both first and second line therapy offer encouragement but the impact on survival of the patient group as a whole cannot as yet be judged. The outlook for the elderly patient with advanced Hodgkin's disease remains poor.

NON-HODGKIN'S LYMPHOMA

Patient stratification

Histological classification

The primary stratification in the non-Hodgkin's lymphomas is based on the histological subtype. The Rappaport classification described in 1966 (Rappaport 1966) was widely used but was increasingly criticised, predominantly because of the use of the term 'histiocytic lymphoma' for large lymphocytic lymphomas and because the diffuse histocytic lymphoma category encompassed a large proportion of patients with a wide spectrum of different histological appearances. In the 1970s numerous other classifications appeared (Lennert et al 1975, Bennett et al 1974, Lukes & Collins 1974) creating considerable confusion amongst physicians trying to analyse results from different centres. In 1982 a National Cancer Institute study was reported in which the clinical value of six classification systems was compared. All were found to be equally useful and a 'Working Formulation' was devised to facilitate translation between the different systems (Table 10.11). The value of this formulation has been independently confirmed (Nissen & Ersboll 1985). It is apparent from Table 10.11 that the categories defined by the Working Formulation are in general very similar to those of Rappaport and also the British National Lymphoma Investigation. It is the terminology rather than concepts that differ.

Details of the prognostic groupings may be debated. In the BNLI series the diffuse small cleaved cell lymphomas have survival curves similar to other low grade lymphomas (Farrer-Brown 1981). In the Finsen Institute series of 602 patients, multivariate analysis was performed to determine an independent hazard ratio for each histological subtype (Nissen & Ersboll 1985). The diffuse small cleaved cell lymphoma would again appear to be a low grade lymphoma. In this series the hazard ratio for large cell follicular lymphomas was very high bracketing it with the high rather than intermediate grade lymphomas.

Table 10.11   NCI Working Formulation

Working formulation (WF)	WF study group (%)	Finsen Institute series (%)	Rappaport classification	Kiel classification
Low grade				
Small lymphocytic	3.6	8.5	Diffuse well differentiated lymphocytic	Lymphocytic, CLL Lymphoplasmacytic/ Lymphoplasmacytoid
Follicular predominantly small cleaved cell	22.5	15.4	Nodular poorly differentiated lymphocytic	Centroblastic-centrocytic (small) follicular ± diffuse
Follicular mixed small cleaved and large cell	7.7	5.6	Nodular mixed lymphocytic histocytic	
Intermediate grade				
Follicular predominantly large cell	3.8	3.8	Nodular histiocytic	Centroblastic-centrocytic (large) follicular ± diffuse
Diffuse small cleaved cell	6.9	5.3	Diffuse poorly differentiated lymphocytic	Centrocytic (small)
Diffuse mixed small and large cell	6.7	8.3	Diffuse mixed lymphocytic and histocytic	Centroblastic-centrocytic (small) diffuse lymphoplasmacytic-cytoid polymorphic
Diffuse large cell	19.7	12.6	Diffuse histocytic	Centroblastic-centrocytic (large) diffuse Centrocytic (large) Centroblastic
High grade				
Large cell immunoblastic	7.9	24.3	Diffuse histocytic	Immunoblastic T zone lymphoma Lymphoepithelioid cell lymphoma
Lymphoblastic	4.2	11.0	Lymphoblastic	Lymphoblastic, convoluted cell type Lymphoblastic unclassified
Small non cleaved	5.0	5.2	Diffuse undifferentiated	Lymphoblastic Burkitt type and other B lymphoblastic
Miscellaneous including: Composite Mycosis fungoides Histiocytic Extramedullary plasmacytoma				Mycosis fungoides Plasmacytic

The formulation does lump together some entities that may be biologically distinct (see Kiel classification). Although the follicular lymphomas are of B cell origin, the diffuse lymphomas may be of B or T cell origin as emphasised by the classification of Lukes & Collins (1974). No account of such immunophenotype is taken in the working formulation. This does not mean that the cell lineage is unimportant. The T cell lymphomas comprise several distinct clinico-pathological entities (Cossman et al 1984) (Table 10.12). The term peripheral T cell lymphoma is applied to other

Table 10.12 T cell lymphomas

1. Mycosis fungoides and Sezary's syndrome
2. HTLV-1 associated leukaemia/lymphoma
3. Large granular lymphocytosis—CD8$^+$
   T cell chronic lymphocytic leukaemia
4. Peripheral T cell lymphomas

T cell lymphomas with a mature phenotype (c.f. T lymphoblastic lymphomas). The histological appearances of the PTL are varied and the heterogeneity of this group may account in part for the controversy over their prognosis. Whereas several groups have reported that the PTL are usually disseminated at presentation and have a very poor prognosis (Lippman et al 1987, Swan et al 1987), other groups have found that the prognosis is not overall different from the aggressive B cell lymphomas (Cossman et al 1984).

With the availability of monoclonal antibodies reactive in paraffin sections and probes for immunoglobulin and T cell receptor gene rearrangements more complete studies of larger numbers of patients treated in similar ways will undoubtedly be reported. It is likely that more precise prognostic stratification will be obtained by a combination of immunophenotype and morphological appearances.

It must also be noted that the different groupings in the working formulation are based on survival outcome and this does not invariably dictate the treatment strategy. Immunoblastic lymphomas (high grade) are usually treated in the same way as the large cell lymphomas (intermediate grade) often without CNS prophylaxis. In the lymphoblastic lymphomas and small non cleaved cell lymphomas the risk of CNS relapse is very high and CNS prophylaxis is essential (Nissen & Ersboll 1985). A histological stratification based on treatment approach is shown in Table 10.13. The term indolent lymphoma is used instead of low grade lymphoma emphasising that the long term survival of these cases is at least as bad as in cases with high grade histology (Fig. 10.4).

Anatomical staging
Anatomical staging does not dictate the treatment to be used in most cases of NHL. For this reason, a staging laparotomy is not justified except in occasional patients or in an investigational setting. Clinical staging identifies disseminated disease in approximately two thirds of patients at presentation and if pathological staging is performed the incidence of disseminated disease is nearly 80% (Anderson et al 1982). This is undoubtedly an underestimate. In approximately 90% of follicular lymphomas there is a t14;18 (q32;q21) which involves reciprocal translocation of the immuno-globulin heavy chain gene and bcl-2 gene. This rearrangement can be detected by DNA hybridisation and Southern blotting, and the polymerase chain reaction

Table 10.13   Therapy based grouping of NHL histological subtypes

Type	Working formulation
Indolent	Small lymphocytic Follicular predominantly small cleaved cell Follicular mixed small cleaved and large cell
	Diffuse small cleaved cell
Aggressive	Follicular large cell Diffuse mixed small and large cell Diffuse large cell Large cell immunoblastic
Aggressive with high risk of CNS and leukaemic relapse	Lymphoblastic Small-non cleaved

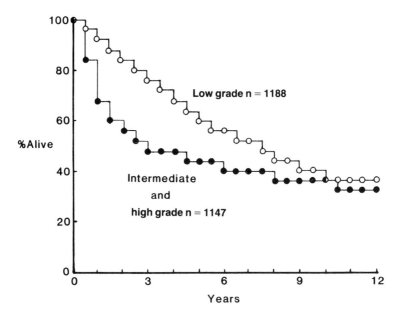

Fig. 10.4   Overall survival in non-Hodgkin's lymphoma divided according to histological type (BNLI).

technique allows detection of one cell with this translocation in 100 000 normal cells. Lee and colleagues (Lee et al 1987) used this technique to analyse the blood of 11 patients with follicular lymphomas and found malignant cells in 10, 4 of whom were thought to be in complete remission at the time of the study. It is thus likely that nearly all follicular lymphomas have stage IV disease although it may frequently be undetected. Conventional clinical staging does none the less provide useful prognostic information, although it must be regarded in general as a reflection of total disease bulk rather than precise anatomical localisation.

The staging procedure should include a bone marrow examination and examination of the cerebrospinal fluid in patients with lymphoblastic or small non cleaved cell lymphomas and in those patients with relevant signs or symptoms.

Other prognostic factors

Apart from histological grade and anatomical stage multivariate analysis of the whole Finsen Institute series showed that age, male sex and B symptoms were independent prognostic variables (Nissen & Ersboll 1985). Age is probably most important in the high grade lymphomas reflecting the difficulty of giving intensive chemotherapy to an elderly population. The sex difference is not apparent in several other series. The presence of B symptoms is a poor prognostic feature in nearly all series, as are other markers of systemic disturbance such as an increased ESR and reduced albumin. In multivariate analysis limited to patients with follicular lymphoma, the major poor prognostic factors in order were found to be splenomegaly, hepatomegaly, abnormal liver function tests, B symptoms and anaemia (Gallagher et al 1986). The importance of bulk abdominal disease and a raised LDH has been shown by others, in both low grade and high grade lymphomas (Fisher et al 1981, Jagannath et al 1985). A recent communication by Anderson et al (1987) emphasises the importance of performance status in determining therapeutic outcome. This is a product of many factors and is difficult to quantify, and for this reason is rarely analysed in detail in large studies. Despite this it is obvious that the outcome of a patient with IVB high grade lymphoma who is having night sweats but working normally might be quite different from the IVB patient moribund from multisystem failure.

Treatment

Indolent disease

It is common practice to treat localised indolent lymphomas with local radiotherapy. In the small group of PS I and II the response is excellent with an 80% disease free survival reported at 10 years (Rosenberg 1982). Late relapses do occur however and it is difficult to be confident of cure. In CS I and II the relapse rate is higher as might be expected. In the Toronto series reported by Bush et al (1982) the relapse rate at 10 years was nearly 50%. In the BNLI series of 141 CS I and II patients the 5 year survival was 81.5% but DFS was only 45.6% (see Fig. 10.5). Chen et al (1979) reported improved disease free survivals with extended field irradiation but this is not confirmed in the Stanford experience (Paryani et al 1983). Radiotherapy alone is thus unsatisfactory in clinically staged local disease but there is no evidence that adjuvant chemotherapy as used to date can improve on the eventual outcome (Nissen et al 1983).

Stage III disease has also been treated initially by extended field radiotherapy. In the Stanford series of 66 such patients (Paryani et al 1984) the actuarial relapse free survival at 5 years was 60% and actuarial survival 78%. A very similar overall survival was reported by Glatstein et al (1977) but the 5 year DFS was considerably lower at 43% and only 33% at 10 years.

More commonly stage III disease is treated by chemotherapy. Stanford compared single agent vs combination chemotherapy (COP) and COP plus radiotherapy. All approaches gave a high remission rate but no difference in disease free survival (median duration of remission approximately 1 year) or overall survival was seen (Portlock 1983). This experience has subsequently been repeated in many other centres. Although the NCI report improved results with C-MOPP in the subgroup of patients with follicular mixed small and large cell lymphomas (Anderson et al 1977) this was

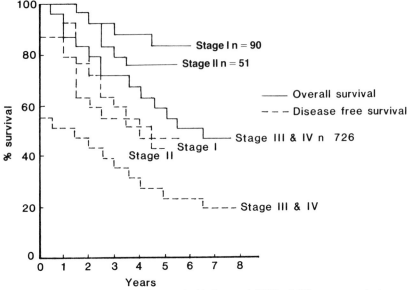

Fig. 10.5 Overall survival and disease free survival in low grade NHL of different anatomical stage (BNLI).

not confirmed in an Eastern Oncology Group Study (Glick et al 1981). These observations showing that combination chemotherapy did not prevent continued relapse prompted Portlock & Rosenberg (1979) to delay chemotherapy until required for the alleviation of symptoms or organ dysfunction. The median period of delay possible was 31 months. The overall survival was not affected. Those patients with symptoms or critical organ dysfunction at presentation have a much worse prognosis (Fig. 10.6) and within the BNLI this group of patients are being randomised to receive chlorambucil or CHOP. CHOP is producing a higher CR rate (53% vs 17%) although the overall survivals are not yet different. Those patients without symptoms or organ dysfunction are randomised to delayed chemotherapy (i.e. observation) or immediate chlorambucil.

Such approaches of delaying treatment are certainly negative in outlook, however reasonable. Implicit in the strategy is the assumption that the disease can only be controlled and not cured and that relapse is inevitable. Most of the studies alluded to above have not used anthracyclines but several limited studies with more intensive regimes have not been encouraging. In the South Western Oncology group 148 patients with follicular lymphomas received CHOP or CHOP Bleo, and although the overall survival at 4 years exceeded 70% there was no evidence that relapse was prevented with nearly half the complete responders having relapsed by 3 years (Jones et al 1983). 18 patients with follicular lymphoma were treated in Boston with M-BACOD. The CR rate was 56% with 60% of the responders relapsing by 5 years (Anderson et al 1984). Young and colleagues at the National Cancer Institute (1987), USA are using ProMACE-MOPP but it will be several years before this strategy can be meaningfully assessed. Another intensive approach to the indolent lymphomas is that of total body irradiation and autologous bone marrow transplantation. At St Bartholomews Hospital this modality of treatment is being assessed in patients in second remission

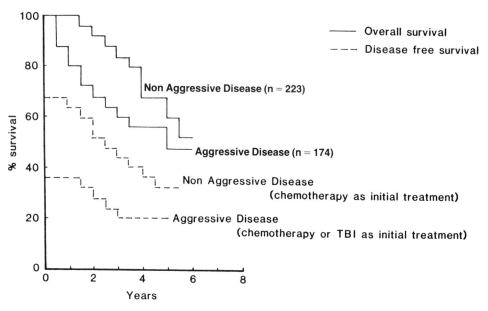

Fig. 10.6   Overall survival and disease free survival in 'aggressive' and 'non-aggressive' low grade non-Hodgkin's lymphoma (BNLI).

or state of minimal disease (Gallagher & Lister 1987). The marrow is purged with an anti-CD20 monoclonal antibody and complement. The selection of this relapsed but chemosensitive group of patients means that again it will be many years before this most interesting approach can be evaluated.

Further comment is necessary on the nature of relapse or drug resistance in the indolent lymphomas. In a significant proportion of patients this is associated with transformation to high grade histology. In the Stanford series in which re-biopsies were frequently performed it has been estimated that approximately 50% of those rebiopsied transform by 10 years (Rosenberg 1985). Transformation to high grade histology is a poor prognostic feature, although response to intensive chemotherapy may be achieved. Some patients may present in this situation, with the composite nature of the lymphoma detected either initially or on follow-up when persistent indolent lymphoma is found in a patient with previously diagnosed high grade disease.

Aggressive histology

LOCALISED DISEASE

Localised lymphomas that are still stage I or IE after pathological staging are most likely to be diffuse large cell and immunoblastic lymphomas. Excellent results may be achieved by local radiotherapy (Miller & Jones 1980). In the Chicago series of 17 patients, all achieved a CR and the disease free survival at 5 and 10 years was 94% and 72% respectively with an overall survival at 10 years of 70% (Vokes et al 1985). Systemic chemotherapy is probably equally effective however and does obviate the need for a laparotomy. In CS I and IE disease the relapse rate is nearly 50% and these patients should receive chemotherapy (Miller & Jones 1980). In CS

II disease the relapse rate following radiotherapy is even higher and initial chemotherapy is mandatory, as the results of such an approach appear to be superior for both freedom from relapse and overall survival (Miller & Jones 1980). This situation is distinct from that in localised Hodgkin's disease where chemotherapy salvage following radiotherapy is as effective as initial chemotherapy and may relate to the rapid growth of high grade NHL.

ADVANCED DISEASE

All patients with high grade histology except those that are PS I should receive combination chemotherapy. By the early 1970s the powerful antilymphomatous effect of the anthracyclines had been appreciated and CHOP had become the standard regime at many centres. Complete remission rates between 44% and 70% were reported for stage III/IV disease (Table 10.14) with about 30% of patients apparently cured of their disease. In more localised disease the results with CHOP chemotherapy are considerably better. In the BNLI experience the long term survival of CS II patients is approximately 50%. Thus the large majority of patients still die of their disease and considerable efforts have been made in the last decade to improve upon these CHOP results.

The first step was the addition of further agents to the CHOP cycle. Initially several groups used CHOP + Bleomycin, but the results have not been superior to CHOP alone. A recent long term follow-up from Lee et al (1986) indicates that Bleomycin plus CHOP at doses above the standard regime did not improve the outcome. The BACOP regime from the NCI and Boston used the same 5 drugs but the cyclophosphamide, vincristine and prednisone were given on day 1 and 8 and the Bleomycin on days 15 and 21 with prednisone from days 15–29 in an attempt to prevent tumour regrowth between cycles. No improvement over CHOP was apparent (Skarin et al 1977). Other groups had demonstrated the efficacy of the antimetabolites in the high grade NHL (Sweet et al 1980) and these were also added to the CHOP cycle without obvious improvement. Skarin had noted a high incidence of CNS relapse in their BACOP study and they therefore added high dose methotrexate (M-BACOD) with the specific intention of providing CNS prophylaxis. Excellent results have been reported in the diffuse large cell lymphomas (Skarin et al 1983, Table 10.14) but formal randomised trials comparing CHOP with M-BACOD have not been reported. The results of M-BACOD in the diffuse mixed lymphomas and diffuse small cleaved lymphomas have been reported separately (Anderson et al 1984). The CR rate is less at 58% and the relapse rate is considerably higher. More recently the dose of methotrexate has been reduced from 3 g every 3 weeks to 200 mg twice every 3 weeks (m-BACOD) with no apparent loss of therapeutic efficacy (Skarin 1986). The SWOG group have also evaluated this regime in 85 stage II–IV patients finding a somewhat lower CR rate of 65% (Dana et al 1987).

Other 6 drug regimes such as COPBLAM I and III (the latter gives vincristine and bleomycin by infusion) and CHOP-Bleo-Procarbazine have also been reported to give good results in small pilot studies although the results with CAP-BOP were disappointing (Table 10.14). Several centres sequentially use two different chemotherapy regimes. In the Pro-MACE-MOPP flexitherapy the ProMACE is given until CR, or until lack of further response, and MOPP and further ProMACE are given as consolidation (Fisher et al 1983). The LNH-80 protocol induces remission with

Table 10.14   Selected chemotherapy regimes in advanced high-grade non-Hodgkin's lymphoma

Type of regime	Regime	Centre	Reference	No. of patients	Stage	CR rate	Overall survival
CHOP	CHOP	SWOG	McKelvey et al (1976)	105	III & IV DS-C included	70%	—
	CHOP	SWOG	Coltman et al (1986)	418	III & IV large cell only	53%	30% (7 y)
	CHOP	BNLI		385	III & IV	47%	39% (5 y)
	CHOP	ECOG	O'Connell et al (1987)	70	III & IV	46%	32% (5 y)
	CHOP	SECSG	Gams et al (1985)	153	III & IV	44%	35% (5 y)
5 Drug regimes	CHOP-Bleo	ECOG	O'Connell et al (1987)	133	III & IV	46%	40% (5 y)
	BACOP	Boston	Skarin et al (1977)	44	93% stage IV all diffuse lymphomas	66%	42% (3 y)
	CHOP-Bleo (high dose)	MD Anderson	Lee et al (1986)	36	94% stage III or IV (large cell lymphomas)	81%	48% (10 y)
6 Drug regimes	M-BACOD	Boston	Skarin et al (1983)	107	15% I or II (diffuse large cell (includes immunoblastic and undifferentiated) only	72%	59% (5 y)
	m-BACOD	Boston	Skarin (1986)	80	Large cell lymphoma	75%	65% (3 y)
	m-BACOD	SWOG	Dana et al (1987)	85	II–IV (poor risk patients excluded)	65%	—
	COP BLAM I	New York	Laurence et al (1982)	33	III & IV (diffuse large cell only)	73%	70% (4 y)
	COP-BLAM III	New York	Coleman et al (1984)	34	6% stage II (diffuse large cell only)	85%	—
	CHOP-Bleo-Procarbazine	Nebraska	Armitage et al (1986)	51	20% stage II (diffuse large cell only)	73%	55% (2 y)
	CAP-BOP	ECOG	O'Connell et al (1987)	129	III & IV	43%	40% (5 y)
Sequential regimes	ProMACE-MOPP flexitherapy	NCI	Fisher et al (1983)	79	23% stage II	74%	65% (4 y)
	LNH-80	Lyon	Coiffier et al (1986)	97	85% stage III & IV	87%	60%+ (4 y)
	CHOP/HOAP-Bleo/IMVP16	MD Anderson	Cabanillas et al (1983)	56	Includes 2 follicular mixed & some stage I and II	82%	71% (4 y)
Alternating regime	CVP/A BP	Milan	Monfardini et al (1984)	60	III & IV large cell only	63%	39% (5 y)
'Hybrid regimes'	ProMACE-MOPP	NCI	Longo et al (1987)	75	II–IV	76%	56% (3 y)
	ProMACE-Cytabom	NCI	Longo et al (1987)	73	II–IV	79%	70% (3 y)
	ProMACE-Cytabom	SWOG	Miller et al (1987)	83	II–IV	58%	—
Weekly regimes	MACOP-B	Vancouver	Klimo & Connors (1987)	125	Approx 40% stage II	84%	68% (5 y)
	MACOP-B	Memorial Sloane Kettering	Lowenthal et al (1987)	31	Approx 30% stage II	39%	—
	MACOP-B	SWOG	Weick et al (1987)	116	28% stage II	50%	—

CHOP-BLEO and then uses the same drugs plus cytosine arabinoside, methotrexate, asparaginase and teniposide in a consolidation/late intensification programme (Coiffier et al 1986). At the M D Anderson Hospital patients not achieving CR with three courses of CHOP received three courses of HOAP-BLEO and if still not in remission three courses of IMVP16 (Cabanillas et al 1983). There have been few studies alternating two different non cross-resistant chemotherapy regimes. This is largely because there is no obvious equally effective alternative regime to CHOP. In the CVP alternating with ABP regime reported by Monfardini et al (1984) the CVP cycle would certainly appear to be suboptimal therapy. A solution to this problem has been the development of so called hybrid regimes which contain elements of two regimes and thus multiple agents are introduced from the beginning of treatment. A hybrid ProMACE MOPP was reported with good results from the NCI and this is being compared with Pro-MACE cytabom in which the day 8 MOPP is replaced by Cytosine arabinoside, bleomycin and methotrexate. The early results are very encouraging (Longo et al 1987) but the South Western Oncology Group using an identical protocol only obtained a CR of 58% which is not dissimilar from their CHOP experience (Miller et al 1987).

A particularly interesting strategy is the use of weekly rotating drug schedules such as MACOP-B which introduce many agents quickly with minimal drug free intervals in accordance with the Goldie–Coldman hypothesis. The preliminary results with this regime from Vancouver are exciting not only because of the high incidence of substained CRs but also because therapy is completed within 3 months (Klimo & Connors 1987). In two pilot studies these good results have unfortunately not been reproduced (Lowenthal et al 1987, Weick et al 1987).

A further approach used in Seattle is that of combined modality therapy. Patients received four courses of CHOP + Procarbazine, radiotherapy, and then four more courses of chemotherapy (Sullivan et al 1983). Radiotherapy consisted of 150 cGy TBI for extensive disease or 3500 cGy for localised disease. In the intermediate and high grade lymphomas (working formulation) the CR rate was 80% with an actuarial survival at 6 years of 47%. If the lymphoblastic and small non cleaved cell lymphomas are excluded the 6 year survival is 55%. Although this is not a randomised study the results are good and combined modality therapy merits further studies.

CNS PROPHYLAXIS

In the high grade lymphomas with a high risk of CNS relapse (lymphoblastic and small non cleaved) CNS prophylaxis is essential. In earlier studies the lymphoblastic lymphomas were reported to have an extremely poor prognosis (Nathwani et al 1981, Nissen & Ersboll 1985). Recently Coleman and colleagues have reported their results using CHOP plus intrathecal methotrexate and cranial irradiation. In those patients without CNS involvement or marrow infiltration at diagnosis the 5 year survival is 94%. For those patients with CNS or marrow disease the prognosis remains dismal. Similar results using CHOP + Asparaginase, cranial prophylaxis and multidrug maintenance therapy have been reported by ECOG (Coglan et al 1987). The lymphoblastic lymphomas are closely related to acute lymphoblastic leukaemia and many centres use leukaemia protocols in this situation (Slater et al 1986). The experience with adult small non cleaved cell lymphomas is small, but extrapolation from results in childhood Burkitt's disease indicates that aggressive multidrug regimes with full cranial prophylaxis may give improved results (Bernstein et al 1986). Burkitt's lymphoma is at least initially very sensitive to cyclophosphamide and thus should be included in any regime.

The need for CNS prophylaxis in other forms of high grade lymphoma is more controversial. Although the CNS relapse rate was high in the Boston BACOP study (25%), in the Finsen Institute series, if lymphoblastic and small non cleaved cell lymphomas are excluded, the CNS relapse rate is 4% with a probably somewhat higher risk in those with bone marrow involvement (Young et al 1979). Most of the CNS relapses are also accompanied by concomitant systemic relapse, so intrathecal cytotoxics and brain irradiation are probably not warranted. This is especially true in the more recent protocols which include drugs such as methotrexate, cytosine arabinoside and procarbazine which cross the blood brain barrier.

In summary, the last decade has seen progressive intensification of the therapy used in advanced high grade disease with introduction of multiple agents early in the course of treatment. The preliminary results with some of those regimes are highly encouraging but no randomised trial has yet proven that any are superior to CHOP.

Salvage therapy in high grade NHL

CHEMOTHERAPY

The results of salvage therapy are poor with complete remission rates of between 5% and 35% reported. The results of several studies were recently reviewed by Singer & Goldstone (1986). The largest studies have been reported from the M D Anderson. In 41 cases of resistant or relapsed high grade NHL treated with ifosphamide, methotrexate and VP16 (IMVP16) the CR rate was 34% but over half of these patients relapsed within 18 months (Cabanillas et al 1982). In a more recent study methyl-gag was added to these agents (MIME) 123 patients with recurrent or relapsed high grade lymphoma received MIME (Cabanillas et al 1987). The CR rate was 32%, with over 75% of complete responders relapsing within 2 years giving an overall survival of less than 20%. The best responses were achieved in patients who had obtained a CR with front line therapy and been off therapy for at least 6 months prior to relapse. Other promising agents in salvage regimes include cisplatin, amsacrine and mitozantrone but with all regimes it must be concluded that only a small minority of patients will obtain prolonged survival. With the more recent induction regimes in which increasing numbers of active agents are used, the problems of salvage become even more difficult. Cabanillas from the M D Anderson has pointed out that whereas many patients failing CHOP type regimes respond to second line therapy there is no effective salvage for patients failing ProMACE-MOPP (Cabanillas 1985).

AUTOLOGOUS BONE MARROW TRANSPLANTATION

Very high dose chemotherapy or radiotherapy followed by autologous bone marrow rescue is an alternative form of salvage therapy. The results from many small pilot studies have been reported in recent years and some selected results are shown in Table 10.15. The survey from the European Bone Marrow Transplant Group shows no clear cut advantage for chemotherapy or total body irradiation in the ablative protocol. Overall there is a high response rate but also a high relapse rate. From the preliminary studies it can be concluded that this approach to salvage is most effective in patients who have had a good PR to first line treatment but not achieved

Table 10.15   Results of salvage therapy in high-grade non-Hodgkin's lymphoma using very high-dose chemo/radiotherapy and autologous bone marrow rescue

Status at time of graft	Centre	Reference	No. of patients	CR rate	Overall survival
Resistant disease*	Toronto	Phillips et al (1984)	24	64%	23% (3 y)
	Bloomsbury	Anderson et al (1986)	11	18%	18% (1½ y)
	Seattle	Appelbaum et al (1987)	20 approx	—	13% approx (2 y)
	Europe/USA Multicentre	Philip et al (1987)	56	34%	6% approx (2 y)
	EBMTG†	Goldstone et al (1987a)	85	36%	22% (3 y)
Chemosensitive disease					
1. PR to first line treatment	France/UK Multicentre	Philip et al (1984)	7	86%	86% (1 y)
	Boston	Takvorian et al (1987)	17	85% approx	65% approx (2 y)
	EBMTG†	Goldstone et al (1987)	24	37%	26% (3 y)
2. Chemosensitive relapse**	Europe/USA Multicentre	Philip et al (1987)	44	86%	38% (2 y)
	Boston	Takvorian et al (1987)	24	85% approx	65% approx (2 y)
	EBMTG†	Goldstone et al (1987)	79	83%	48% (3 y)

* Includes primary treatment failures (no response) and resistant relapses.
** Includes many patients already in 2nd CR.
† The EBMTG registry includes patients reported by Anderson et al and Philip et al.

CR and in patients who have relapsed from CR, especially if the tumour still demonstrates sensitivity to chemotherapeutic agents at conventional doses. It is also apparent that patients with bulky disease at the time of transplant fare less well than those without bulk disease. Those patients who respond well to ABMT are thus a similar group to those in whom the best results are achieved with conventional salvage therapy. This must be borne in mind when considering the excellent results reported from Boston (Takvorian et al 1987) and emphasises the need for randomised controlled trials. In the Boston study the marrow was purged with an anti CD 20 monoclonal antibody and complement lysis, but it is not possible to analyse the contribution of purging to their results. From the European Bone Marrow Transplant Group registry it is apparent that over 80% of relapses occur at sites of previous disease (especially if bulky), and until the conditioning regimes are improved it will be difficult to demonstrate any therapeutic improvements due to removal of minimal residual disease from the harvested marrow.

It has been argued that very intensive chemo/radiotherapy and ABMT may have a role in first remission in the lymphoblastic lymphomas. If the patient did not present with disease of the bone marrow or central nervous system however, the results with conventional treatment appear good (see earlier section), and ABMT should probably be limited to those with marrow or CNS disease at presentation (Table 10.16). In other categories of high grade lymphomas it is equally difficult to define a group of patients in first CR who merit ABMT. In the BNLI CHOP series, although many factors predict for failure to achieve CR, once CR has been obtained it appears that

Table 10.16 Possible indications for intensive therapy and autologous bone marrow transplantation in the non-Hodgkin's lymphoma

A. High-grade disease
   1. First CR if:
      a. Lymphoblastic lymphoma with marrow infiltration at presentation
      b. CNS disease at presentation
   2. Partial response to first line chemotherapy (not patients with no response)
   3. First relapse from CR especially if tumour still chemosensitive to drugs at conventional doseage

B. Low grade disease
   Therapy failures without bulk disease

only the presence of B symptoms at presentation predict (weakly) for relapse. Patients with CNS disease at presentation may be a small but appropriate group for ABMT once in remission. It is generally agreed that these patients fare badly with conventional treatment, and a report from the EBMTG (Gribben et al 1987a) suggests that CNS disease at presentation may not adversely effect the outcome of an ABMT performed in remission. This must be interpreted with some caution however as this small series included several children with Burkitt's lymphomas.

Few patients with non-Hodgkin's lymphoma have a matched sibling and are young enough to be considered for an allogeneic transplantation. The experience of allogeneic transplants is thus small but the results have not been better than autologous bone marrow transplantation with a high level of treatment related toxicity (Appelbaum et al 1987, Phillips et al 1986).

The use of biological agents

SEROTHERAPY

Monoclonal antibodies have been used in the treatment of malignant lymphomas since the beginning of the decade (Nadler et al 1980, Miller & Levy 1981). There have been few satisfactory responses due to the inherent limitations of this therapeutic approach (Table 10.17). The lack of tumour specificity is relative, and not as major

Table 10.17 Limitations of serotherapy in malignant lymphomas

1. Lack of tumour specificity
2. Tumour heterogeneity and variable antigen expression
3. Presence of free antigen in serum
4. Antigenic modification of tumour cells
5. Finite capacity of host effector systems
6. Immunogenicity of xenogenic immunoglobulin

a problem as in chemotherapy or radiotherapy. Nonetheless, Miller et al (1982) produced an antiidiotypic antibody to increase tumour specificity. The response was so good that control by idiotype networks was advocated. Unfortunately further patients treated with antiidiotypic antibodies did not have significant responses (Meeker et al 1985). A major limitation is undoubtedly the finite capacity of host cells to infiltrate the tumour tissue and partake in the antibody dependent lysis of tumour cells. This may be overcome by using antibodies conjugated to toxins, drugs or radioactive substances. The latter has the advantage that cells with low antigen expression will still receive radioactive exposure from conjugates bound to neighbouring cells with higher antigen densities. Several promising preliminary reports using radioactive antibody conjugates have been reported (Lenhard et al 1985, De Nardo et al 1986, Rosen et al 1987), particularly in mycosis fungoides. The use of radioactive conjugates will be accompanied by some increased toxicity to normal tissues. The immunogenicity of the conjugates remains a major problem but this may be reduced by the use of hybrid antibodies containing mouse or rat antigen binding domains with human constant region domains (Morrison et al 1984).

INTERFERONS

Experience with α-interferon has been obtained by many lymphoma groups, initially with crude impure material and more recently with the recombinant product. These recent studies show a response in approximately 50% of patients with indolent B cell lymphomas or cutaneous T cell lymphomas (Foon et al 1986) although the complete remission rate is only 10–15%. Present studies are investigating the role of combined chemotherapy and α-interferon in these settings. In the high grade lymphomas the response rate to α-interferon has been less than 20% (Canellos et al 1985) and as the responses are of brief duration it is unlikely that this agent will have a significant role in this disease.

LYMPHOKINES

Lymphokines might have two possible uses in the malignant lymphomas. Firstly they could be used to stimulate host antitumour activity in the way IL-2 or IL-2 stimulated lymphokine activated killer cells (LAK-cells) have been used in resistant solid tumours (Rosenberg 1988). The toxicity is however considerable and IL-2 might actually stimulate growth of a non-Hodgkin's lymphoma. Nonetheless Rosenberg has treated 4 patients with non-Hodgkin's lymphoma. One achieved a complete and two a partial remission. The second strategy is to deliberately stimulate the tumour with the aim of putting lymphoma stem cells into cell cycle and thus render them more chemosensitive. The array of stimulating lymphokines available in recombinant form is increasing rapidly (Dinarello & Mier 1987) and with appropriate synergistic combinations of factors it may be possible to stimulate most NHL cells in this way.

COLONY STIMULATING FACTORS

Clinical studies are in progress with both granulocyte-colony stimulating factor (G-CSF) and granulocyte-monocyte colony stimulating factor (GM-CSF) and will soon commence with interleukin 3. It is apparent that both G-CSF and GM-CSF accelerate haemopoietic recovery following chemotherapy and thus may enable increased doses of chemotherapeutic agents to be given over a shorter period of time. In our own studies of high dose chemotherapy and autologous bone marrow transplantation in advanced relapsed Hodgkin's disease it is apparent that GM-CSF reduces the period of neutropenia by nearly 1 week, and it is to be hoped that this will reduce the morbidity and mortality of the procedure.

OVERALL CONCLUSIONS

Patients with malignant lymphomas fall into three broad categories. One group of patients can be readily cured and these patients were being successfully treated 15–20 years ago. A further disappointingly large group of patients, the elderly sick with advanced disease, was and still remains predominantly incurable. The battleground in recent years has been for a relatively small intermediate group of younger patients who might be rescued by more intensive therapy, and it is therefore not surprising that a major impact on overall survival is difficult to demonstrate from these efforts. This does not mean that such efforts are in vain. Although the malignant lymphomas are rare they are the 4th most common malignant disease in the Western World accounting for absence from work. There have been sufficiently encouraging developments in the last decade to believe that this situation may change in the next.

ACKNOWLEDGEMENTS

We are indebted to Dr G. Vaughan-Hudson for providing unpublished data from the BNLI and for assistance in the preparation of this chapter. We would like to thank Miss J. Bonner for typing the manuscript.

REFERENCES

Ahmed T, Ciavarella D, Feldman E et al 1987 Blood 70 (Suppl 1): 1010
Anderson C C, Goldstone A H, Souhami R L et al 1986 Cancer Chemother Pharmacol 16: 170–175
Anderson H, Deakin D P, Wagstaff J et al 1984 Br J Cancer 49: 695–707
Anderson J R, Glick J, Ginsberg S, Gottlieb A, Harrington D, O'Connell M 1987 Proc ASCO: 782
Anderson K C, Skarin A T, Rosenthal D S et al 1984 Cancer Treat Rep 68: 1343–1350
Anderson T, Bender R A, Fisher R I et al 1977 Cancer Treat Rep 61: 1057–1066
Anderson T, Chabner B A, Young R C et al 1982 Cancer 50: 2699–2707
Appelbaum F R, Sullivan K M, Buclever C D et al 1987 J Clin Oncol 5: 1340–1347
Armitage J O, Weisenberger D D, Hutchins M et al 1986 J Clin Oncol 4: 160–164
Bakemeier R F, Anderson J R, Costello W et al 1984 Annals of Int Med 101: 447–456
Barrett A, Gregor A, McElwain T J, Peckham M J 1984 Clin Radiol 32: 221–224
Bartl R, Frisch B, Burckhardt R, Huln D, Pappenberger R 1982 Brit J Haematol: 345–360
Bennett M H, Farrer-Brown G, Henry K et al 1974 Lancet ii: 405–406
Bennett M H, MacLennan K A, Easterling M J, Vaughan Hudson B, Vaughan Hudson G, Jelliffe A M
    1985 In: Quagliono D, Hayhoe F G J (eds) Proc int symp on cytobiology of leukaemias and lymphomas.
    Vol 20. Raven, New York, p 15–32
Bernstein J I, Coleman C N, Stricker J G, Dorfman R F, Rosenberg S A 1986 J Clin Oncol 4: 847–858
Blackledge G, Best J J K, Crowther D, Isherwood I 1980 Clin Radiol 31: 143–147
Bonadonna G 1985 Seminars in Oncology 12 (suppl 6): 1–14
Bonadonna G, Santora A, Valagussa P et al 1985 In: Cavalli F, Bonadonna G, Rozencweig M (eds)
    Malignant lymphomas and Hodgkin's disease: experimental and therapeutic advances. Martinus Nijhoff,
    Boston, p 299–307
Bonadonna G, Valagussa P, Santoro A 1986 Annals Int Med 104: 739–746
Brada M, Easton D F, Horwich A, Peckham M J 1986 Radiotherapy and Oncology 5: 15–22
Brada M, Nicholls J, Ashley S, Coleman M, Peckham M J, Horwich A 1988 Proc ECCO: 1037
Bush R S, Gospodarowics M 1982 In: Rosenberg S, Kaplan H S (eds) Malignant lymphomas. Academic
    Press, New York, p 452–502
Cabanillas F 1985 In: Dicke K A, Spitzer G, Zander A R, Gorin N C (eds) Proceedings of the First
    International Symposium. University of Texas, Houston, p 125–128
Cabanillas F, Hagemeister F B, Bodey G P, Freireich E J 1982 Blood 60: 693–697
Cabanillas F, Burgess M A, Bodey G P, Freireich E J 1983 Amer J Med 74: 382–388
Cabanillas F, Hagemeister F B, McLaughlin P et al 1987 J Clin Oncol 5: 407–412
Canellos G P 1985 Semin Oncol 12: 25–32
Canellos G P, Young R C, De Vita V T 1972 Clin Pharmacol Therapeutics 13: 750–754
Carbone P P, Kaplan H S, Musshoff K, Smithers D W, Tubiana M 1971 Cancer Res 31: 1860–1861
Carde P, MacKintosh F R, Rosenberg S A 1983 J Clin Oncol 1: 146–153
Case D C, Young C W et al 1977 Cancer 39: 1382–1386
Castellino R A, Hoppe R T, Blank N et al 1984 Am J Roentgenol 143: 37–41
Chen M C, Prosnitz L R, Gonzales Serva A, Fisher D B 1979 Cancer 43: 1245–1254

Coglan J, Anderson J, Glick J, O'Connell M, Earle J 1987 Proc ASCO: 764
Coiffier B, Sebban C, Ffrench M et al 1986 J Clin Oncol 4: 147–153
Coleman C N, Picozzi V J, Cox R S et al 1986 J Clin Oncol 4: 1628–1637
Coleman M, Boyd D B, Bernhardt B et al 1984 Proc ASCO: C–964
Coltman C A, Dahlberg S, Jones S E et al 1986 Proc ASCO: 774
Cossett J M, Henry-Amar M, Carde P, Clarke D, Le Bourgeois J P, Tubiana M 1984 Haematol Oncol
    2: 33–43
Cossman J, Jaffe E S, Fisher R I 1984 Cancer 54: 1310–1317
Dady P J, McElwain T J, Austin D E et al 1982 Brit J Cancer 45: 841–859
Dana B, Jones S, Fisher R I et al 1987 Proc ASCO: 777
De Nardo S J, De Nardo G L, O'Grady L F et al 1986 J Nuc Med 27: 903–909
Diggs C H, Wiernik P H, Sutherland J C 1981 Cancer 47: 224–228
Dinarello C A, Mier J W 1987 N Engl J Med 317: 940–945
Dutcher J P, Wiernik P H 1985 In: Cavalli F, Bonadonna G, Rozencweig M (eds) Malignant lymphomas
    and Hodgkin's disease: experimental and therapeutic advances. Martinus Nijhof, Boston, p 317–327
Farrer-Brown G 1981 Clin Rad 32: 501–504
Ferme C, Teillet F, D'Agay M F, Gisselbrecht C, Marty M, Boiron M 1984 Cancer 54: 2324–2329
Fisher R I, Hubbard S M, De Vita V T et al 1981 Blood 58: 45–51
Fisher R I, DeVita V T, Hubbard S M 1983 Ann Int Med 98: 304–309
Foon K A, Roth M S, Bunn P A 1986 Semin Oncol 13 (suppl 2): 35–42
Fox K A, Lippman S M, Cassady J R, Heusinkveld R S, Miller T B 1987 J Clin Oncol 5: 38–45
Gallagher C J, Lister T A 1987 Clinical Haematology 1.1: 141–155
Gallagher C J, Gregory W M, Jones A E, Stansfield A G, Richards M A, Dhaliwal H S, Malpas J S, Lister
    T A 1986 J Clin Oncol 4: 1470–1480
Gams R A, Rainey M, Dandy M, Bartolucci A A, Silberman H, Omura G 1985 J Clin Oncol 3: 1188–1195
Glatstein E 1977 Cancer 39: 837–842
Glatstein E 1984 Proc 2nd Int Conference on Malignant Lymphoma (Abstract pg 28), Lugano
Glatstein E, Fuks S Z, Goffinet D R et al 1976 Cancer 37: 2806–2812
Glees J P, Taylor K J W, Gazet J C et al 1977 Clin Rad 28: 233–238
Glick J H, Barnes J M, Ezdinli E Z et al 1981 Blood 58: 920–925
Goldie J H, Coldman A J 1984 Cancer Res 44: 3643–3653
Goldstone A H, Gribben J G, Dones L 1987a Bone Marrow Transplantation, 2 (suppl 1): 200–203
Goldstone A H, Gribben J G, Linch D C, Hooper P, Souhami R L 1987b Blood 70 (suppl 1): 837
Gribben J G, Giles F, Dones L, Goldstone A H, Philip T 1987a Bone Marrow Transplantation 2
    (suppl 1): 220
Gribben J G, Vaughan Hudson B, Linch D C 1987b Haematol Oncol 5: 281–293
Hagemeister F B, Fuller L M, Velasquez W S et al 1982 Cancer Treat Rep 66: 789–798
Hancock B W 1986 Radiotherapy and Oncology 7: 215–221
Harker W G, Kushlan P et al 1984 Ann Int Med 101: 440–446
Haybittle J L, Hayhoe F G J, Easterling M J et al 1985 Lancet i: 967–972
Hellman S, Mauch P 1982 Cancer Treat Rep 66: 915–923
Hoppe R T, Coleman C N, Cox R S, Rosenberg S A, Kaplan H S 1982 Blood 59: 455–465
Horwich A, Easton D, Nogueira-Costa R, Liew K H, Coleman M, Peckham M J 1986 Radiotherapy and
    Oncology 6: 1–14
Jagannath S, Velasquez W S, Tucker S L et al 1985 J Clin Oncol 4: 859–865
Jagannath S, Armitage J A, Dicke K A et al 1988 J Clin Oncol (in press)
Jairam R, Vrints L W, Breed W P M, Wijlhuizen T J, Wijnen J T M 1987 The importance of the
    histological subclassification of the nodular sclerotic type of Hodgkin's Disease for the prognosis
    (in press)
Jelliffe A M 1979 Clin Radiol 30: 121–137
Jelliffe A M, Vaughan Hudson G 1987 In Selby P, McElwain T J (eds) Hodgkin's disease. Blackwell
    Scientific, Oxford
Jones S E, Haut A, Weick J K et al 1983a Cancer 51: 1339–1347
Jones S E, Grozea P N, Metz E N et al 1983b Cancer 51: 1083–1090
Klimo P, Connors J M 1985 J Clin Oncology 3: No 9 (Sept)
Klimo P, Connors J M 1987 Abstract 67. Third International Conference on Malignant Lymphoma,
    Lugano
Laurence J, Coleman M, Allen S L, Silver R T, Pasmantier M 1982 Ann Int Med 97: 190–195
Lee M, Cabanillas F, Chang K S, Freireich E, Trujillo J, Stass S 1987 Blood 70 (suppl 1): 724
Lee R, Cabanillas F, Bodey G P, Freireich E J 1986 J Clin Oncol 4: 1455–1461
Lenhard R E, Order S E, Spunberg J J et al 1985 J Clin Oncol 3: 1296–1300
Lennert K, Mohri N, Stein H et al 1975 Brit J Haematol (suppl) 31: 193–203

Liew K H, Ding J C, Matthews J P et al 1983 Aust NZ J Med 13: 135–140
Liew K H, Easton D, Horwich A, Barrett A, Peckham M J 1984 Haematol Oncol 2: 45–49
Lippman S M, Miller T P, Spier C M, Slyman D J, Grogan T P 1987 Blood 70 (suppl 1): 727
Longo D L, Young R C, Wesley M et al 1986 J Clin Oncol 4: 1295–1306
Longo D, De Vita V, Duffey P et al 1987 Proc ASCO: 811
Lowenthal D A, White A, Koziner B, Straus D J, Lee B J, Clarkson B D 1987 Proc ASCO 6: 794
Lukes R J, Craver L F, Hall T C, Rappaport H, Ruben P 1966 Cancer Res 26: 1311
Lukes R J, Collins R D 1974 Cancer 34: 1488–1503
Macintyre E A, Vaughan Hudson B, Linch D C, Vaughan Hudson G, Jelliffe A M 1987 Eur J Haematol
    39: 66–70
McKelvey E M, Gottlieb J A, Wilson H E et al 1976 Cancer 38: 1484–1493
Mauch P, Goffman T, Rosenthal D S, Cannellos G P, Come S E, Hellman S 1985 J Clin Oncol 3: 1166–1173
Mauch P, Tarbell N, Skarin A, Rosenthal D, Weinstein H 1987 J Clin Oncol 5: 544–549
Meeker T, Lowder J, Maloney D G et al 1985 Blood 65: 1349–1363
Miller R A, Levy R 1981 Lancet ii: 226–229
Miller R A, Maloney D J, Warnke R, Levy R 1982 New Eng J Med 306: 517–522
Miller T P, Jones S E 1980 Cancer Chemother Pharmacol 4: 67–70
Miller T P, Dahlberg S, Jones S E, Fisher R I, Coltman C A 1987 Proc ASCO: 776
Monfardini S, Rilke F, Valagussa P et al 1984 Eur J Cancer Clin Oncol 20: 609–617
Morrison S L, Johnson M J, Herzenberg L A et al 1984 Proc Nat Acad Sci (USA) 81: 6851–6855
Nadler L M, Stashento P, Hardy R et al 1980 Cancer Res 40: 3147–3154
Nathwani B N, Diamond L W, Winberg C D et al 1981 Cancer 48: 2347
National Cancer Institute sponsored study of classifications of Non Hodgkin's Lymphomas 1982 Cancer
    49: 2112–2135
Nissen N I, Ersboll J 1985 In: Wiernik P H (ed) Leukaemia and lymphomas. Churchill Livingstone,
    New York, p 97–126
Nissen N I, Ersboll J, Hamen H S et al 1983 Cancer 52: 1–7
Nissen N I, Nordentoft A M 1982 Cancer Treatment Rep 66: 799–803
Nissen N I, Pajak T F, Glidewell O et al 1979 Cancer 43: 31–40
O'Connell M J, Harrington D P, Earle J D et al 1987 J Clin Oncol 5: 1329–1339
O'Reilly S, Connors J, Vass N et al 1987 Proc ASCO: 774
Paryani S B, Hoppe R T, Cox R S et al 1983 Cancer 52: 2300–2307
Paryani S B, Hoppe R T, Cox R S, Colby T V, Kaplan H S 1984 J Clin Oncol 2: 841–848
Pavlovsky S, Maschio M, Garcia F et al 1987 Proc ASCO: 785
Peckham M J, Ford H T, McElwain T J, Harmer C L, Atkinson K, Austin D E 1975 Brit J Cancer
    32: 391–400
Philip T, Biron P, Maranunchi D et al 1984 Lancet i: 391
Philip T, Durmont J, Teillet F et al 1986 Brit J Cancer 53: 737–742
Philip T, Armitage J A, Spitzer G et al 1987 N Engl J Med 316: 1493–1498
Phillips G L, Herzig R H, Lazarus H M et al 1984 N Eng J Med 310: 1557–1561
Phillips G L, Herzig R H, Lazarus H M, Fay J W, Griffith R, Herzig G P 1986 J Clin Oncol 4: 480–488
Portlock C S 1983 Sem Haematol 20: 25–34
Portlock C S, Rosenberg S A 1979 Ann Int Med 90: 10–13
Prosnitz L R, Montalvo R L, Fischer D B 1978 Int J Radiat Oncol Biol Phys 4: 781–787
Rappaport H 1966 Atlas of Tumour Pathology Section 3, Fascicle 8. Washington DC US Armed Forces,
    Institute of Pathology
Reddy S K, Gomez G A, Panahon L et al 1986 Proc ASCO: 781
Roach M, Kapp D S, Rosenberg S A, Hoppe R T 1987 J Clin Oncol 5: 550–555
Rosen S T, Zimmer A M, Goldman-Leiken R et al 1987 J Clin Oncol 5: 562–573
Rosenberg S A 1982 In: Wiernik P H (ed) Controversies in oncology. Wiley, New York, p 45–60
Rosenberg S A 1985 In: Cavalli F, Bonadonna G, Rosencweig M (eds) Malignant lymphomas and
    Hodgkin's disease: experimental and therapeutic advances. Martinus Nijhof, Boston, p 455–464
Rosenberg S A 1988 Immunology Today 9: 58–62
Rubin P, Keys H, Mayer E, Antemann R 1974 Am J Roentgenol Rad Therapy and Nuclear Med 120: 536–
    548
Russell K J, Hoppe R T, Colby T V, Burns B F, Cox R S, Kaplan H S 1984 Radiother Oncol 3: 197–205
Santoro A, Bonfante V et al 1982 Ann Int Med 96: 139–143
Santoro A, Bonadonna G, Valagussa P et al 1987 J Clin Oncol 5, No 1 (Jan): 27–37
Selby P, McElwain T J 1987 In: Selby P, McElwain T J (eds) Hodgkin's disease. Blackwell Scientific,
    Oxford UK, p 94–125
Singer C R J, Goldstone A H 1986 Clinics in Haematol 15: 105–150
Skarin A T 1986 Seminars in Oncol 13, No 4 (suppl 5): 10–25

Skarin A T, Rosenthal D S, Moloney W C, Foci E 1977 Blood 49: 759–770
Skarin A T, Canellos G P, Rosenthal D S 1983 J Clin Oncol 1: 91–98
Slater D E, Nertelsmann R, Koziner B et al 1986 J Clin Oncol 4: 57–67
Sloane J P 1987 In: Selby P, McElwain T J (eds) Hodgkin's disease. Blackwell Scientific, Oxford, p 4–30
Straus D J, Myers J, Lee B J et al 1984 Amer J Med 76: 270–278
Sullivan K M, Neiman P E, Kadin M E et al 1983 Blood 62, No: 1: 51–61
Sutcliffe B, Wrigley P F M, Peto J et al 1978 BMJ 1: 679–683
Sutcliffe S B, Gospodarowicz M K, Bergasel D E et al 1985 J Clin Oncol 3: 393–401
Swan F, Cabanillas F, Velasquez W et al 1987 Proc ASCO: 769
Sweet D L, Golomb H M, Vitmann J E et al 1980 Annals of Int Med 92: 785–790
Takvorian T, Canellos G P, Ritz J et al 1987 N Engl J Med 316: 1499–1505
Timothy A R, Sutcliffe S B J, Wrigley P F M et al 1979 Int J Rad Onc Rad Biol Phys 5: 165–169
Tubiana M, Henry-Amar M, Hayat M 1979 Eur J Cancer 15: 645–657
Tubiana M, Hayat M, Henry-Amar M, Breur K, Werf Messing B, Burgess M 1981 Eur J Cancer 1: 355–363
Tubiana M, Henry-Amar M, Hayat M et al 1984 Int J Rad Oncol 10: 197–210
Tubiana M, Henry-Amar M, Werf Messing B et al 1985 Int J Rad Onc Biol Phys 11: 23–30
Vaughan Hudson B, MacLennan K A, Easterling M J, Jelliffe A M, Haybittle J L, Vaughan Hudson G 1983 Clin Rad 34: 503–506
Vokes E E, Ultmann J E, Golomb H M et al 1985 J Clin Oncol 3: 1309–1317
Wagener D J T, Burgess J M V, Dekter A D W et al 1983 Cancer 52: 1558–1562
Weick J, Fisher R I, Dahlberg S, Hartsock R 1987 Blood 70 (suppl 1): 852
Willett C G, Lingwood R M, Meyer J et al 1987 Cancer 59: 1107–1111
Young R C, Canellos G P, Chabner B A, Hubbard S M, DeVita V T 1978 Cancer 42: 1001–1007
Young R C, Howser D M, Anderson T et al 1979 Am J Med 66: 435–443
Young R C, Longo D L, Glatstein E 1985 In: Cavalli F, Bonadonna G, Rozencweig M (eds) Malignant lymphomas and Hodgkin's disease: experimental and therapeutic advances. Martinus Nijhoff, Boston, p 293–298
Young R C, Longo D L, Glatstein E et al 1987 Proc ASCO: 790
Zittoun R, Audebert A, Boerru B et al 1985 J Clin Oncol 3: 207–214

11. Hemophilia A in man: molecular defects in the factor VIII gene

S. E. Antonarakis   H. H. Kazazian

INTRODUCTION

Hemophilias are X-linked hereditary disorders of blood coagulation due to deficiency of clotting factors VIII and IX. Hemophilia A is associated with abnormality of factor VIII and affects about 1 in every 10 000 males; hemophilia B is associated with abnormality of factor IX and affects about 1 in every 50 000 males (McKee 1983). Both clotting factors are involved in the intermediate steps of the intrinsic clotting cascade which consists of several proteases and cofactors that are serially activated in response to an initial stimulus. Factor VIII in its activated form serves as a cofactor to factor IX in the activation of factor X (Jackson & Nemerson 1980). In this short review the molecular basis of factor VIII deficiency will be discussed. The cloning and characterization of factor VIII gene and the identification of several gene defects have provided a better understanding of the pathogenesis of hemophilia A and the nature of mutations that occur in a non-selectable X-linked locus.

FACTOR VIII GENE

The human factor VIII gene was cloned by researchers from two biotechnology companies (Genentech, Inc. and Genetics Institute). Both groups used synthetic oligonucleotides as probes to clone and characterize the factor VIII gene from genomic and cDNA libraries (Gitschier et al 1984, Toole et al 1984). The oligonucleotide sequences used were deduced from small sequenced peptides of human and porcine factor VIII. The gene spans 186 kilobases (kb) of DNA and is divided into 26 exons and 25 introns. The coding DNA (exon length) is 9 kb which codes for 2351 amino acids. The complete nucleotide sequence of the coding regions, the promoter elements, and the intron exon boundaries have been determined, and the amino acid sequence of the protein has been deduced (Vehar et al 1984). The first 19 amino acids of the protein sequence comprise the secretory leader peptide of the precursor factor VIII. Computer analysis of the factor VIII protein sequence revealed that there are three homologous sequences (A domain) at amino acid positions 1–329, 380–711, and 1649–2019 of the mature polypeptide. The A domains have about 30% homology. The second and third A domains are separated by the B domain of 983 amino acids which is extremely rich in potential asparagine-linked glycosylation sites. After the third A domain there are two C domains of 150 amino acids with about 40% homology. Most of the 23 cysteine residues of mature factor VIII are located in the A and C domains. The mature polypeptide has the structure A_1-A_2-B-A_3-C_1-C_2. The A domains are homologous (about 30%) with the three domains of the copper binding protein ceruloplasmin. There is also considerable homology between the A domains of factor VIII and factor V and between the C domains of these two factors and discoidin

Table 11.1   Factor VIII gene defects in hemophilia A The Johns Hopital Hospital experience

Patients studied	240	
Mutations identified	28	(11.7%)
Deletions	14	(5.8%)
Insertions	2	(0.8%)
Point mutations	12	(5.0%)
Mutations not yet identified	212	(88.3%)

I (Kane & Davie 1986). The B domain is encoded by the unusually long (3106 nucleotides) exon 14.

Factor VIII circulates in plasma in conjunction with von Willebrand factor, a large polymer of a polypeptide encoded by an autosomal gene on human chromosome 12 (Ginsburg et al 1985). Factor VIII isolated from plasma is usually degraded because it undergoes proteolytic cleavages during its activation (Rotblat et al 1985). It is thought that the 'activated' form of factor VIII is a 90 000 Da polypeptide composed of the first two A domains (N-terminus) and an 80 000 Da polypeptide which contains the third A and both C domains (C-terminus). These polypeptides are the result of thrombin cleavage of the whole factor VIII molecule. Furthermore, the large B domain is cleaved off during the activation of factor VIII, and it appears to have no role in procoagulation (Toole et al 1986). A detailed discussion of the factor VIII protein biochemistry (proteolytic cleavages, 'activation' of the molecule, von Willebrand binding site, factor IX binding site, factor X binding site, phospholipid binding site, etc.) is beyond the scope of this review, and many of these issues remain as yet unclear.

MUTATIONS IN THE FACTOR VIII GENE IN HEMOPHILIA A

Hemophilia A patients can be divided according to clinical severity into mild, moderate, and severe, and this clinical classification relates closely to factor VIII clotting activity. In the great majority of patients, the biological activity of factor VIII closely parallels the amount of protein in plasma as measured by an immunological method. In addition, about 6–12% of patients with hemophilia A develop antibodies against factor VIII (inhibitor patients) after therapy with exogenous factor VIII. Inhibitors develop almost exclusively in patients that have no detectable factor VIII in their plasma (Hoyer 1984).

In the past 3 years we have examined the DNA of 240 different patients with hemophilia A and found molecular defects in 28 patients (Table 11.1). Deletions, single nucleotide changes, and, more recently, insertions in the factor VIII gene were found as causes of hemophilia A. These mutations have provided new insights into the pathogenesis of hemophilia A, including the existence of 'hotspots' for mutation and further evidence that a considerable number of mutations occur de novo. In addition, they have provided evidence for a new mechanism of mutation in man, i.e., retrotransposition of L1 or LINE sequences. Other investigators have also identified deletions and point mutations in the factor VIII gene. Most of the following discussion will focus on the Johns Hopkins findings, but information on the findings and the experience from other laboratories will be provided.

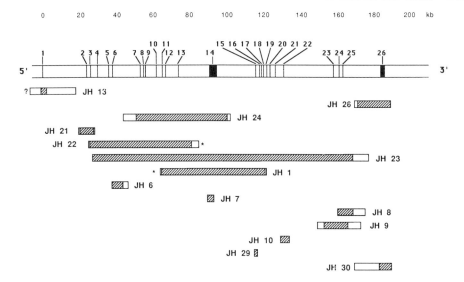

Fig. 11.1   Deletions of the factor VIII gene in patients with hemophilia A studied at The Johns Hopkins Hospital. The top of the figure shows the factor VIII gene. Kb numbers from the first exon of the gene are shown. Each exon is represented by a vertical line or filled box. Exons are numbered from 1 to 26. Each horizontal bar represents a different deletion within the factor VIII gene. Open bars at the ends of deletions denote the uncertainty of the extent of the deletion. The patient number is given. Asterisk after the deletion represents the presence of inhibitors in that particular patient.

Deletions of the factor VIII gene

We have observed 14 different deletions within the factor VIII gene. Figure 11.1 shows the extent of the deletions and the presence of factor VIII inhibitors (Antonarakis et al 1985, Gitschier et al 1985b, Higuchi et al 1988, Youssoufian et al 1987b, 1988b). No two unrelated patients share the same endpoints of these deletions. All but one of the partial factor VIII gene deletions are associated with severe hemophilia A. The deletion in patient JH 10 which involves exon 22 and results in an in-frame deletion of 52 amino acids is associated with moderately severe disease. Other laboratories have identified several other partial gene deletions and Casarino et al have studied a total factor VIII gene deletion without inhibitors. No association between inhibitors and size or location of deletions has been found. The ends of two deletions that occur in IVS-13 and exon 14 have been cloned and sequenced. In neither case did the deletion involve an Alu or other repetitive element or unequal crossing over within homologous sequences. The study of more breakpoints may provide insights on the mechanism of deletions in factor VIII. Finally, it is of interest that 14/240 patients (5.8%) with hemophilia A examined have sizable deletions within the factor VIII gene which can be recognized by simple restriction analysis.

Insertion of L1 repetitive elements in the factor VIII gene

L1 sequences are a human-specific family of long interspersed repetitive elements present in about 10^5 copies dispersed throughout the genome (Skowronski & Singer 1986). The full length L1 sequence is 6.1 kb, but the majority of L1 elements are truncated at the 5′ end resulting in a five-fold higher copy number of 3′ sequences. (Skowronski & Singer 1986). The nucleotide sequence of L1 elements includes an

A-rich 3' end and two long open reading frames (ORF-1 and ORF-2), the second of which encodes a potential polypeptide with homology to reverse transcriptases (Skowronski & Singer 1986). This structure suggests that L1 elements represent a class of non-viral retrotransposons (Scott et al 1987). A number of L1 cDNAs, including a nearly full-length element, have been isolated from an undifferentiated teratocarcinoma cell line (Skowronski & Singer 1986). We have found insertions of L1 elements into exon 14 of the factor VIII gene in 2 of 240 unrelated patients with hemophilia A (Kazazian et al 1988). In both cases the parent did not have the insertion and, therefore, the event occurred de novo. Both of these insertions (3.8 kb and 2.3 kb) contained 3' portions of the L1 sequence, including the poly A tract, and created target site duplications of at least 12 and 13 nucleotides of the factor VIII gene (Fig. 11.2). In addition, their 3'-trailer sequences following ORF-2 are nearly identical

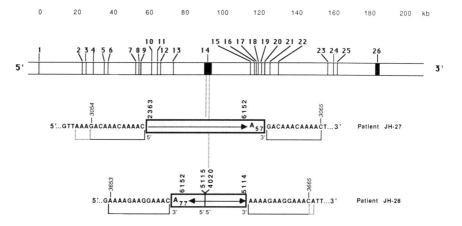

Fig. 11.2   Diagram of L1 insertions in exon 14 of the factor VIII gene. The 3.8 kb L1 insertion from patient JH-27 is flanked by a 12 bp target site duplication of factor VIII cDNA sequence (nucleotides 3054–3065 where nucleotide 1 is the A of the initiator codon). Residues 3051–3053 of the factor VIII cDNA are adenylic acids and could also be duplicated (shown by the hatched bracket). The rearranged 2.3 kb insertion from patient JH-28 is shown and is flanked by a 13 bp target site duplication. Residue 3666 of the factor VIII cDNA is an A and could also be duplicated. Filled boxes represent the L1 elements, and the arrows within the boxes point toward the 3' end of the L1 sequence. Both L1 insertions showed 98% similarity to the consensus genomic L1 sequence outside of the 3'-trailer region.

to the consensus sequence of L1 cDNAs. The data indicate that in man certain L1 sequences can be dispersed presumably via an RNA intermediate and cause disease by insertional mutation.

Insertion of L1 elements, involving retrotransposition of DNA sequences through an RNA intermediate into a new and distant location in the genome, represents a fundamentally different mechanism of mutation producing human disease from those previously described. Because we do not know when these L1 insertion events occur, whether in the sperm or ovum, after fertilization, or during early stages of embryogenesis, the proportion of such insertions that are heritable is unknown. Yet finding two L1 insertions among 240 patients with hemophilia A suggests that this mechanism of mutation is not uncommon.

Single nucleotide mutations within the factor VIII gene

Although the gene for factor VIII is very large and it seemed unlikely that single nucleotide changes would be identified using restriction analysis, a large number of point mutations have actually been identified by us and others (Fig. 11.3).

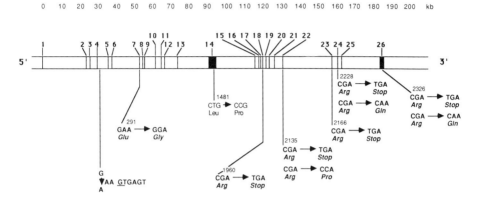

Fig. 11.3 Single nucleotide mutations within the factor VIII gene. The nucleotide changes and the amino acid changes are shown. Arg, Arginine; Gln, glutamine; Leu, leucine; Pro, proline; stop, nonsense codon. It is unknown if the mutation at codon 1481 Leu→ Pro (B domain) causes hemophilia A. The mutations at codon 2326 and the Arg→ Pro mutation at codon 2135 were described by Gitschier et al, 1985a,b, 1986. The mutation in intron 4 probably creates a new donor splice site.

Screening the factor VIII gene using restriction analysis with Taq I has turned out to be fruitful in discovering point mutations, many of which are CpG-TpG substitutions. Ten different substitutions of this type were discovered among the 240 patients at 5 Taq I sites in exons (Antonarakis et al 1985, Youssoufian et al 1986, 1988a). Nine of these mutations were CpG-TpG substitutions and the tenth was not in the CpG dinucleotide. CpG dinucleotides are thought to be 'hotspots' for mutations because C can be methylated at the 5' position of the pyrimidine ring and subsequently deaminated spontaneously to thymine. This accounts for CG-TG and CG-CA mutations. That CpG dinucleotides are 'hotspots' for mutations is also supported by the fact that a considerable number of DNA polymorphic sites are in restriction endonuclease recognition sequences which contain CpG (Taq I and Msp I for example). The factor VIII gene contains 7 Taq I sites in its coding region, 5 of which have CGA as a codon for arginine. Mutations have been observed in all of these 5 Taq I sites (Antonarakis et al 1985, Gitschier et al 1985, 1986, Higuchi et al 1988, Levinson et al 1987, Youssoufian et al 1986, 1988a).

It is of interest that examples of recurrent mutation have been observed for 5 different mutations among the first 600 defective factor VIII genes examined. One can calculate that up to a few thousand recurrences of these same exact mutations may have occurred in man in the last 2000 years. The estimated mutation rate of C-T in CG dinucleotides in the factor VIII gene is calculated to be 10–20 times more than the average mutation rate for any dinucleotide. It appears that, on average, a mutation in each of the 5 Taq I sites in exons is observed in every 170 hemophilia A patients examined.

Table 11.2   DNA polymorphic markers useful in carrier detection and prenatal diagnosis of hemophilia A.

DNA polymorphic site	Location	Comments
DNA polymorphisms within the factor VIII gene		
Bcl I	IVS 18	Excellent marker for carrier detection and prenatal diagnosis in Caucasians. Complete linkage disequilibrium with Hind III and Msp I. Relatively small fragments to score (Gitschier et al 1985a)
Hind III	IVS 19	Complete linkage disequilibrium with the Bcl I site (Ahrens et al 1987)
Xba I	IVS 22	Second marker of choice in Caucasians. About $\frac{1}{4}$ of females homozygous for Bcl I are heterozygous for Xba I (Wion et al 1986)
Bgl I	IVS 25	Good marker for American Blacks (Antonarakis et al 1985)
Msp I	3′ Flanking	Excellent marker for Caucasians and other ethnic groups. Complete linkage disequilibrium with Bcl I and Hind III. Very easy to score (Youssoufian et al 1987a)
DNA polymorphisms linked to the factor VIII gene		
Taq I VNTR	DXS52 (probe ST14)	Excellent marker (Oberle et al 1985) 3–5% recombination with factor VIII gene
Bgl II	DXS15 (probe DX13)	3–5% recombination with factor VIII gene (Harper et al 1984). The locus order is DXS15–DXS52 — factor VIII

Origin of the mutations

Thirteen of the 28 mutations identified in our patient population occurred de novo within 2 generations. (In 5 families, it was not possible to determine whether the mutation had arisen within 2 generations or the proband.) In 11 of these 13 de novo mutations, the origin (mother or maternal grandfather or maternal grandmother) has been identified. Both deletions and point mutations occurred de novo in maternal grandfathers (5/11). The remaining 6 mutations occur de novo in mothers or maternal grandmothers. The question of the association of advanced paternal age and de novo mutation to hemophilia A cannot be addressed as yet, since a larger number of cases in which the mutation is known needs to be collected and analyzed.

DNA polymorphisms in the factor VIII gene

Since each family with hemophilia A usually has a different mutation in the factor VIII gene, it is almost impossible to detect directly the molecular defect using restriction endonuclease analysis and, therefore, provide accurate carrier detection and prenatal diagnosis. On the other hand, indirect detection of the abnormal factor VIII gene (regardless of the nature of the abnormality) can be achieved using as markers DNA polymorphisms within or adjacent to the factor VIII gene. In the past 3 years there has been considerable effort to identify DNA polymorphisms within the factor VIII gene, but the yield has been relatively poor. The high frequency polymorphic sites within the factor VIII gene identified to date are shown in Table 11.2. If one uses these polymorphic sites as markers for the normal and abnormal factor VIII alleles in families, the error in carrier detection and/or prenatal diagnosis is negligible because the recombination rate between a given marker and the actual site of mutation is extremely low. Recently, using gene amplification techniques, it has become possible to score the most informative of these polymorphic sites within a few days without Southern blotting (Kogan et al 1987).

Other extragenic DNA polymorphic markers have been described which are tightly linked to the factor VIII gene and the hemophilia A phenotype (Table 11.2). There is about 3–5% recombinational distance between these markers and factor VIII and, therefore, an unavoidable 3–5% error in the DNA diagnosis of the presence or absence of the mutant allele in a given family.

SUMMARY

The cloning of the factor VIII gene has provided a great impetus to the molecular analysis of hemophilia A. The large number of deletions and point mutations character-ized to date have produced further basic insights into the variety and nature of muta-tions. In particular, the first instances of mutation via retrotransposition have been observed in the factor VIII gene. In addition, the knowledge gained from these studies has improved the accuracy of prenatal diagnosis and carrier detection in hemophilia. Further studies will include the identification of further mutations and polymorphisms, the correlation of mutations with the severity of disease and inhibitor production, a complete characterization of de novo mutations and their parental origins, and the use of heterologous cell systems to study abnormalities of RNA processing.

ACKNOWLEDGEMENTS

The authors thank Drs H. Youssoufian, C. Wong, and Ms P. Woods Samuels and D. Phillips, all members of their laboratories for data collection, enthusiasm and helpful discussions. We also thank Drs J. Toole, J. Wozney, J. Gitschier, R. Lawn, K. Davies, J. L. Mandel, and Ms D. Pittman for providing molecular probes. We are also indebted to Drs D. Fass, G. Bowie, S. Aronis, C. Kasper, W. Bell, and many other physicians and genetic counselors for providing us with the appropriate patients and families. Finally, we thank Ms E. Pasterfield for expert secretarial assist-ance and J. Strayer for the art work. This work has been supported in part by NIH grants to SEA and HHK.

Reproduced with permission from Trends in Genetics 1988

REFERENCES

Ahrens et al 1987 Human Genetics 26: 127
Antonarakis S E, Waber P G, Kittur S D et al 1985 New England Journal of Medicine 313: 842–848
Ginsburg D, Handin R I, Bonthron D T et al 1985 Science 228: 1401–1406
Gitschier J, Wood W I, Goralka T M et al 1984 Nature: 312: 326–330
Gitschier J et al 1985a Nature 314: 738
Gitschier J, Wood W I, Tuddenham E G D et al 1985b Nature 315: 427–430
Gitschier J, Wood W I, Shuman M A, Lawn R M 1986 Science 232: 1415–1416
Harper et al 1984 Lancet 2: 6
Higuchi M, Kochhan L., Schwaab R et al 1988 Blood (in press)
Hoyer L W (ed) 1984 Factor VIII inhibitors. Liss, New York
Jackson C M, Nemerson Y 1980 Annual Review of Biochemistry 49: 765–811
Kane W H, Davie E W 1986 Proceedings of the National Academy of Sciences USA 83: 6800–6804
Kazazian H H, Wong C, Youssoufian H, Scott A F, Phillips D, Antonarakis S E 1988 Nature 332:
    165–166
Kogan S C, Doherty M, Gitschier J 1987 New England Journal of Medicine 317: 985–990
Levinson B B, Janco R, Phillips J A, Gitschier 1987 American Journal of Human Genetics 41: 225A
    (abstract)

McKee P A 1983 In: Stanbury J B, Wyngaarden J B, Fredrickson D S, Goldstein J L, Brown M S (eds) The metabolic basis of inherited disease 5th edn. McGraw-Hill, New York. p 1531–1560
Oberle et al 1985 New England Journal of Medicine 312: 682
Rotblat F, O'Brien D P, O'Brien F J, Goodall A H, Tuddenham E G 1985 Biochemistry 24: 4294–4300
Scott A F, Schmeckpeper B J, Abdelrazik M et al 1987 Genomics 1: 113–125
Skowronski J, Singer M F 1986 Cold Spring Harbor Symposium on Quantitative Biology 51: 457–464
Toole J J, Knopf J L, Wozney J M et al 1984 Nature 312: 342–347
Toole J J, Pittman D D, Orr E C, Mortha P, Wasley L C, Kaufman R J 1986 Proceedings of the National Academy of Sciences USA 83: 5939–5942
Vehar G A, Keyt B, Eaton D et al 1984 Nature 312: 337–342
Wion et al 1986 Nucleic Acids Research 14: 4535
Youssoufian H, Kazazian H H Jr, Phillips D G et al 1986 Nature 324: 380–382
Youssoufian H et al 1987a Nucleic Acids Research 15: 6312
Youssoufian H, Antonarakis S E, Phillips D G, Aronis S, Tsiftis G, Kazazian H H Jr 1987b Proceedings of the National Academy of Sciences USA 84: 3772–3776
Youssoufian H, Antonarakis S E, Bell W, Griffin A M, Kazazian H H Jr 1988a American Journal of Human Genetics (in press)
Youssoufian H, Kasper C K, Phillips D G, Kazazian H H Jr, Antonarakis S E 1988b Human Genetics (in press)

12. Haemophilia B: a review of patient defects, diagnosis with gene probes and prospects for gene therapy

G. G. Brownlee

INTRODUCTION

Haemophilia has been known since Biblical times to be an inherited bleeding disorder, because boys born into affected families were excluded from ritual circumcision (quoted by McKee 1983). It was, but is fortunately no longer, present in the English Royal Family, since Queen Victoria was a carrier of the disease. Clinical symptoms were life-threatening before effective replacement therapy was introduced. Bleeding occurs often without any obvious trauma and patients could die at a young age from internal haemorrhage into muscles and joints. The pattern of inheritance of the disease, in which males were affected but females were not (although they could transmit this disease to future generations), intrigued the 19th century biologists and was not adequately explained until the genetic basis of sex was understood. Before 1952 it was not realised that there were two forms of haemophilia since both diseases present with similar clinical symptoms and both show an X-linked, recessive, pattern of inheritance. The differential diagnosis of haemophilia A (classical haemophilia) and haemophilia B (Christmas disease) depends on laboratory tests of the clotting time of indicator plasma. The former, haemophilia A, is the more common disease occurring at a frequency of about 1 in 6000 males in Caucasian populations, whereas haemophilia B occurs in about 1 in 30 000 males (see Table 12.1). In haemophilia A patients there is a defect in the clotting factor VIII(C), whilst in haemophilia B patients the defect is in clotting factor IX. Both factors are essential proteins in the middle phase of the intrinsic clotting cascade, summarised in a simplified form in Figure 12.1.

Factor IX circulates in blood as an inactive zymogen. Only when converted to factor IXa by the activation of the clotting cascade and in particular factor XIa, does factor IX undergo the conformational change necessary to unmask its own latent proteolytic activity. Factor IXa, in turn, converts the factor X, in the presence of platelets, factor VIII and Ca^{2+}, into factor Xa, which ultimately results in the formation of the fibrin clot. Although the overall pathway shown in Figure 12.1 is an accepted fact, many details of the steps await a finer dissection, which will only become possible when the 3-dimensional structure of the macromolecules involved is known.

In this review I will concentrate on 4 areas in which progress has been particularly evident in the last 2–3 years. These areas are: (1) studies to define the precise molecular defects in patients; (2) protein engineering of factor IX; (3) improved diagnosis of the disease both antenatally and in carriers; and (4) prospects for gene therapy. I have recently reviewed expression of recombinant factor IX (Brownlee 1987). For other reviews on factor IX and haemophilia B, the reader is referred to Thompson (1986), McGraw et al (1985a) and Giannelli (1988). For reviews covering both

Table 12.1 Vital statistics of the haemophilias

Name	Synonym	Chromosomal location	Frequency (male)	No. UK patients	Protein defect
Haemophilia A	Classical haemophilia	Xq28	Approx. 1 in 6000	4500	Factor VIII(C)
Haemophilia B	Christmas disease	Xq27	Approx. 1 in 30 000	900	Factor IX

haemophilia A and B the reader can consult Brownlee (1986) or Antonarakis (1988). Genetic linkage between the factor IX locus and other disease loci on the X chromosome, e.g. the Martin-Bell syndrome (mental retardation with fragility at Xq27) is outside the scope of this review. The interested reader is referred to Giannelli et al (1987).

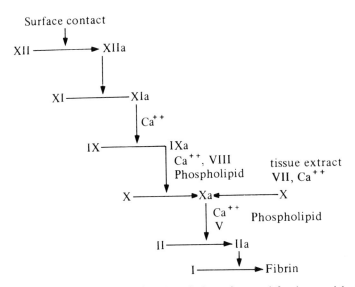

Fig. 12.1 The clotting cascade. The intrinsic pathway is shown from top left to bottom right. The extrinsic pathway (activation of factor X by activated factor VII) is also shown. This is a simplified version showing the main features, but it omits feedback loops and a step, e.g. factor VIIa activation of IX, interconnecting the two pathways. (From Austen & Rhymes 1975.)

STRUCTURE OF THE FACTOR IX GENE AND PROTEIN

The human factor IX gene is 33 kbases long and both it and the cDNA copy of the factor IX mRNA were cloned and sequenced in several laboratories in the period 1982–85 (Choo et al 1982, Kurachi & Davie 1982, Jaye et al 1983, Anson et al 1984, Yoshitake et al 1985). Figure 12.2 shows the arrangement of the 8 exons, labelled a–h, and illustrates the fact that they encode separate domains in the factor IX protein, which are: (a) a hydrophobic *signal* peptide which targets the protein for secretion from the hepatocyte into the blood stream; (b) a propeptide and *gla* domain, needed for the vitamin K-dependent carboxylase modification of 12 N-terminal glutamyl residues to γ-carboxyglutamyl residues. This modification occurs during biosynthesis in the endoplasmic reticulum of the hepatocyte and is required for calcium binding

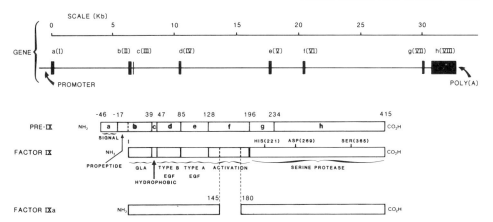

Fig. 12.2 Scheme of the factor IX gene and protein, showing its domain structure. The exon regions a–h (or I–VIII) are shown above, and the protein domains a–h below defined by amino acid position. 'Gla' is an abbreviation for the γ-carboxyglutamyl-containing region and EGF an abbreviation for epidermal growth factor-like domains. Also shown is the relationship between precursor (PRE-IX), factor IX and factor IXa molecules. The two chains of factor IXa are held together by an interstrand disulphide bridge.

to ensure the correct factor IX conformation for activity; (c) a small *hydrophobic* domain, which was formerly considered part of the gla domain since it contains one of the 12 gla residues. However, recent crystallographic data on prothrombin indicates, by analogy, that it might have a different function promoting heterodimerisation of gla domains of unrelated clotting factors (Harlos et al 1987); (d) *a type B, epidermal growth factor-like domain*, which shows homology to epidermal growth factor (EGF) and, in addition, contains conserved carboxylate residues including a β-hydroxyaspartate at amino acid 64. This domain may bind additional Ca^{2+} with high affinity and may also bind to factor VIII (see below, under Protein engineering); (e) *a type A, epidermal growth factor-like (EGF) domain* which shows homology to EGF, but lacks the homologous carboxylate residues of the EGF type B domain. Its function is unknown; (f) an *activation* domain, within which factor XIa cleaves twice, converting factor IX to IXa; (g and h) the *serine protease domain*, responsible for the proteolysis of factor X to Xa. This region is homologous to other well studied serine proteases (e.g. chymotrypsin) and it is thought likely that his (221), asp (269) and ser (365), all participate in the classical catalytic mechanism.

The factor IX protein is initially synthesised as a precursor molecule, some 40 amino acids longer at its N-terminus than the 415 long mature factor IX, which is found in plasma. The processing steps, which sequentially remove the hydrophobic signal peptide and the propeptide, occur in the hepatocyte prior to secretion. In addition to the γ-carboxylation of the N-terminal glutamyl residues, and the β-hydroxylation of aspartate 64, N-linked carbohydrate side chains are added at residues 157 and 167.

In summary, the active site of factor IX is contained within the serine protease domain, which is supported by 6 other signalling regions. For all except the type A EGF domain, we have information suggesting these domains are essential either for correct biosynthesis, for modification, for activation by XIa, or for ensuring maximal catalytic activity.

MOLECULAR DEFECTS IN HAEMOPHILIA B

Evidence of heterogeneity exists in haemophilia B as there is variation in the clinical severity of the disease in different pedigrees. There is also a corresponding variation in the laboratory tests of clotting activity and in the antigen concentration measured in samples of blood taken from different patients. We therefore expect a wide range of molecular defects. Haemophilia patients may be conveniently subdivided into those in whom protein is present as detected by immunological methods, referred to as antigen positive, and those in whom it is absent, referred to as antigen negative. The former might be expected to have point mutations in those regions of the gene coding for the factor IX protein and studies of such patients should pinpoint critical functional regions of the protein. The antigen negative patients are likely to have either deletions or point mutations critical for the correct biosynthesis of the messenger RNA or the protein. A small subgroup of patients of the antigen negative type are referred to as 'inhibitors', because these patients, in response to injection of factor IX protein in the course of therapy, produce specific anti-factor IX antibodies.

Point mutations

Only a few patients have been characterised fully at the molecular level although new methods for amplifying and sequencing DNA (Saiki et al 1985, Wong et al 1987, Saiki et al 1988, Stoflet et al 1988) are beginning to be used and should speed up their analysis in future. All currently fully characterised *point* mutations are listed in Table 12.2. I include two factor IX antigen positive patients factor $IX_{Chapel\ Hill}$ and factor $IX_{Cambridge}$ in whom the defect has been characterised by a study of the abnormal protein.

Point mutations in the antigen positive patients (Table 12.2) clearly demonstrate that there are critical amino-acid residues in the signalling regions of factor IX. Propeptide mutations in haemophilia $B_{Oxford\ 3}$ and factor $IX_{San\ Dimas}$ and factor $IX_{Cambridge}$ cause severe haemophilia, while other mutations e.g. asp (145) of factor $IX_{Chapel\ Hill}$ and asp (47) of factor $IX_{Alabama}$ are milder allowing some residual clotting activity. Three mutations in the catalytic domain (at amino acids 252, 333 and 397) have now been defined in an unnamed patient, in factor $IX_{Vancouver}$ and in factor $IX_{London\ 2}$, respectively, demonstrating that residues other than those proposed as directly participating in the catalytic mechanism (see above) are critical for function. The precise reason why a particular mutated factor IX fails to mediate clotting is often unclear in detail; what is known is beyond the scope of this review. Suffice it to say that a 3-dimensional structure of normal factor IX would materially assist our understanding.

The fact that both haemophilia $B_{Oxford\ 3}$ and factor $IX_{San\ Dimas}$ are identical $G \rightarrow A$ mutations found in independent pedigrees, suggests that this nucleotide is a 'hot spot' for mutation. It is probably significant that this mutation is contained within a CG sequence. This C residue is likely to be methylated giving 5 methylcytosine in the gene. The origin of the identical mutations in these 2 patients could well be the deamination of 5 methylcytosine to thymine in the non-coding strand of DNA. A second 'hot spot' may occur at or near to amino acid 252, since there is preliminary

Table 12.2 Characterised point or frameshift mutations. Antigen positive have >0.5% of normal factor IX antigen negative <0.5%. Mild has >5% clotting activity, moderate 0.5–5% and severe <0.5% of normal plasma.

Subgroup	Patient	Severity	Defect**	Nucleotide change**	Reference
Antigen positive	Factor IX$_{Chapel Hill}$	Mild	Arg → His (145)	G → A* (20 414)	Noyes et al (1983)
	Factor IX$_{Alabama}$	Mild	Asp → Gly (47)	A → G (10 392)	Davis et al (1984)
	Haemophilia B$_{Oxford 3}$	Severe	Arg → Gln (−4)	G → A (6365)	Bentley et al (1986)
	Factor IX$_{San Dimas}$	Severe	Arg → Gln (−4)	G → A (6365)	Ware et al (1986)
	Factor IX$_{Cambridge}$	Severe	Arg → Ser (−1)	G → C or T* (6375)	Diuguid et al (1986)
	Factor IX$_{Vancouver}$	Moderate	Ile → Thr (397)	T → C (31 311)	Geddes et al (1987)
	Unnamed	Not stated	Arg → Leu (252)	G → T (30 876)	Chen et al (1987)
	Factor IX$_{London 2}$	Severe	Arg → Gln (333)	G → A (31 119)	Tsang et al (1988)
	Haemophilia B$_{Leyden}$	Varies†	normal	T → A (−20)	Reitsma et al (1987)
Antigen negative	Haemophilia B$_{Oxford 1}$	Severe	Unstable mRNA and/or truncated protein	G → T (20 566) (affecting donor splice junction, exon f)	Rees et al (1985)
	Haemophilia B$_{Oxford 2}$	Severe	?	T → G (6704) (affecting donor splice junction, exon c)	Winship (1986)
	Factor IX$_{Seattle 2}$	Severe	Frameshift with translation stop codon at amino acid 86	$\triangle A^6$ (17 669)	Schach et al (1987)
	Unnamed	Severe	Arg → Stop (252)	C → T (30 875)	Siguret et al (1988)

* These nucleotide changes were predicted from the observed amino acid mutation.

** For amino acid numbering see Anson et al (1984); for nucleotide numbering, Yoshitake et al (1985).

† Severe before puberty, then becoming increasingly mild to asymptomatic with age, producing normal factor IX.

evidence that a patient studied by Poon et al (1987) may have one or other of the mutations described by Chen et al (1987) or Siguvet et al (1988), both of which affect amino acid 252 (see Table 12.2). Furthermore, 5 of the 8 antigen positive protein defects (Table 12.2) involve mutations within CG dinucleotides in arginine codons, again illustrating their mutability, presumably due to methylation.

The defect in haemophilia B_{Leyden} is particularly interesting since patients improve markedly at puberty in response to testosterone. Such patients have an abnormality in the regulation of transcription of factor IX and the factor IX which is produced is normal. Fortunately some patients improve so markedly that, within a few years of puberty, they may have nearly normal levels of normal factor IX (Briet et al 1982). Reitsma et al 1987 have recently reported that one such patient has 2 point mutations, but this has been corrected (see Tsang et al 1988) to a single mutation at residue −20 (see Table 12.2), which is close to the presumed promoter (Anson et al 1984).

Two of the antigen negative patients, haemophilia $B_{Oxford\ 1}$ and $_{Oxford\ 2}$ show mutations (Table 12.2) at different donor splice sites. The other antigen negative patient factor $IX_{Seattle\ 2}$ is a frameshift mutation.

No antigen positive mutations have yet been defined in the gla domain (see Fig. 12.3) although it has been suggested that factor $IX_{Zutphen}$ occurs here (Thompson

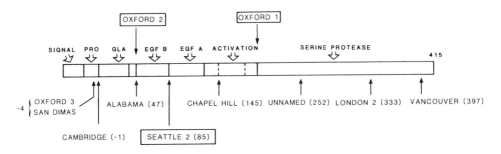

Fig. 12.3   Scheme showing the name and location of point and frameshift mutations within the factor IX protein. Also included, although not strictly within the protein, are the positions of the 2 splice mutations, $_{Oxford\ 1}$ and $_{Oxford\ 2}$. Haemophilia B_{Leyden} — a promoter mutant, is omitted.

1986). Rees et al 1988 have predicted that factor $IX_{Eindhoven}$ is a mutant of the EGF B domain. The defect in haemophilia B_m is still unknown, although it was described many years ago (Hougie & Twomey 1967).

Deletions and inhibitor patients
We originally suggested (Giannelli et al 1983) that inhibitor patients (fortunately rare, comprising <1% of all patients), who respond to factor IX replacement therapy by mounting a specific anti-factor IX immune response, did so because they lacked immune tolerance to factor IX. Clearly, gene deletions mean absence of factor IX, which could lead to lack of tolerance. Indeed 4 out of the 5 original UK patients had partial or complete deletions (Giannelli et al 1983, Peake et al 1984) supporting the hypothesis. It is now clear, following studies in many centres, that only 50–60%

HAEMOPHILIA B: A REVIEW 257

of all inhibitor patients show deletions as assayed by Southern blots, although it remains possible that small deletions could be missed and the actual % is somewhat higher than 50–60%.

The extent of the deletions in the deletion-type inhibitor patients varies from 2.5 kb to over 250 kb and is summarised in Figure 12.4, along with deletions observed in 5 non-inhibitor cases, and one case of unknown status. Only in a single case, haemophilia B$_{London\ 1}$, are both endpoints of the deletion precisely known. In this patient a non-homologous (or illegitimate) recombination has occurred between an Alu repeat in the 3' flanking DNA of the factor IX gene and DNA within an intron of the gene, at the same time generating 16 base pairs of 'new' DNA (see Fig. 12.4). Green et al (1988) propose that such deletions occur during DNA replication. Haemophilia B$_{Chicago}$ and an unnamed Australian patient show, respectively, a 'complex' deletion (Matthews et al 1987) and evidence of both deletion and insertion (Trent 1987), although no sequence details are available yet. Many other deletions shown in Figure 12.4 may be longer than shown as they have not yet been tested against gene probes from the 270 kb cloned DNA around and including the factor IX gene (Anson et al 1988). A point of particular interest is that 4 of the patients, specifically $_{Manchester\ 1}$ and $_{2,\ Jersey}$ and $_{Boston}$, lack an adjacent transforming gene called mcf2 as well as the factor IX gene. There are no obvious clinical complications common to these 4 patients that can be correlated with a lack of the mcf2, as well as the factor IX gene. It seems likely that mcf2 is non-essential, at least in males.

Among the deletion patients (Fig. 12.4) there is only one patient, factor IX$_{Strasbourg}$, who produces a large amount of antigen (30%). Despite lacking exon d, this patient probably synthesizes a shortened inactive factor IX by alternative splicing between the donor splice site of exon c and the acceptor splice site of exon e (Vidaud et al 1986).

Many authors have emphasised that not all deletions, even large ones, result in high-titre antibodies when patients are treated (Chen et al 1985, Taylor et al 1988, Thompson 1986, Wadelius et al 1986). Thus other factors must be involved in the immune response to therapeutic factor IX. Highly polymorphic immune response genes within the HLA locus in Man are known to be involved in the presentation of processed complex antigens by macrophages and other accessory cells to T helper lymphocytes, as part of the process by which the proliferation of a specific B cell occurs producing antibody. Thus, immune response phenomena in haemophilia B therapy are not surprising, and, indeed, were noted many years ago (Shapiro 1979). Nevertheless, it would be interesting to establish the nature of the critical epitopes in factor IX, and find out which HLA haplotypes (and genes) are involved. Recently Wadelius et al (1988) have reported that the HLA2B12 haplotype is shared by 2 patients who are cousins and who have a complete deletion of the factor IX gene, yet fail to produce inhibitors in response to therapeutic factor IX. It will be interesting to learn whether unrelated patients share this haplotype (see Taylor et al 1988). An examination of the variety of deletions in Figure 12.4 suggests no *one* exon of factor IX is critical for tolerance. On the theoretical grounds that the 'signalling' regions of factor IX, with the exception of the activation region, all show some similarity in amino acid sequence, either to other clotting factors or to extracellular proteins, it seems possible that some degree of cross-tolerance to these regions of factor IX might exist. From such arguments, it may be predicted that the more critical determi-

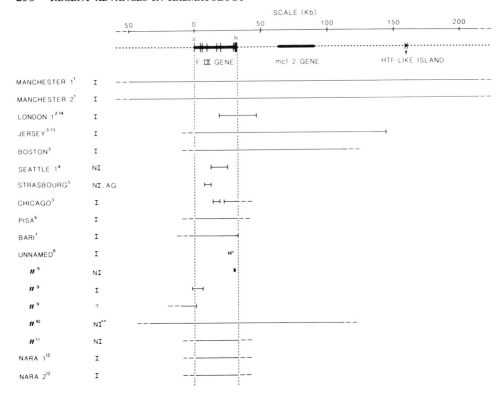

Fig. 12.4   Diagram of the extent of gene deletions in 18 haemophilia B patients. A vertical bar indicates that the end point of the deletion has been defined roughly by Southern blots, or in the case of factor IX$_{London\ 1}$, precisely, by sequence analysis; a dashed line that it remains undefined. I, inhibitor patient; NI, non-inhibitor patient; AG, antigen positive. mcf2 and HTF-like island are 2 adjacent structures. The long vertical dashed line delimits the extent of the factor IX (FIX) gene, and the 8 exons (only a and h are labelled) of the factor IX gene are indicated by vertical bars. Superscript numbers refer to detailed references as follows: (1) Anson et al (1988), (2) Giannelli et al (1983), (3) Matthews et al (1987), (4) Chen et al (1985), (5) Vidaud et al (1986), (6) Bernardi et al (1985), (7) Hassan et al (1985), (8) Trent (1987), (9) Ludwig (1987), (10) Taylor et al (1988), (11) Wadelius et al (1986), (12) Mikami et al (1987), (13) Matthews et al (1988), (14) Green et al (1988). Seattle 1 produces detectable truncated factor IX in urine.

Key: ★ Believed to contain both a deletion and insertion. ★★ This patient is unusually mildly affected producing no antibodies, but an affected male relative has formed antibodies, transiently.

nants for tolerance to factor IX might be in the more variable activation region or in the serine protease domain. Indeed, a preliminary classification of determinants suggests that several epitopes are involved, including some located towards the carboxy-terminus of factor IX (Thompson 1987). Thompson has further suggested that, if a limited number of defined linear epitopes were present, one might be able to neutralize inhibitory immunoglobulin with synthetic peptides in a specific manner. If this were possible, it might, in principle, be a new therapeutic method for inhibitor patients.

Nilsson et al (1986) have improved earlier, largely unsuccessful protocols for inducing tolerance to therapeutic factor IX in inhibitor patients, by the combined use of immunoglobulin, factor IX and cyclophosphamide (an immunosuppressant). Three out of 4 high titre inhibitor patients eliminate, at least in a period of 6 months, their inhibitory antibodies, apparently because they form a 'modified factor IX — new antibody' immune complex, which acts as a tolerogen. No long term complications were reported, although the patient treated longest had received this treatment for only 4 years.

PROTEIN ENGINEERING

Protein engineering allows an investigation of the effect of mutations introduced by design into factor IX cDNA clones by recombinant DNA methods. Such studies can complement information derived from naturally occurring defects in patients. Only rather limited studies on two signalling domains, specifically the propeptide domain and one of the EGF domains, have been performed so far. Jorgensen et al (1987) deleted the entire propeptide domain. The modified factor IX is inactive in clotting activity, because it lacks a correctly modified gla domain. Point mutations of amino acids -16 and -10 within the propeptide resulted in a factor IX with a defective gla domain also. These observations supported the hypothesis that the N-terminal part of the propeptide domain serves as a γ-carboxylase recognition site (γCRS), which is required for correct γ-carboxylation of glutamyl residues in the adjacent gla domain. Galeffi & Brownlee (1987) mutated arginine at -4 of the propeptide and observed that γ-carboxylation was seriously impaired. They suggested that the γCRS should include all the propeptide domain. Thus protein engineering supported the patient studies on factor IX$_{Cambridge}$ and $_{San\ Dimas}$, but partly contradicted the study of factor IX$_{Oxford\ 3}$, in which the propeptide -4 mutation had interfered with propeptide processing, although the extent of γ-carboxylation was near normal (Bentley et al 1986). Further work is needed to clarify this discrepancy.

The EGF domain is particularly interesting because of its homology to epidermal growth factor and the existence of related domains in a wide range of proteins of varying function. The EGF type B domain was mutated at the amino acids containing a carboxylate side chain, specifically aspartate (47), aspartate (49), β-hydroxyaspartate (64) and glutamate (78), because these residues are homologous in many different type B EGF domains (Rees 1986, Rees et al 1988). The mutant factor IX molecules were all $<10\%$ as active as normal, except for glutamate (78). The factor IX mutants were activated normally by factor XIa but failed to convert factor X to Xa, when assayed in the presence of factor VIII. We propose that this type B EGF domain binds calcium structurally; in some way this aids recognition of factor VIII during the enzymic conversion of factor X to Xa. Whether or not this is correct, these results demonstrate the importance of amino acid residues 47, 49 and 64 in the type B EGF domain for the correct function of factor IX.

CARRIER AND ANTENATAL DIAGNOSIS USING GENE PROBES

Because of heterogeneity of the molecular defect in haemophilia B, the exact molecular cause is usually unknown in families seeking diagnosis, making specific diagnosis of the patient defect impossible. Therefore, linkage analysis using a polymorphic factor IX probe is the method of choice. Six intragenic, and several reasonably closely linked extragenic polymorphisms are now known in Caucasian families (Table 12.3). Despite significant linkage disequilibrium (or association) between the intragenic markers, we estimated that 80% of families can be diagnosed with an accuracy of 99% or better (Winship & Brownlee 1986), if intragenic markers are used. For the remaining uninformative pedigrees, extragenic markers such as DXS99, DXS51 or DXS102 (see Table 12.3) may be considered for diagnosis, but here the chance of recombination is significant (up to 5%, depending on the marker used). There is also the uncertainty that recombination could be as high as 15% in some pedigrees (see Davies et al 1985). Moreover, the overall error rate in a diagnosis may be greater than the recombination fraction if there is any inaccuracy in 'phase determination'. Nevertheless for persons requesting information, so long as the chance of error is understood, this accuracy of diagnosis will often be better than, or can be combined with, traditional methods of carrier diagnosis based on measurements of factor IX concentrations in plasma (reviewed in Brownlee 1986). Nevertheless error rates of 5–15% are unsatisfactory and clearly, more closely linked and therefore more accurate diagnostic polymorphic markers are required. These should be sought in the mcf2 gene region, or beyond the HTF-island like sequence in the 3' flanking region, or in the 5' flanking region of factor IX (Anson et al 1988).

Unfortunately, the known intragenic polymorphisms of Caucasians are absent, or in much lower frequency, in other ethnic groups. For example, the TaqI intragenic polymorphism exists at allelic frequencies of 0.35/0.65 in Caucasians, 0.11/0.89 in Thais, 0.06/0.94 in Australian aborigines and 0/1.0 (i.e. not polymorphic at all) in Papua New Guineans, Han Chinese and Asians (Summers 1987, Scott et al 1987). The use of a monoclonal antibody, specific for one form of the intragenic Ala/Thr protein polymorphism of Caucasians (Table 12.3) (Smith et al 1987), demonstrated a lack of this polymorphism in 52 chromosomes derived from Chinese, Filipino and Japanese people (Thompson et al 1987). However, other factor IX intragenic polymorphisms were present in Japanese populations, albeit at lower frequencies than in Caucasians. Specifically 4/10 Japanese families could be diagnosed with either the TaqI, XmnI or DdeI polymorphisms (Mikami et al 1987). Fortunately for American (and presumably other) negroes the BamHI and MspI polymorphisms are highly informative intragenic probes. So is the DXS99 extragenic probe for American negroes and Asians (Hay et al 1986, Cullen et al 1986, Scott et al 1987). What is badly needed for all ethnic groups, including Caucasians, is a hypervariable 'mini-satellite' locus, like that occurring near the α-globin or insulin gene (Weatherall 1985), because there is still a proportion of families uninformative for all known polymorphisms. So far, only two such multiallelic polymorphisms have been found on the X chromosome although both are unlinked to haemophilia B (Mandel et al 1986, Fraser et al 1987). Despite these difficulties, many carrier diagnoses and antenatal diagnoses of haemophilia B have been carried out worldwide, including a therapeutic abortion in Shanghi, where a patient-specific intragenic deletion gave rise to an abnormal XmnI restriction fragment, which was used as the disease marker (Zeng et al 1987). Chinese parents are very concernced for the well-being of the, often, sole child of a marriage. I predict eventually a wide use of such diagnositic techniques, in a country of 10^9 people.

There is, however, an obvious need to search for polymorphisms in Chinese and other ethnic groups. Disease prevention by therapeutic abortion should in time decrease the incidence of the disease, as has apparently occurred with thalassaemia

Table 12.3 Intra- and extragenic polymorphisms in Caucasian populations

Polymorphisms	Factor IX locus (nucleotide position)	Other locus (θ = recombination fraction with factor IX)	Frequency of rarer allele(s) in population	Heterozygote frequency (2pq)	Comments	Reference
1. **BamHI RFLP**	−587	—	0.05	0.09		Hay et al (1986) Winship (1986) Winship et al (1984)
2. **DdeI RFLP**	Deletion 5505–5554	—	0.24	0.37		Winship et al (1984)
3. **XmnI RFLP**	7076 (G→C)	—	0.29	0.41		Winship et al (1984)
4. **TaqI RFLP**	11 111	—	0.35	0.45	In linkage disequilibrium	Giannelli et al (1984) Camerino et al (1984)
5. **MspI RFLP**	Near 16 000	—	0.22	0.34		Camerino et al (1985) Freedenberg et al (1987) Winship (1986)
6. **OP1 [Ala/Thr* (amino acid 148)]**	20 422 (G→A)	—	0.33	0.44		Winship & Brownlee (1986) McGraw et al (1985b) Mulligan et al (1987)
7. SstI	—	DXS99 (θ = 0.05)	0.43	0.49		
8. TaqI	—	DXS51 (θ = 0.02)**	0.5	0.5		Drayna et al (1984)
9. TaqI	—	DXS102 (θ = 0.02)	0.15	0.26		Arveiler et al (1988)

* The Ala/Thr dimorphism at amino acid 148 of the protein may be detected by a monoclonal antibody (Smith et al 1987).
** A value of θ of >0.15 has been reported by another group (Davies et al 1985).

major in some parts of Italy and Cyprus (Weatherall 1985), but cannot eliminate it entirely because of newly arising mutations.

GENE THERAPY OR CURE

The ultimate cure for patients with inherited genetic defects would involve replacing their defective or absent gene with a normal active gene giving a permanent supply of factor IX endogenously. As factor IX is not needed at 100% of normal level, it is a favourable model system. 10–20% of the normal factor IX concentration might suffice for a haemophiliac except for major surgery. We can envisage a methodology based on removing a part of some tissue from a patient, introducing recombinant factor IX genes efficiently, perhaps by the use of retroviruses, and then reintroducing the factor IX-producing cells into the patient. The main problem in connection with gene therapy is that it is an untried procedure when compared to the present symptomatic replacement treatment. This means that there is a need for laboratory experiments to test procedures, efficacy and, more importantly, safety, before any such gene therapy is contemplated in humans (see Weatherall 1985 for a fuller review).

There are still many problems associated with gene therapy and a cure for haemophilia patients is still some way away. Nevertheless a start has been made using the retrovirus approach in cells and in mice. Factor IX helper-free stocks of a retrovirus, based on the Moloney leukaemia virus LTRs, have been constructed and after infection of transformed human hepatocytes, and fibroblasts, small quantities of biologically active factor IX were purified from conditioned medium (Anson et al 1987). By contrast, a lymphoblast cell line, on infection, failed to produce factor IX. These experiments suggested that skin transplants of infected cells might be used for therapy. This tissue has the advantage of being more accessible and more easily monitored than transplants of liver where factor IX is normally synthesized. Using an improved factor IX retrovirus producing higher yields of factor IX, St Louis & Verma (1988) have implanted normal mouse fibroblasts subcutaneously in syngeneic mice. They showed that biologically active human factor IX accumulates in the blood stream, soon inducing an immune response. These experiments demonstrate that factor IX can move from the extracellular matrix into plasma, and they open the way to testing longer term transplants, improved factor IX vectors and other transplantation methods. Another important step will be to attempt to cure haemophilia B by gene therapy in the colony of dogs who have this disease. Only if it proves possible to cure this disease in this animal model will it, I suggest, be ethically possible to consider such treatment in patients with haemophilia. In attempting to cure haemophilia, one must not initiate a tumour inadvertently due to the insertion of the retrovirus, by chance, in an oncogene. Ideally, correction of the genetic defect would be carried out by homologous recombination of the incoming DNA with the defective factor IX gene, or at least with a defined non-essential region of the genome, which is transcriptionally active. However the frequency of such homologous recombination is still very low (Thomas & Capecchi 1987) and methods must be improved considerably if this is to be a viable option.

ACKNOWLEDGEMENTS

I thank Drs Verma, Trent, Ludwig, Mandel, Giannelli, Lillicrap, Peake, Summers, Thompson, Blake, Rees, Lavergne and Winship for supplying me with preprints or unpublished information which they have allowed me to quote, Drs Handford and Winship for constructive criticism of the manuscript, Barbara Paxman for secretarial assistance, and the Medical Research Council for support.

REFERENCES

Anson D S, Choo K H, Rees D J G et al 1984 European Molecular Biology Organization Journal 3: 1053–1064

Anson D S, Hock R A, Austen D et al 1987 Molecular Biology and Medicine 4: 11–20

Anson D S, Blake D J, Winship P R, Birnbaum D, Brownlee G G 1988 European Molecular Biology Organization Journal 7: 2795–2799

Antonarakis S E 1988 Chapter 11, this volume

Arveiler B, Oberle I, Vincent A, Hofker M H, Pearson P L, Mandel J L 1988 American Journal Human Genetics 42: 380–389

Austen D E G, Rhymes I L 1975 A laboratory manual of blood coagulation. Blackwell Scientific, Oxford

Bentley A K, Rees D J G, Rizza C, Brownlee G G 1986 Cell 45: 343–348

Bernardi F L, del Senno L, Barbieri R et al 1985 Journal Medical Genetics 22: 305–307

Briet E, Bertina R M, van Tilburg N H, Veltkamp J J 1982 New England Journal Medicine 306: 788

Brownlee G G 1986 Journal Cell Science supplement 4: 445–458

Brownlee G G 1987 Biochemical Society Transactions 15: 1–8

Camerino G, Grzeschik K H, Jaye M et al 1984 Proceedings National Academy Sciences USA 81: 498–502

Camerino G, Oberle I, Drayna D, Mandel J L 1985 Journal Human Genetics 71: 79–81

Chen S-H, Yoshitake S, Chance P F et al 1985 Journal Clinical Investigation 76: 2161–2164

Chen S-H, Freedenberg D L, Kurachi K, Scott C R 1987 American Journal Human Genetics 41 (suppl): 211 (abstract)

Choo K H, Gould K G, Rees D J G, Brownlee G G 1982 Nature 299: 178–180

Cullen C R, Hubberman P, Kaslow D C, Migeon B R 1986 European Molecular Biology Organization Journal 5: 2223–2229

Davies K E, Mattei M G, Mattei J F et al 1985 Human Genetics 70: 249–255

Davis L M, McGraw R A, Graham J B, Roberts H R, Stafford D W 1984 Blood 64: 262a (suppl 1) (abstract)

Diuguid D L, Rabiet M J, Furie B C, Liebman H A, Furie B 1986 Proceedings National Academy Sciences USA 83: 5803–5807

Drayna D, Davies K, Hartley D et al 1984 Proceedings National Academy Sciences USA 81: 2836–2839

Fraser N J, Boyd Y, Brownlee G G, Craig I W 1987 Nucleic Acids Research 15: 9616

Freedenberg D L, Chen S-H, Kurachi K, Scott C R 1987 Human Genetics 76: 262–264

Galeffi P, Brownlee G G 1987 Nucleic Acids Research 15: 9505–9513

Geddes V A, Louie G V, Brayer G D, MacGillivray R T A 1987 Thrombosis Haemostasis 58 (suppl): 294 (abstract)

Giannelli F 1988 In: Atti del Congresso: From man to gene, from gene to man. Firenze City of Culture, 1986, Ed. Permanent Committee for the Identification of Genetic Syndromes in Paediatrics

Giannelli F, Choo K H, Rees D J G, Boyd Y, Rizza C R, Brownlee G G 1983 Nature 303: 181–182

Giannelli F, Choo K H, Winship P R et al 1984 Lancet i: 239–241

Giannelli F, Morris A H, Garrett C, Daker M, Thurston C, Smith C A B 1987 Annals Human Genetics 51: 107–124

Green P M, Bentley D R, Mibashan R S, Giannelli F 1988 Molecular Biology and Medicine 5: 95–106

Harlos K, Holland S K, Boys C W G, Burgess A I, Esnouf M P, Blake C C F 1987 Nature 330: 82–84

Hassan H J, Leonardi A, Guerriero R et al 1985 Blood 66: 728–730

Hay C W, Robertson K A, Yong S L et al 1986 Blood 67: 1508–1511

Hougie C, Twomey J J 1967 Lancet i: 699

Jaye M, de la Salle H, Schamber F et al 1983 Nucleic Acids Research 11: 2325–2335

Jorgensen M J, Cantor A B, Furie B C, Brown C L, Shoemaker C B, Furie B 1987 Cell 48: 185–191

Kurachi K, Davie E W 1982 Proceedings National Academy Sciences USA 79: 6461–6464

Ludwig M 1987 Personal communication

Mandel J L, Arveiler B, Camerino G et al 1986 Cold Spring Harbor Symposia on Quantitative Biology 51: 195–203

McGraw R A, Davis L M, Lundblad R L, Stafford D W, Roberts H R 1985a Clinics in Haematology 14: 359–383

McGraw R A, Davis L M, Noyes C M, Graham J B, Roberts H R, Stafford D W 1985b Proceedings National Academy Sciences USA 82: 2847–2851

McKee P A 1983 In: Stanbury J B, Wyngaarden J B, Fredrickson et al (eds) The metabolic basis of inherited disease, 5th edn. McGraw-Hill, New York, p 1531–1560

Matthews R J, Anson D S, Peake I R, Bloom A L 1987 Journal of Clinical Investigation 79: 746–753

Matthews R J, Peake I R, Bloom A L, Anson D S 1988 Journal Medical Genetics (in press)

Mikami S, Nishino M, Nishimura T, Fukui H 1987 Japanese Journal Human Genetics 32: 21–31

Mulligan L, Holden J J A, White B N 1987 Human Genetics 75: 381–383

Nilsson I M, Berntorp E, Zettervall O 1986 Proceedings National Academy Sciences USA 83: 9169–9173

Noyes C M, Griffith M J, Roberts H R, Lundblad R L 1983 Proceedings National Academy Sciences USA 80: 4200–4202

Peake I R, Furlong B L, Bloom A L 1984 Lancet i: 242–243

Poon M-C, Chui D H K, Patterson M, Starozik D M, Dimik L S, Hoar D I 1987 Journal Clinical Investigation 79: 1204–1209

Rees D J G 1986 Studies on the gene coding for the anti-haemophiliac factor IX. D.Phil. thesis, Oxford University

Rees D J G, Rizza C R, Brownlee G G 1985 Nature 316: 643–645

Rees D J G, Jones I M, Handford P A et al 1988 European Molecular Biology Organization Journal 7: 2053–206

Reitsma P H, Riemens A M, Bertina R M, Briet E 1987 Thrombosis Haemostasis 58 (suppl): 294 (abstract)

Saiki R K, Scharf S, Faloona F et al 1985 Science 230: 1350–1354

Saiki R K, Gelfand D H, Stoffel S et al 1988 Science 239: 487–491

St Louis D, Verma I M 1988 Proceedings National Academy Sciences USA 85: 3150–3154

Schach B G, Yoshitake S, Davie E W 1987 Journal of Clinical Investigation 80: 1023–1028

Scott C R, Chen S H, Schoof J, Kurachi K 1987 American Journal of Human Genetics 41: A262 (abstract)

Shapiro S S 1979 In: Rizza C R (ed) Clinics in Haematology 8: 207–214. Saunders, London

Siguret V, Amselem S, Vidaud M et al 1988 18th International Congress of the World Federation of haemophilia p 72 (abstract)

Smith K, Thompson A R, McMullen B A et al 1987 Blood 70: 1006–1013

Stoflet E S, Koeberl D O, Sarkar G, Sommer S S 1988 Science 239: 491–494

Summers K M 1987 Annals of Human Biology 14: 203–217

Taylor S A M, Lillicrap D P, Blanchette V, Giles A R, Holden J J A, White B N 1988 Human Genetics (in press)

Thomas K R, Capecchi M R 1987 Cell 51: 503–512

Thompson A R 1986 Blood 67: 565–572

Thompson A R 1987 Thrombosis Research 46: 169–174

Thompson A R, Chen S-H, Smith K J 1987 Blood 70 (suppl 1): 382a

Trent R J A 1987 Personal communication

Tsang C T, Bentley D R, Mibashan R S, Giannelli F 1988 European Molecular Biology Organizational Journal (in press)

Vidaud M, Chabret C, Gazengel C, Grunebaum L, Cazenave J P, Goossens M 1986 Blood 68: 961–963

Wadelius C, Goonewardena P, Blombäck M et al 1986 7th International Congress of Human Genetics 654 (abstract)

Wadelius C, Blomback M, Pettersson U 1988 Molecular studies of haemophilia B in Sweden: Identification of patients without inhibitory antibodies although having a total deletion of the factor IX gene (submitted)

Ware J, Liebman H, Kasper C et al 1986 Blood 68 (suppl): 343a (abstract)

Weatherall D J 1985 The new genetic and clinical practice 2nd edn. Oxford University Press

Winship P R 1986 Carrier detection and patient studies in haemophilia B. D.Phil. thesis, Oxford University

Winship P R, Brownlee G G 1986 Lancet ii: 218–219

Winship P R, Anson D S, Rizza C R, Brownlee G G 1984 Nucleic Acids Research 12: 8861–8872

Wong C, Dowling C E, Saiki R K, Higuchi R G, Erlich H A, Kazazian H H 1987 Nature 330: 384–386

Yoshitake S, Schach B G, Foster D C, Davie E W, Kurachi K 1985 Biochemistry 24: 3736–3750

Zeng Y, Zhang M, Ren Z et al 1987 Journal of Medical Genetics 24: 632–633

13. Thrombolytic therapy

D. Collen   D. C. Stump   H. K. Gold

INTRODUCTION

The key event which most frequently triggers the clinical syndrome of acute myocardial infarction or stroke, is the thrombotic occlusion of a critically situated blood vessel. Pharmacological dissolution of the blood clot by intravenous infusion of plasminogen activators, which activate an enzyme system in the blood known as the fibrinolytic system, has been attempted for over 30 years, yet it has only recently become an accepted treatment for evolving myocardial infarction. This has resulted from the fact that the presently available thrombolytic agents, streptokinase and urokinase, lack clot-specificity, resulting in relative inefficiency and associated blood coagulation system breakdown. The relatively recent recognition that acute myocardial infarction is triggered by thrombosis of an atherosclerotic coronary artery and that early administration of streptokinase may reduce mortality, has however rekindled interest in thrombolytic therapy and in research of improved thrombolytic agents.

COMPONENTS OF THE FIBRINOLYTIC SYSTEM

The fibrinolytic system, schematically represented in Figure 13.1, contains a proenzyme, plasminogen, which is converted to the active enzyme plasmin by the action of several different types of plasminogen activators. Plasmin hydrolyzes fibrin to soluble degradation products. Inhibition of the fibrinolytic system in blood occurs both at the level of plasminogen activators and at the level of plasmin (Collen & Lijnen 1986, Bachmann 1987, Collen 1987).

Plasminogen

Plasminogen, a single chain glycoprotein consisting of 790 amino acids, is converted to plasmin by cleavage of the Arg^{560}-Val^{561} peptide bond. The plasminogen molecule contains structures, called lysine binding sites, which mediate its binding to fibrin and which accelerate the interaction between plasmin and its physiological inhibitor α_2-antiplasmin. As further illustrated below, the lysine binding sites play a key role in the regulation of fibrinolysis (Wiman & Collen 1978a, Collen 1980).

Plasminogen activators

Plasminogen activators hydrolyze the Arg^{560}-Val^{561} peptide bond in plasminogen, yielding the active enzyme plasmin. Streptokinase is a protein with a molecular weight of 47 000, produced by beta-hemolytic streptococci, which activates the fibrinolytic system indirectly. It forms a 1:1 stoichiometric complex with plasminogen which then undergoes a conformational change whereby an active site in the modified plasminogen

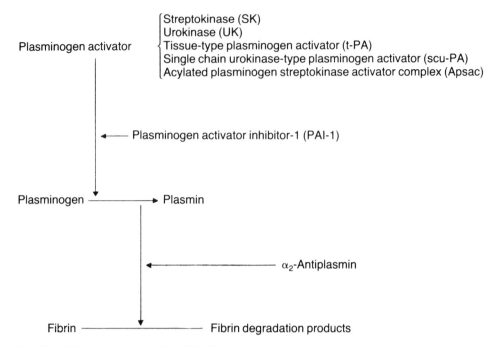

Fig. 13.1   Schematic representation of the fibrinolytic system

moiety is exposed and whereby the complex becomes a potent plasminogen activator (Kosow 1975).

Urokinase is a trypsin-like serine protease composed of two disulfide bonded polypeptide chains, which activates plasminogen directly to plasmin (White et al 1966). Single-chain urokinase-type plasminogen activator (scu-PA) or pro-urokinase is a single chain glycoprotein containing 411 amino acids, which is converted to urokinase by hydrolysis of the Lys^{158}-Ile^{159} peptide bond (Holmes et al 1985). scu-PA has intrinsic plasminogen activating potential, with a catalytic efficiency about 5% of that of urokinase (Lijnen et al 1986a).

Tissue-type plasminogen activator (t-PA) is a trypsin-like serine protease composed of 527 amino acids (Pennica et al 1983). It occurs either as a single chain glycoprotein or as a two chain proteolytic derivative, but both forms have comparable enzymatic properties. t-PA is a poor plasminogen activator in the absence of fibrin, but it binds specifically to fibrin and activates plasminogen at the fibrin surface several hundredfold more efficiently than in the circulation (Hoylaerts et al 1982).

α_2-Antiplasmin

α_2-Antiplasmin is a glycoprotein of the serine protease inhibitor (Serpin) superfamily, composed of 452 amino acids with Arg^{364}-Met^{365} as the reactive site (Holmes et al 1987). α_2-Antiplasmin reacts very rapidly with plasmin, to form an inactive but reversible complex, which is then slowly converted into an irreversible complex. The first step of the reaction is dependent on the presence of free lysine binding sites and a free active center in the plasmin molecule (Wiman & Collen 1978b).

Plasminogen activator inhibitor-1

Plasminogen activator inhibitor-1 (PAI-1) is a serpin, composed of 379 amino acids with Arg^{364}-Met^{347} as the reactive site (Bachmann 1987). It is a fast acting inhibitor of t-PA and urokinase (Kruithof et al 1984) occurring at very low concentration in the blood, but which may be significantly increased in several disease states including venous thromboembolism and ischemic heart disease.

MECHANISM OF FIBRIN-SPECIFIC THROMBOLYSIS

Plasmin has a low substrate specificity and in purified systems hydrolyzes fibrinogen almost as well as fibrin. When circulating freely in the blood, it degrades a number of plasma proteins including fibrinogen and the blood coagulation factors V and VIII. Plasmin generated in blood, however, is rapidly neutralized by α_2-antiplasmin via interaction with both its lysine-binding sites and active center. Extensive plasminogen to plasmin conversion results in α_2-antiplasmin consumption, free plasmin generation in the circulation and hemostatic breakdown. In contrast, plasmin which is generated at the fibrin surface to which it is bound via its lysine-binding sites is only very slowly inactivated by α_2-antiplasmin (Collen 1980). Clot-specific thrombolysis thus requires plasminogen activation at the surface of the fibrin clot.

The two physiological plasminogen activators, t-PA and scu-PA exert clot-specificity in a plasma environment, however via different molecular mechanisms (Collen 1987). t-PA is relatively inactive in the absence of fibrin, but it binds specifically to fibrin, whereby it acquires a high affinity for plasminogen, resulting in efficient plasminogen activation at the fibrin clot. With scu-PA, relatively fibrin-specific clot lysis in a plasma milieu can be obtained within a rather narrow concentration range whereas in the absence of fibrin, no significant plasminogen activation occurs. Apparently, plasma exerts a competitive inhibitory effect which is reversed by fibrin. In addition, fibrin-bound plasminogen may be more sensitive to activation by scu-PA.

THROMBOLYTIC THERAPY

The agents used for thrombolytic therapy in man can be classified in two main categories: (1) the 'classical' thrombolytic agents, streptokinase and urokinase and (2) the 'second generation' thrombolytic agents presently under clinical investigation, now including t-PA, scu-PA and acylated plasminogen-streptokinase activator complex (Apsac).

Early experience with streptokinase and urokinase

Administration of the classical thrombolytic agents streptokinase and urokinase is generally associated with a systemic fibrinolytic state and extensive fibrinogen degradation. Uncertainty about the optimal dose and the benefit versus bleeding risk ratio has hampered their use, particularly after invasive procedures. In addition, there is a very poor correlation between the laboratory parameters of the hemostatic system on one hand and the thrombolytic efficacy and the incidence of bleeding on the other (Verstraete & Collen 1986).

Timely administration of streptokinase and urokinase results in lysis of massive pulmonary emboli and improvement of the hemodynamics (Urokinase-Streptokinase

Pulmonary Embolism Trial Study Group 1974), and in a reduced incidence of chronic pulmonary hypertension (Sharma et al 1980), but the reported studies were too small to allow investigation of the impact of thrombolysis on mortality.

Several randomized studies with streptokinase in patients with deep vein thrombosis, using phlebography, have been reported. None of these trials were large enough to determine the efficacy and safety with adequate confidence (Marder 1979). Pooled data of 6 randomized trials revealed that thrombolysis was achieved 3.7 times more often in the streptokinase group than in the heparin-treated controls (p < 0.001) but bleeding was 2.9 times greater during streptokinase therapy (p < 0.04) (Goldhaber et al 1984). The beneficial effect of thrombolysis on vascular function and chronic venous insufficiency is not well established.

The investigation of streptokinase in acute myocardial infarction has been severely hampered by bleeding complications (often as high as 1% fatality rates), and by the lack of identification of thrombosis as the key event in coronary artery occlusion. An analysis of pooled data of the earlier trials has however revealed a significant reduction in mortality of about 20% (Stampfer et al 1982). The first large scale study to establish the benefit of early coronary reperfusion on 1 year mortality was reported by the Dutch Interuniversity Study Group (Simoons et al 1985).

The experience with urokinase has largely paralleled that with streptokinase, although it has been very much less extensively investigated (Mathey 1987).

Early experience with second generation thrombolytic agents

Tissue-type plasminogen activator
Following a series of antecedent studies in animals, the first two patients with renal vein thrombosis were treated with natural t-PA, purified from a human melanoma cell culture line, in 1981 (Weimar et al 1981). Successful lysis was obtained with 5 and 7.5 mg of t-PA, which in retrospect were unusually small doses. The first pilot study in patients with acute myocardial infarction was carried out in 1983 and demonstrated timely coronary reperfusion in 6 of 7 patients given intravenous t-PA without marked systemic fibrinolytic activation (Van de Werf et al 1984).

Single-chain urokinase-type plasminogen activator
The recent recognition of a single chain form of urokinase, designated scu-PA, with relative fibrin specificity in vitro and clot selectivity in animal models of thrombosis (Stump et al 1986), has led to its preliminary investigation as a fibrin-specific thrombolytic agent.

The first pilot study in 6 patients with acute myocardial infarction revealed efficient coronary artery reperfusion with 40 mg of intravenous scu-PA isolated from a cultured human cell line (Van de Werf et al 1986a). This was however associated with fibrinogen depletion in one patient.

Acylated plasminogen streptokinase activator complex (Apsac)
When plasminogen forms a complex with streptokinase, it undergoes a conformational change whereby an active site is exposed, converting plasminogen to plasmin with a high degree of specificity and efficiency (Kosow 1975). This active site can be reversibly acylated and thereby transiently inactivated (Smith et al 1982). Apsac, when

injected into the blood stream, is catalytically inert but may bind to fibrin via the lysine binding sites of its plasminogen moiety. It was hypothesized that fibrin-bound Apsac might deacylate at the fibrin surface, yielding an active enzyme which would locally induce clot-specific fibrinolysis (Smith et al 1982).

The original hypothesis that Apsac would produce thrombolysis with a higher degree of fibrin-specificity than streptokinase has not been confirmed (Marder et al 1986). In several uncontrolled small studies in patients with acute myocardial infarction, Apsac when given at a sufficiently high dose (30 mg intravenous bolus) was found to be an efficient coronary thrombolytic agent (de Bono 1987).

THROMBOLYSIS IN ACUTE MYOCARDIAL INFARCTION

In the late 1970s, it was recognized that thrombosis within the infarct related coronary artery played a major pathological role in pathogenesis of acute myocardial infarction (De Wood et al 1980). It was further recognized that early administration of either intracoronary or intravenous streptokinase resulted in reperfusion of 75% and 45% of patients, respectively (Rentrop 1985). This has formed the basis for several larger scale studies employing intravenous thrombolytic agents with the intention to (1) define the real impact of early coronary reperfusion on patient survival and (2) establish patterns of efficacy and safety for new and potentially improved thrombolytic agents.

Streptokinase

The first major study employing intravenous streptokinase in early acute myocardial infarction and demonstrating relative improvement in survival was carried out in 11 806 patients and reported as the GISSI Study (GISSI 1986). Patients randomized to receive 1.5 million units of SK over 60 minutes were found to have an overall reduction in 21 day mortality from 13% to 10.7% (p = 0.0002) relative to untreated controls. The most profound impact was observed in patients treated within less than 6 hours, and especially less than 3 hours, from onset of symptoms. Life-threatening bleeding was only observed in 0.2% of patients receiving streptokinase and judged not to be a limitation for therapy.

The positive results of the GISSI trial were not confirmed in a very similar but somewhat smaller study of the ISAM study group (ISAM 1986). Patients receiving streptokinase within 6 hours of symptoms, although having better left ventricular function, did not achieve significantly improved survival relative to controls (21 day mortality 6.3% vs 7.1%). In addition, life-threatening bleeding was more common, occurring in 0.8% of patients. However, a recent preliminary report from the still ongoing ISIS-2 study has confirmed the GISSI findings in the first 4000 patients of a planned 20 000 patient study, with an in-hospital mortality reduction from 12–8% in patients receiving streptokinase within 4 hours of onset of symptoms (ISIS 1987). Data on adverse effects are not yet available.

In aggregate, these studies are suggestive of two conclusions. First, the intravenous administration of streptokinase early (preferably within 4 hours but up to 6 hours from the onset of symptoms) in acute myocardial infarction is of benefit to patient survival within the first month of follow-up. Second, the life-threatening side effects, predominantly intracranial hemorrhage, are not negligible but still consistently less frequent than 1%.

Tissue-type plasminogen activator

Following the demonstration of the potential of natural t-PA as a thrombolytic agent, an intensive effort was launched to enhance its production by recombinant DNA technology (Pennica et al 1983, Collen 1985). This successful effort has now culminated in its study in over 4000 patients.

Intravenous recombinant t-PA (rt-PA) has now been shown to be superior to both placebo (Verstraete et al 1985a) and streptokinase (TIMI 1985, Verstraete et al 1985b, Chesebro et al 1987) for coronary artery reperfusion. When given at a sufficiently high dose (40–80 mg over 1–2 hours), rt-PA produced reperfusion of approximately 65% of infarct-related arteries (Collen et al 1984, TIMI 1985, Verstraete et al 1985a, Verstraete et al 1985b, Chesebro et al 1987, Topol et al 1987b), and was associated with much less extensive systemic fibrinogen breakdown than observed with streptokinase (Collen 1986a, Garabedian et al 1987, Stump et al 1987b, Mueller et al 1987). Reocclusion rates following successful thrombolysis with rt-PA have varied between 10–15% in large trials (Topol et al 1987b, Verstraete et al 1987) but up to 40% in smaller trials (Gold et al 1986a). Reocclusion can however adequately be prevented by a brief duration maintenance infusion of rt-PA (Gold et al 1986a, Gold et al, 1986b). Successful sustained reperfusion was associated with improved regional wall motion of the infarcted zone (Jang et al 1986, Sheehan et al 1987, O'Rourke et al 1987, Guerci et al 1987). The reported studies to date have been carried out with two different preparations of rt-PA: initially with a predominantly two chain form (G11021) produced on a pilot scale for initial clinical evaluation, and subsequently with a predominantly single chain form (G11035, G11044) produced for commercial use. The single chain material is cleared 30–40% more rapidly than the initial material (Garabedian et al 1987), but when the dose is increased correspondingly, its thrombolytic efficacy and fibrin-specificity is similar if not better (Garabedian et al 1987, Mueller et al 1987, Topol et al 1987c). The thrombolytic efficacy of rt-PA seems to be maintained for several hours after the onset of symptoms (Chesebro et al 1987), whereas the efficacy of streptokinase both in terms of thrombolytic efficacy (Chesebro et al 1987) and impact on mortality (GISSI, 1986) declines rapidly.

Life-threatening bleeding was not observed in the initial small scale comparative studies. In a recent larger study (TAMI 1) in 386 patients receiving 150 mg of single chain rt-PA over 5–8 hours (Topol et al 1987b), coronary arteries were patent at 90 minutes in 75% of individuals. In this study, 0.5% of patients experienced life-threatening intracranial hemorrhage, while mean nadir fibrinogen levels decreased to about 50% of baseline, reflecting a relative degree of clot-selectivity at this effective dose (Stump et al 1987, Topol et al 1987b). However, in a second large study (TIMI 2) at a dose of 150 mg of rt-PA of which 90 mg was administered in the first hour, a higher rate of intracranial hemorrhage has been observed, 1.6% in 311 patients (Braunwald et al 1987). The study is continuing at a reduced dose of 100 mg, but clinical data is not yet available.

Thus, initial evaluation of rt-PA in myocardial infarction has been promising, suggesting its potential role as an improved thrombolytic agent. However, its use is clearly not risk-free despite its relatively higher clot-selectivity than streptokinase. Further large scale clinical studies are needed to determine its exact impact on patient survival and its therapeutic index.

Single-chain urokinase-type plasminogen activator

The first pilot study in 17 patients treated with intravenous recombinant scu-PA obtained from *E. coli* demonstrated good coronary arterial thrombolytic efficacy at a dose of 70 mg given over 1 h, but fibrinogen degradation to below 50% of baseline occurred in over one-half and extensive fibrinogen depletion in about one-fourth of the patients (Van de Werf et al 1986b). A larger multicenter trial with natural scu-PA in 63 patients has demonstrated coronary reperfusion in 50–70% of patients receiving intravenous doses of 50–70 mg (Welzel & Wolf 1987). Mean fibrinogen levels fell on average by 25% and no severe bleeding was observed. In addition, the inclusion of a small bolus of supplemental urokinase apparently shortened reperfusion times without deleterious effects on plasma fibrinogen levels. Thus, at present scu-PA shows promise in limited studies, but its clinical value for thrombolysis remains to be defined.

Acylated plasminogen streptokinase activator complex

In controlled studies comparing intravenous Apsac with intravenous or intracoronary streptokinase, Apsac was found to cause reperfusion at a frequency intermediate between that of intravenous and intracoronary streptokinase (Brochier 1987, Bonnier 1987, Anderson et al 1987). The available data do not yet allow to state whether Apsac is comparable to or more efficacious than intravenous streptokinase (de Bono 1987).

THROMBOLYTIC THERAPY IN OTHER FORMS OF THROMBOEMBOLIC DISEASE

Of the newer thrombolytic agents, only rt-PA has been studied to date in other forms of thromboembolic disease than myocardial infarction, including unstable angina (Gold et al 1987), pulmonary embolism (Bounameaux et al 1985, Goldhaber et al 1986, Verstraete 1987), peripheral arterial occlusion (Graor & Risius 1987, Verhaeghe et al 1987), deep vein thrombosis (Turpie 1987) and a single case of lysis of an artificial tricuspid valve thrombosis (Cambier et al 1987). Although the available data suggest a useful role of rt-PA in the management of these diseases, much more clinical research will be required.

SYNERGISM BETWEEN THROMBOLYTIC AGENTS

Because the mechanisms which regulate the fibrin-specificity of t-PA and scu-PA are different, combined infusions of both agents might act synergistically, to produce enhanced efficacy with reduced side effects on the hemostatic system. In an in vitro system, composed of a ^{125}I-fibrin labeled plasma clot, immersed in citrated plasma, t-PA, scu-PA and urokinase, in molar ratios between 4:1 and 1:4, do not display significant synergism (Collen et al 1986b, Lijnen et al 1986b, Gurewich & Pannell 1987). In vivo, however, in a jugular vein thrombosis model in the rabbit, significant synergism between t-PA and scu-PA and between T-PA and urokinase for thrombolysis was observed (Collen et al 1986c). When t-PA and scu-PA were infused in a molar ratio of approximately 1:3, the specific thrombolytic activity of the mixture was approximately 3-fold higher than was anticipated on the basis of additive effects of both agents. The synergistic effect of t-PA and urokinase was only borderline significant. A synergistic effect of at least a factor 2 between t-PA and scu-PA was also found on coronary arterial thrombolysis in dogs (Ziskind et al 1987).

Preliminary results in patients with acute myocardial infarction (Collen et al 1986d, Collen & Van de Werf 1987) suggest that t-PA and scu-PA and t-PA and urokinase also act synergistically in man. Indeed, combination of t-PA and scu-PA at approximately $\frac{1}{5}$ of their individual thrombolytic doses produced coronary artery reperfusion in patients with acute myocardial infarction without associated systemic fibrinogen breakdown. Although these results are still preliminary and need to be confirmed in larger studies, they are potentially of significant clinical importance. The synergistic effect of t-PA and urokinase on coronary reperfusion has, however, not been confirmed in a large scale study, although the use of the combination was associated with a significant reduction of the frequency of reocclusion (Topol et al 1987a).

CONCLUSIONS

Thrombotic complications of cardiovascular diseases are a main cause of death and disability and consequently one might assume that thrombolysis could favourably influence the outcome of such life-threatening diseases as myocardial infarction, cerebrovascular thrombosis and venous thromboembolism.

Although streptokinase was first administered to man over 30 years ago, it is not yet widely used, mainly as a result of uncertainty about the optimal dose, fear of bleeding complications and a poor correlation between the results of laboratory parameters and the incidence of either therapeutic success or of bleeding complications. Interest in thrombolytic therapy has been renewed by the demonstration that acute myocardial infarction is most frequently caused by thrombotic occlusion of an atherosclerotic coronary artery and that the early administration of streptokinase significantly reduces mortality. The efficacy of streptokinase is however limited and rapidly decreases with time after the onset of coronary artery thrombosis. In addition, it has no fibrin-selectivity and its use is associated with extensive breakdown of the hemostatic system; yet the occurrence of life-threatening bleeding in association with high-dose short-duration therapy is consistently less than 1%.

A better understanding of the molecular mechanisms which regulate fibrinolysis in vivo, the identification of the physiological activators in t-PA and scu-PA with higher degrees of fibrin-selectivity and the development of recombinant DNA technology which allows large scale production of these proteins, have fuelled the hope that newer and better thrombolytic drugs might become available. One of these new generation thrombolytic agents, t-PA, has now been studied in over 4000 patients. These studies have indicated that it is more efficacious, more fibrin-specific, and when used in adequate dose, at least as safe as streptokinase. Important issues such as its impact on morbidity and mortality and its cost-benefit ratio remain to be resolved. The physiological plasminogen activators t-PA and scu-PA, however, still suffer shortcomings, including the need for large doses to be therapeutically efficient, a limited fibrin-specificity and residual toxicity in terms of bleeding complications. Consequently, research into the development of still further improved therapeutic regimes or thrombolytic agents is intensifying.

In summary, thrombolytic therapy, despite a 30 year period of relatively slow development, will probably become routine therapy for early acute myocardial infarction and possibly for other thrombotic cardiovascular diseases. Further improvements of thrombolytic agents to maximize efficacy, minimize side effects and optimize cost-benefit ratios are needed.

REFERENCES

Anderson J L, Rothbard R L, Hackworthy R A et al 1986 Circulation 74: I I-6
Bachmann F 1987 In: Verstraete M, Vermylen J, Lijnen R, Arnout J (eds) Fibrinolysis. Leuven University Press, Leuven, Belgium, p 227–265
Bonnier J J R M 1988 Drugs (in press)
Bounameaux H, Vermylen J, Collen D 1985 Ann Intern Med 103: 64–65
Braunwald E, Knatterud G L, Passamani E 1987 J Am Coll Cardiol 9: 467
Brochier M L 1988 Drugs (in press)
Cambier P, Mombaerts P, De Geest H, Collen D, Van de Werf F 1987 Eur Heart J 8: 906–909
Chesebro J H, Knatterud G, Roberts R et al 1987 Circulation 76: 142–154
Collen D 1980 Thromb Haemost 43: 77–89
Collen D 1985 Circulation 72: 18–20
Collen D 1987 J Cell Biochem 33: 77–94
Collen D, Lijnen H R 1986 CRC Crit Rev Hemat Oncol 4: 249–301
Collen D, Van de Werf F 1987 Am J Cardiol 60: 431–434
Collen D, Topol E J, Tiefenbrunn A J et al 1984 Circulation 70: 1012–1017
Collen D, Bounameaux H, De Cock F, Lijnen H R, Verstraete M 1986a Circulation 73: 511–517
Collen D, De Cock F, Demarsin E, Lijnen H R, Stump D C 1986b Thromb Haemost 56: 35–39
Collen D, Stassen J M, Stump D C, Verstraete M 1986c Circulation 74: 838–842
Collen D, Stump D C, Van de Werf F 1986d Am Heart J 112: 1083–1084
de Bono D 1987 In: Verstraete M, Vermylen J, Lijnen R, Arnout J (eds) Thrombosis and Haemostasis. Leuven University Press, Leuven, Belgium, p 267–280
De Wood M A, Spores J, Notske R et al 1980 N Engl J Med 303: 897–902
Garabedian H D, Gold H K, Leinbach R C et al 1987 J Am Coll Cardiol 9: 599–607
GISSI (Grupo Italiano per lo studio della streptochinasi nell'infarto miocardico) 1986 Lancet 1: 397–401
Gold H K, Leinbach R C, Garabedian H D et al 1986a Circulation 73: 347–352
Gold H K, Leinbach R C, Johns J A, Yasuda T, Garabedian H D, Collen D 1986b Circulation 74: II-368
Gold H K, Johns J A, Leinbach R C et al 1987 Circulation 75: 1192–1199
Goldhaber S Z, Buring J E, Lipnick R J, Hennekens C H 1984 Am J Med 76: 393–397
Goldhaber S Z, Vaughan D E, Markis J E et al 1986 Lancet 2: 886–889
Graor R A, Risius B 1987 In: Sobel B E, Collen D, Grossbard E B (eds) Tissue plasminogen activator in thrombolytic therapy. Marcel Dekker, New York, p 171–204
Guerci A, Gerstenblith G, Brinker J A et al 1988 N Eng J Med (in press)
Gurewich V, Pannell R 1987 Thromb Haemost 57: 372
Holmes W E, Pennica D, Blaber M et al 1985 Biotechnology 3: 923–929
Holmes W E, Nelles L, Lijnen H R, Collen D 1987 J Biol Chem 262: 1659–1664
Hoylaerts M, Rijken D C, Lijnen H R, Collen D 1982 J Biol Chem 257: 2912–2919
ISAM Study Group 1986 N Engl J Med 314: 1465–1471
ISIS Steering Committee 1987 Lancet 1: 502
Jang I, Vanhaecke J, De Geest H, Verstraete M, Collen D, Van de Werf F 1986 J Am Coll Cardiol 8: 1455–1460
Kosow D P 1975 Biochemistry 14: 4459–4465
Kruithof E K O, Tran-Thang C, Ransijn A, Bachmann F 1984 Blood 64: 907–913
Lijnen H R, Van Hoef B, Collen D 1986a Biochim Biophys Acta 884: 402–408
Lijnen H R, Zamarron C, Blaber M, Winkler M E, Collen D 1986b J Biol Chem 261: 1253–1258
Marder V J 1979 Ann Intern Med 90: 802–808
Marder V J, Rothbard R L, Fitzpatrick P G, Francis C W 1986 Ann Intern Med 104: 304–310
Mathey D G 1987 In:Topol E J (ed) Acute coronary intervention. Liss, New York, p 25–33
Mueller H S, Rao A K, Forman S A 1987 J Am Coll Cardiol 10: 479–490
O'Rourke M, Baron D, Keogh A et al 1987 Randomized, placebo-controlled, double blind trial of intravenous recombinant tissue-type plasminogen activator initiated within $2\frac{1}{2}$ hours of symptom onset in acute coronary occlusion. Presented in association with the 60th Scientific Sessions of the American Heart Association, Anaheim CA, November 15, 1987
Pennica D, Holmes W E, Kohr W J et al 1983 Nature 301: 214–221
Rentrop P 1985 Circulation 71: 627–631

Sharma G V R K, Burleson V A, Sasahara A A 1980 N Engl J Med 303: 842–845
Sheehan F H, Braunwald E, Canner P et al 1987 Circulation 75: 817–829
Simoons M L, van de Brand M, de Zwaan C et al 1985 Lancet 1: 578–581
Smith R A G, Dupe R J, English P D, Green J 1982 Nature (London) 47: 132–135
Stampfer M J, Goldhaber S Z, Yusuf S, Peto R, Hennekens C H 1982 N Engl J Med 307: 1180–1182
Stump D C, Lijnen H R, Collen D 1986 Cold Spring Harbor Symp Quant Biol 51: 563–569
Stump D C, Topol E J, Califf R, Chen A J, Hopkins A, Collen D 1987 Thromb Haemost 58: 259 (abstract 947)
TIMI Study Group 1985 N Engl J Med 312: 932–936
Topol E J, Califf R M, O'Neill W W et al 1987a Circulation 76: IV-307 (Abstract 1219).
Topol E J, Califf R M, George B S et al 1987b N Engl J Med 317: 581–588
Topol E J, Morris D, Smalling R et al 1987c J Am Coll Cardiol 9: 1205–1213
Turpie A G G 1987 In: Sobel B E, Collen D, Grossbard E B (eds) Tissue plasminogen activator in thrombolytic therapy. Marcel Dekker, New York, p 131–146
Urokinase-Streptokinase Pulmonary Embolism Trial Study Group 1974 J Am Med Assoc 229: 1606–1613
Van de Werf F, Ludbrook P A, Bergmann S R et al 1984 N Engl J Med 36: 609–613
Van de Werf F, Nobuhaera M, Collen D 1986a Ann Intern Med 104: 345–348
Van de Werf F, Vanhaecke J, De Geest H, Verstraete M, Collen D 1986b Circulation 74: 1066–1070
Verhaeghe R, Wilms G, Mombaerts P, Vermylen J, Baert A, Verstraete M 1987 Thromb Haemost 58: 299 (Abstract 1093)
Verstraete M 1987 Thromb Haemost 58: 299 (Abstract 1094)
Verstraete M, Collen D 1986 Blood 67: 1529–1541
Verstraete M, Bleifeld W, Brower R W et al 1985a Lancet 2: 965–969
Verstraete M, Bernard R, Bory M et al 1985b Lancet 1: 842–847
Verstraete M, Arnold A E R, Brower R W et al 1987 Am J Cardiol 60: 231–237
Weimar W, Stibbe J, Van Seyen A J, Billiau A, De Somer P, Collen D 1981 Lancet 2: 1018–1020
Welzel D, Wolf H 1987 Thromb Haemost 58: 47 (Abstract 160)
White W F, Barlow G H, Mozen M M 1966 Biochemistry 5: 2160–2169
Wiman B, Collen D 1978a Nature (London) 272: 549–550
Wiman B, Collen D 1978b Eur J Biochem 84: 573–578
Ziskind A A, Gold H K, Yasuda T et al 1987 Clin Res 35: 337A

14. Protein C pathways

J. S. Greengard J. H. Griffin

INTRODUCTION AND OVERVIEW

The blood coagulation pathways consist of series of sequential activations of serine protease zymogens culminating in the generation of thrombin and the formation of a fibrin clot. Several stoichiometric protease inhibitors are known to have roles in the control of this process by acting as suicide substrates for the active enzymes (Travis & Selvesen 1983). Protein C (PC) plays a different role in regulating thrombosis (Fig. 14.1). Upon activation by thrombin bound to the endothelial cell membrane

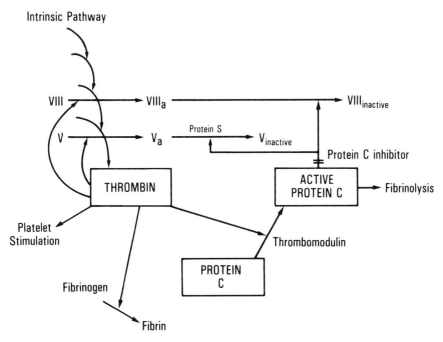

Fig. 14.1 Interactions of protein C important to regulation of its function and to overall regulation of hemostasis.

protein thrombomodulin (TM), activated protein C (APC) proteolytically inactivates the cofactor proteins of the intermediate and terminal stages of the intrinsic pathway, factors Va and VIIIa (Walker et al 1979, Suzuki et al 1983a, Kisiel et al 1977, Marlar et al 1982, Fulcher et al 1983, Vehar & Davie 1980). APC also displays profibrinolytic activity (Seegers et al 1972, Comp & Esmon, 1981), both through neutralization of PAI-1, a major inhibitor of plasminogen activation (Sakata et al 1985, 1986, van

Hinsbergh et al 1985, Taylor & Lockhart 1985), and possibly by other mechanisms. Protein S (PS), another vitamin K-dependent plasma protein, potentiates the anti-coagulant activity of APC (Walker 1980). The importance of the PC pathway in controlling hemostasis is underscored by the wide variety of mechanisms that control APC activation and activity. These mechanisms include modulation of PC activation through alteration of thrombin specificity by thrombomodulin, by control of APC by activation or inhibition of PS, and by specific APC inhibitors. In biology, as in engineering, critical control systems are protected from failure by a high degree of redundancy, thus affording better opportunities for fine tuning. Defects in the PC system are associated with a variety of thrombotic conditions, both acquired and hereditary, and various disease complications are correlated with altered levels of various components of the system. Thus, an understanding of this important regulator of hemostasis will be potentially very helpful for the design of new therapies for such conditions.

STRUCTURES OF THE COMPONENTS OF THE PC SYSTEM

PC is a vitamin K-dependent zymogen plasma protein of MW 62 000 Da predominantly consisting of a heavy and light chain (41 000 Da and 21 000 Da) connected by disulfide bridge (Stenflo 1976, Mammen et al 1960, Kisiel 1979). It contains 23% carbohydrate (Kisiel 1979), as well as nine-γ-carboxyglutamic acid residues (DiScipio & Davie 1979) and one-β-hydroxyaspartic acid (Drakenberg et al 1983). Both of these post-translational modifications appear to be involved in calcium ion binding. Additionally, PC is unusual among the serine proteases in displaying a requirement for monovalent cations (Steiner et al 1980). PC is synthesized in liver as a single polypeptide chain with 5–15% of the circulating form remaining in this nascent form (Miletich et al 1983). After synthesis, a signal peptide is removed, leaving a prozymogen whose propeptide contains the γ-carboxylation signal (Foster et al 1987). The majority of the single chain form is cleaved to two chains prior to secretion.

The PC molecule is divided into several domains: the leader sequence, followed by the γ-carboxylated domain, two epidermal growth factor-like domains containing the β-hydroxyaspartic acid, an activation peptide released upon thrombin cleavage, and the serine protease domain (Beckman et al 1985, Long et al 1984, Foster & Davie 1984). Its gene structure is quite similar to that of factor IX, thus underscoring the evolutionary relatedness of these proteins (Plutzky et al 1986).

PS, the cofactor for PC anticoagulant activity, is also a vitamin K-dependent plasma protein. As such, it bears many resemblances to the other proteins of this type, including PC. However, unlike PC and most other vitamin K-dependent plasma proteins, PS is not an enzyme. Its primary structure is known from the cloning and sequencing of its cDNA (Lundwall 1986, Hoskins et al 1987, Dahlback et al 1986). The N terminus is typical of other vitamin K-dependent proteins, including the leader sequence, γ-carboxylase recognition site (Foster et al 1987), a Gla-containing region, the thrombin-sensitive region unique to PS, and an epidermal growth factor-like region containing β-hydroxy Asp and β-hydroxy Asn (Dahlback et al 1986, Stenflo et al 1987). The COOH-terminal protease domain present in, for example, PC and factor IX has been replaced by a domain homologous to rat androgen binding protein (Baker et al 1987). The functional significance of this domain is not understood, but the anticoagulant cofactor activity of PC is not altered by androgen (Richter & Griffin, unpublished observations).

Thrombomodulin (TM) is an endothelial cell lipoprotein which acts as a cofactor in the thrombin activation of PC (Esmon et al 1982a). Its apparent MW is 78 000 Da, appearing slightly larger after reduction (Esmon et al 1982a). The structure of TM has been determined through analysis of cDNA clones (Suzuki et al 1987a, Wen et al 1987, Jackman et al 1986). TM consists of a signal peptide, an amino-terminal ligand-binding domain, six epidermal growth factor-like domains, a serine/threonine-rich region containing possible sites of O-linked glycosylation, a membrane-spanning region, and a short cytoplasmic tail. The C-terminal two-thirds of the molecule show homology to the LDL receptors. The N terminal cysteine-rich region of the latter is not present in TM. There are five potential sites of N-linked glycosylation, and the difference between the calculated (60 000 Da) and observed (75 000 Da) MWs suggest heavy glycosylation. The transmembrane domain shows unusual interspecies conservation of sequence, suggesting an important role for this region. Two overlapping copies of the octanucleotide consensus sequence TTATTTAT characteristic of inflammatory mediators (Caput et al 1986) are found, suggesting that like other such proteins, TM regulation may be under posttranscriptional control. Interestingly, analysis of genomic clones of TM (Jackman et al 1987) shows that no introns are present, a highly exceptional finding which may indicate that unusual mechanisms are employed in the control of TM expression.

A specific inhibitor of APC (Marlar & Griffin 1980) has been isolated from plasma, known as PC inhibitor (PCI). This inhibitor has a MW of 57 000 Da and displays multiple isoelectric forms (Suzuki et al 1983b). Its primary structure has been determined through cloning of the cDNA (Suzuki et al 1987b). PCI is a typical member of the serine protease inhibitor superfamily with strong homology to α_1-antitrypsin and antithrombin III. PCI is highly glycosylated with five potential N-linked glycosylation sites. A 33 amino acid COOH-terminal peptide is released upon incubation with APC or thrombin. Alignment of the putative heparin-binding region of antithrombin III with PCI did not detect a homologous sequence, which was interpreted to mean that the location of the heparin-binding sites on the two proteins differ (Suzuki et al 1987b).

REGULATION OF PC ACTIVITY

The PC pathway is regulated at several levels, most of which are not fully understood. PC, PS and PCI are all produced in liver cells (Foster & Davie 1984, Long et al 1984, Beckmann et al 1985, Lundwall et al 1986, Suzuki et al 1987b). PS has also been observed in platelets (Schwarz et al 1985, Harris & Esmon 1985). TM is an endothelial cell protein (Wen et al 1987, Maruyama et al 1985, Jackman et al 1986). There has been no systematic assessment of factors influencing the biosynthesis of these proteins. The fact that pregnancy, gender, and oral contraceptive use can affect the levels of PC or of PS under some circumstances (see below) suggests some degree of hormonal control of synthesis (Boeger et al 1987, Gonzalez et al 1985, Comp et al 1986a), as does the effect of anabolic steroids (see below) (Melissari et al 1986, Broekmans et al 1987, Kluft et al 1984, Mannucci et al 1984, Gonzalez et al 1985).

The participation of TM is required for efficient activation of PC. It stimulates the thrombin-catalyzed activation of PC at least 800–1000-fold (Esmon et al 1982, 1983, Salem et al 1984, Ishii & Majerus 1985). The number of TM molecules on the cell surface is regulated by thrombin and PC in that endocytosis of TM increases in the presence of thrombin, but is inhibited by PC but not APC (Maruyama & Majerus 1985, 1987). Endothelial cells stimulated with interleukin 1, tumor necrosis factor, or endotoxin exhibit reduced rates of PC activation due to decreased exposure of TM on their surfaces (Nawroth & Stern 1986, Nawroth et al 1986, Moore et al 1987). Enhanced internalization of TM could account for this observation. Although TM does function in solution, its environment influences its efficacy. TM appears to exist in three functional states. The Km for PC of TM on the endothelial cell is 10-fold lower than in solution (Owen & Esmon 1981, Salem et al 1984, Esmon et al 1983a). Incorporation of TM into phospholipid vesicles lowers the Km for PC to that found for TM on the cell surface (Galvin et al 1987). Interestingly, a form of TM antigen is found in plasma and urine which apparently lacks the membrane binding domain (Ishii & Majerus 1985). This truncated TM has the cellular Km for PC in the absence of phospholipid, although its Km for thrombin is high. It is tempting to speculate in light of these results that the activity of TM on the cell surface may be in part regulated by factors that alter the conformation of the cell-bound form of TM. A recent report described the presence of TM on platelets (Ogura et al 1987). It has also been reported that factor Va and its light chain enhance PC activation by thrombin on the endothelial surface (Maruyama et al 1984). The potential physiologic significance of this in vitro activity of factor Va remains to be defined.

Once activated, APC activity is modulated by the cofactor PS (Walker 1980), which in turn is regulated by the complement protein C4b-binding protein (Dahlback & Stenflo 1981) with which PS associates reversibly and noncovalently. Only the free form of PS is effective in enhancing APC activity (Dahlback 1986, Comp et al 1984). Free PS enhances inactivation of factor Va by APC (Walker 1981) in a phospholipid and Ca^{++} dependent reaction. As discussed below, there is considerable interest in possible changes of the ratio of free PS to C4BP-bound PS in various disease states. A bovine PS-binding protein has been reported to enhance the activity of APC (Walker 1986) but as yet no human analog has been reported.

PS also enhances binding of APC to phospholipids (Suzuki et al 1983c) and platelets (Harris & Esmon 1985) and is found in platelets (Schwarz et al 1985a). Additional control mechanisms for PS enhancement of APC activity are shown by the finding that thrombin-cleaved PS not only inhibits APC inactivation of factor Va, but promotes the dissociation of APC from phospholipid surfaces (Mitchell et al 1986, Suzuki et al 1983c, Walker 1984a). There is no effect of PS on cleavage of peptide substrates by APC (Suzuki et al 1983c).

The enzymatic activity of APC can be controlled directly through the action of the heparin-dependent serine protease inhibitor, PCI (Suzuki et al 1983b). PCI inhibits a spectrum of other plasma proteases in addition to APC (Suzuki et al 1984a, España et al, submitted 1988), and it has been suggested that it may be an important inhibitor of factor XIa (España et al, submitted 1988). PCI has been found in urine (Geiger et al 1988) as well as in plasma and is immunologically identical to the plasminogen activator inhibitor-3 (Heeb et al 1987a).

APC is able to form complexes with PAI-1, the major inhibitor of tissue plasminogen activator (Sakata et al 1985) which may be the root of its profibrinolytic activity.

A second heparin-dependent PCI exists in plasma that appears to form significant levels of APC complexes in different disease states (Heeb et al 1987b,c, 1988 submitted, van der Meer et al 1987).

THE ROLE OF THE PC PATHWAYS IN HEMOSTASIS AND THROMBOSIS

APC potentially plays a dual role in the maintenance of hemostasis: it may be both profibrinolytic and anticoagulant. The direct anticoagulant effect of APC is mediated through its cleavage of factors Va and VIIIa (Suzuki et al 1983a, Kisiel et al 1977, Marlar et al 1982, Fulcher et al 1983, Vehar & Davie 1980, Walker et al 1979). These substrates are cleaved much more readily than the procofactors factors V and VIII (Marlar et al 1981, Nesheim et al 1982). These reactions require the equimolar binding of PS to a phospholipid surface in the presence of Ca^{++} ions (Suzuki et al 1983c, Walker 1984b, Gardiner et al 1984).

APC cleaves factor Va in two locations, one of which (in the E chain) is identical to a factor Xa cleavage site which does not result in loss of factor Va activity (Odegaard & Mann 1987). The D chain cleavage is responsible for factor Va inactivation. Inactivation of factor Va by APC reduces the affinity of the cofactor for both prothrombin and factor Xa (Guinto & Esmon 1984), presumably explaining the loss of procoagulant activity. Conversely, factor Va bound to factor Xa is protected from cleavage (Suzuki et al 1983a) and, indeed, APC and factor Xa compete for binding to factor Va (Nesheim et al 1982). APC also destroys the factor Va in the prothrombinase complex on the platelet surface (Dahlback & Stenflo1980, Comp & Esmon 1979). PS plays a crucial role in this reaction (Suzuki et al 1984b, Harris & Esmon 1985). Factor Xa protects platelet-associated factor Va from APC (Comp & Esmon 1979).

APC was first shown to exhibit profibrinolytic activity in whole blood samples taken following infusion into dogs (Seegers et al 1972, Comp & Esmon 1981). No direct plasminogen activation by APC occurred, but rapid clot lysis was observed without degradation of fibrinogen or consumption of plasminogen. APC fibrinolytic activity was shown to require both plasma and cellular compartments of blood, which was interpreted to mean that APC generates a second messenger which caused elevation of blood plasminogen activation. Increased fibrinolytic activity as well as anticoagulation was observed after APC infusion into cats (Burdick & Schaub 1986), but only anticoagulation occurred in infused squirrel monkeys (Colucci et al 1984). The fibrinolytic system of a patient with homozygous PC deficiency who suffered from skin lesions which were successfully treated with fresh plasma infusion was found to be normal (Aznar et al 1986). It was suggested that only low levels (~1% normal) of PC are needed to control local fibrinolysis and avoid such skin lesions, while a higher level of PC is required to generate anticoagulant activity and avoid conditions such as deep vein thrombosis. At least one molecular mechanism for APC-induced profibrinolytic activity has been determined: the inactivation of plasminogen activator inhibitor I (PAI-1) by APC (Sakata et al 1985, 1986, van Hinsbergh et al 1985, Taylor & Lockhart 1985). The role of APC in this system is thought to be to prevent inhibition of plasminogen activator by PAI-1. It has also been suggested that complexation of PAI-1 by APC has a minor role, and that the major effect of APC is to reduce the thrombin concentration available to clot fibrinogen and to stimulate platelets to release PAI-1 (de Fouw et al 1987). A role for leukocytes in APC-mediated clot lysis has also been proposed (Taylor et al 1981).

The action of APC at the platelet surface merits special mention. As discussed above, APC exerts negative feedback on its own thrombin-catalyzed activation by destroying the factor Va portion of the prothrombinase complex on the platelet surface, with PS as a cofactor. PS is contained in and released by platelets (Schwarz et al 1985a), yielding ~20% of the PS in blood, possibly more in the local area. Presumably the newly released PS is all in the free active form as well. PS binds to platelets (Schwarz et al 1985b) and promotes the binding of APC but not PC to stimulated platelets (Harris & Esmon 1985). Since platelet releasate is also a source of PAI-1 since it inhibits APC, the local concentration of this protease inhibitor may be high enough to cause a significant drop in APC concentrations. PS has been reported to act as a cofactor for the interaction of PAI-1 in platelet releasate with APC (D'Angelo et al 1987), although another report did not find this (de Fouw et al 1987).

The role of TM extends beyond that of cofactor in the activation of PC. TM induces sweeping changes in the activity of thrombin, so that it changes an overall procoagulant into an overall anticoagulant enzyme. Thrombin bound to TM on the endothelial cell retains <1% of the fibrinogen clotting activity of free thrombin, a change which is not dependent upon the availability of divalent cations, unlike the activation of PC. The rate of factor V activation by thrombin likewise decreases ~100-fold in the presence of TM (Esmon et al 1982b). The activation of factor XIII is also decreased (Polgar et al 1986). The ability of thrombin to stimulate platelets is blocked by TM (Esmon et al 1983b). However, the mechanism does not involve simple blockage of the thrombin active site, since as discussed above, the activation of PC by thrombin-TM increases several hundred-fold over that by thrombin alone, and since thrombin in the complex displays increased susceptibility towards antithrombin III inhibition (Preissner et al 1987b). This latter reaction does not occur due to the participation of heparin-like structures in the TM molecule. In addition, the ability of TM-bound thrombin to cleave small synthetic substrates is unchanged (Esmon et al 1982). These alterations in the substrate specificity of thrombin are reversed upon dissociation from TM. Such large alterations in the specificity of an enzyme upon binding to a cofactor are most striking. A crystallographic analysis of the conformational differences involved should yield great insights into the structural requirements for enzyme-substrate interactions and may lead to the construction of clinically useful molecules.

NORMAL LEVELS OF COMPONENTS OF THE PC PATHWAY

The range of PC in normal plasma is from about 2.8–5.4 µg/ml (Griffin et al 1982, Marlar et al 1985, Bertina et al 1982) with pooled normal plasma containing 4 µg/ml (Griffin et al 1982). The antigen levels are reduced in patients on oral anticoagulants (Marlar et al 1985, Griffin et al 1981) to a median of approximately 2.7 µg/ml (Griffin et al 1981, Bertina et al 1982, Marlar et al 1985). Since many thrombotic patients take oral anticoagulants, PC antigen levels are compared to the levels of other vitamin K-dependent factors that are also decreased to infer heterozygous PC deficiency when ratios of PC to several other vitamin K-dependent factors fall below a normal range (Griffin et al 1981, Bertina et al 1982). Neonates express low levels (0.3–0.6 unit/ml) of PC with lower levels in premature infants (Mannucci & Vigano 1982,

Manco-Johnson et al 1985). Several groups have found no difference in levels related to age or sex in adults (Mannucci & Vigano 1982, Bertina et al 1982). A recent study of 800 normal subjects found a small steady increase with age yielding a 15% difference between young subjects under 30 and older adults over 59 years of age (Miletich & Broze 1986). No significant effect of oral contraceptives on PC antigen has been observed (Huisveld et al 1987).

PS antigen levels range from $0.71-1.34$ unit/ml with a median of 24 μg/ml (Schwarz et al 1984, Comp & Esmon 1984, Schwarz et al 1987). As detailed above, the level of total PS antigen may not necessarily correlate with the degree of PS function due to the effect of the positive and negative regulator proteins C4b-binding protein and PS-binding protein. Functional assays have been used to estimate the levels of active PS at about 8 μg/ml (Comp & Esmon 1984). As with PC, PS antigen is reduced during treatment with oral anticoagulants and therefore the ratio of PS antigen to other vitamin K-dependent protein antigens is often measured to infer a heterozygous deficiency of PS (Schwarz et al 1984). Oral contraceptive use also reduces total PS levels (Huisveld et al 1987, Boerger et al 1987). Low levels of PS are found in the fetus and neonate, all of which is in the free state since C4b-binding protein is undetectable (Mellissari et al 1987, Malm et al 1987, Schwarz & Muntean 1987). Men have a higher total PS antigen than women (Boerger et al 1987a) with the level of PS decreasing in women during pregnancy (Comp et al 1986).

The plasma PCI reported by Suzuki et al (1983b) is present at about 5 μg/ml (Suzuki et al 1983b, Heeb et al 1987a) with a range of approximately $0.65-1.35$ unit/ml (Marlar et al 1985). The urinary and plasma urokinase inhibitor known as PAI-3 (Stump et al 1986) is identical to PCI (Heeb et al 1987a) and was reported as present in plasma at 2.0 μg/ml with a range of $0.65-1.35$ unit/ml (Stump et al 1986). No age or sex related differences in PCI activity were observed in one study (Marlar & Endres-Brooks 1983).

PC HEREDITARY DEFICIENCY

The clinical picture associated with heterozygous congenital PC deficiency is similar to that seen in familial deficiency of antithrombin III, a major inhibitor of the procoagulant hemostatic enzymes. Patients present with venous thromboses in adolescence or young adulthood, sometimes following trauma or other stresses of the hemostatic system, with thrombophlebitis, deep vein thrombosis, and/or pulmonary emboli as typical findings (reviewed by Gardiner & Griffin 1985). Arterial thrombosis does not appear to be associated with this condition. Half of these symptomatic PC deficient patients suffer thrombotic episodes before the age of 30 (Broekmans et al 1983b, Marlar et al 1985). However, a number of heterozygotes from these families remain asymptomatic throughout life, emphasizing that heterozygous PC deficiency should be considered a risk factor rather than a purely causative factor in venous thrombosis. Two major clinical patterns are associated with hereditary PC deficiency, an autosomal dominant disease and an autosomal recessive disease. Clinically symptomatic type I hereditary PC heterozygous deficiency has been estimated to occur in the general population at a frequency of 1 in 16 000 to 1 in 30 000 (Broekmans et al 1983a, Gladson et al 1988), and in patients under 45 years old with venous thrombosis with a frequency of about 4–8%. At least two modes of transmission have been deduced in different kindreds: an autosomal recessive mode (Seligsohn et al 1984, Soria et al 1985) and an autosomal dominant mode which exhibits variable expressivity (Griffin et al 1981, Bertina et al 1982, Marlar et al 1985, Broekmans et al 1983b).

Autosomal recessive PC deficiency is clinically manifested only in homozygous deficient infants. Severe homozygous PC deficiency is associated with undetectable (<1% normal) levels of PC antigen (Seligsohn et al 1984, Sills et al 1984, Marciniak et al 1985, Gladson et al 1987, Branson et al 1983). This condition was first detected in a neonate who developed purpura fulminans (Branson et al 1983). The condition is life-threatening without plasma replacement followed by oral anticoagulant treatment. One neonate has been described with undetectable levels of PC antigen who had deep vein thrombosis without skin lesions, and two siblings of this patient had previously died shortly after birth of hemorrhage (Seligsohn et al 1984). None of the PC heterozygous deficient parents of the currently known homozygous deficient infants has a history of venous thrombotic disease, emphasizing the recessive nature of this syndrome in such families. 0.03% of a large population of blood donors measured for PC antigen were found to have low levels, i.e. approximately half-normal, with no evidence of thrombotic disease (Miletich & Broze 1986). This finding further demonstrates the recessive mode of transmission of PC deficiency (Seligsohn et al 1984).

A further variation of PC deficiency is identified in a group of patients with very low but detectable PC levels (5–15% of normal) and severe venous thrombotic disease (Sharon et al 1985, Soria et al 1985, Monabe & Matsuda 1985, Kakker et al 1987). These patients should be considered doubly heterozygous deficient rather than homozygous deficient. Purpura fulminans is not reported in these families, and the propositi first show symptoms of venous thromboembolic disease at age 11–25. The symptoms most commonly consist of recurring deep vein thrombosis and pulmonary emboli. In some of the families the heterozygotes with half-normal PC levels are asymptomatic (Sharon et al 1985, Monabe & Matsuda 1985) whereas in others they show possible thrombotic tendencies (Soria et al 1985).

Several patients have been identified with circulating abnormal PC molecules. The frequency of such type II PC deficiencies in one population was estimated as 1 in 70 000 (Briet et al 1987). Two patients have been identified in whom thromboembolic disease is associated with reduced anticoagulant activity of PC but normal antigen levels and amidolytic activity (Vigano-D'Angelo et al 1986). Other patients have a reduced ratio of amidolytic activity to antigen (Bertina et al 1984, Griffin et al 1983, Tirindelli et al 1986). A PC which could release activation peptide after treatment with thrombin-TM complex yet displayed no serine protease activity has been found (Sala et al 1987). The propositus in this family has a thrombotic tendency but his two daughters who have the same abnormal molecule have been asymptomatic. A second family in which the propositus and his father had a PC molecule with abnormal migration in immunoelectrophoresis showed no familial history of thrombosis (Barbui et al 1984). A third family has been reported in which an apparent double heterozygosity is present in which a similar abnormal molecule coexists with a reduction in total antigen. Interestingly, treatment with Danazol raised circulating levels only of the non-functional PC antigen (Gruppo et al 1987). Additionally, a family with inherited thrombotic problems has been described in which PC antigen could not be detected using polyclonal antiserum but which had near normal anticoagulant PC-like activity (Melissari et al 1985). The PC-like activity has yet to be further characterized but may yield some insights into the variability seen in PC deficiency. One DNA study has been performed in which variant restriction patterns were found in two unrelated heterozygotic patients (Romeo et al 1987). Their abnormal PC genes were cloned and sequenced. Each had a single point mutation. In one case a missense mutation caused the conversion of a tryptophan at position 402, which is conserved in all eukaryotic serine proteases, to a cysteine. The mutation in the other patient caused the arginine at position 406 to mutate to a stop codon. Both of these mutations led to lack of circulating antigen derived from the affected allele (Romeo et al 1987).

PS HEREDITARY DEFICIENCY

Once hereditary PC deficiency associated with thrombosis was described (Griffin et al 1981) and PS was identified as a cofactor for APC (Walker 1981, 1982), it was a trivial prediction that hereditary PS deficiency would be found in thrombophilia. Several families with heterozygous PS deficiencies associated with venous thrombosis have been reported (Schwarz et al 1984, Comp et al 1984, Comp & Esmon 1984, Broekmans et al 1985a, Gladson et al 1987, Comp et al 1986, Kamiya et al 1986). The pattern of inheritance appears to be autosomally dominant (Kamiya et al 1986, Broekmans et al 1985a, Sas et al 1985). The frequency of PS deficiency among patients under 45 years old with venous thrombosis is about 5% (Gladson et al 1987). A level of about 50% normal PS total antigen can lead to severe thrombotic difficulties (Broekmans et al 1985a, Schwarz et al 1984) as has been observed with PC deficiency and antithrombin III deficiency. However, even some individuals with severe deficiency of functional PS can be asymptomatic (Kamiya et al 1986). The protective mechanism operating in these latter individuals is unclear, especially in light of the fact that they may have relatives with similar functional PS levels (<20% of normal) who do have thrombotic tendencies (Kamiya et al 1986). Functional and antigenic levels of PS are not always correlated in these patients (Kamiya et al 1986, Comp et al 1986b, Comp & Esmon 1984, Comp et al 1984). It has been shown that in such cases the antigenic reduction is due to a loss of the free PS in plasma. This is the active component. It was suggested that in the individuals with normal PS levels but decreased PS functional activity that the root cause may be an increase in the level of C4b-binding protein (Comp et al 1986b). The clinical manifestations of heterozygous PS deficiency are similar to those of symptomatic heterozygous PC deficiency (Schwarz et al 1984, Broekmans et al 1985b). The most common symptoms are venous thromboembolism, often recurrent superficial thrombophlebitis, deep vein thrombosis, and pulmonary embolism. The mean age at the first event is about 25 years (Broekmans et al 1985a,b), most often without discernible cause. Occasionally thrombosis occurs at unusually young ages (Schwarz et al 1984, Sas et al 1985, Mannucci et al 1986a). No infantile purpura fulminans has been reported associated with PS deficiency.

THE PC SYSTEM AND ACQUIRED DEFICIENCIES

Disseminated intravascular coagulation (DIC) is characterized by the activation of many of the proteins of the coagulation and fibrinolytic systems. As regulators of both systems, it is not surprising that PC and other proteins of the PC pathway are also activated or consumed. More than half of hospitalized patients with DIC have reduced levels of PC antigen (Griffin et al 1982, Mannucci & Vigano 1982, Marlar et al 1985, Vigano-D'Angelo et al 1986). This can arise in part from decreased synthesis due to liver damage (Griffin et al 1982, Mannucci & Vigano 1982), since PC antigen is more reduced in patients with DIC and liver inadequacy (Griffin et al 1982, Mannucci & Vigano 1982, Vigano-D'Angelo et al 1986). However, reduced levels of PC antigen also result from increased rates of clearance. Evidence that PC is activated and cleared comes from the following observations. The plasma concentration of PC activation peptide rises during DIC (Bauer et al 1984) while the ratio of PC activity to antigen drops (Marlar et al 1985). This suggests that inactivated molecules may be accumulating. The levels of PCI drop during DIC in concert with the drop in PC antigen (Marlar et al 1985, Francis & Thomas 1984). In nonfatal cases of DIC, PCI antigen rises faster than PC activity while in fatal DIC both drop to undetectable levels (Marlar et al 1985). Increased levels of APC-PCI complexes are found in plasma of DIC patients (Heeb et al 1987b). PS antigen is decreased in DIC and a greater than normal percentage of it is present in a cleaved form (Heeb et al 1987b). These data imply that activation of coagulant pathways in vivo is accompanied by consumption of PC and PCI consistent with the concept that they play significant roles as hemostatic regulators.

Increased levels of PC and PS antigen have been found in the blood of patients with nephrotic syndrome (Cosio et al 1985, Mannucci et al 1986b, Sala et al 1985, Marlar et al 1983). This appears to be at least in part due to increased synthesis with little loss into the urine relative to total protein loss.

Lupus anticoagulants are antibodies that prolong phospholipid-dependent coagulation assays. Patients who produce these anticoagulants exhibit thrombotic episodes. Plasmas from several patients with such anticoagulants have been found to inhibit the enhancement of thrombin activation of PC by TM free in solution, on phospholipid vesicles, or on the surfaces of endothelial cells (Carriou et al 1986, Freyssinet et al 1986, Comp et al 1983). Presumably this inhibition of PC activation may help explain the thrombotic tendency in such patients.

The effect of normal and eclamptic pregnancy on PC and PS levels has been reviewed elsewhere (Berrettini & Griffin 1987). Little effect is seen on PC antigen in normal pregnancy, but PS activity and antigen decrease. Decrease of PS antigen is observed in eclamptic syndromes.

TREATMENT OF DEFICIENCY STATES

Heterozygous PC or PS deficiency has been treated with oral anticoagulants or heparin (reviewed in Marlar 1985, Berrettini & Griffin 1987). Thrombosis has been treated with thrombolytic therapy (Kakker et al 1987). Homozygous PC deficiency is much more difficult to manage. For this condition PC replacement is an essential first step. Fresh frozen plasma (Branson et al 1983, Marlar 1985), cryoprecipitate-poor plasma (Branson et al 1983), and PC-rich commercial factor IX concentrate (Marlar 1985, Sills et al 1984) have all been used to alleviate the symptoms of purpura fulminans in homozygotic PC deficient infants. The use of oral anticoagulants in these patients has had significant success and it is recommended that an initial plasma replacement be followed by long-term anticoagulation (Berrettini & Griffin 1987). The use of oral anticoagulation in heterozygotic PC deficiency is to be approached with caution.

PC has a short plasma half life compared to several of the procoagulant vitamin K-dependent factors (on the order of 7 hours). Therefore, at the start of anticoagulant therapy PC function drops faster than that of the coagulant factors (Vigano et al 1984) possibly leading to an induced hypercoagulable state. In patients with hereditary PC deficiency the differential between procoagulant and anticoagulant factors transiently may become too great. Coumarin-induced skin necrosis due to diffuse thrombosis of the small venules followed by bleeding has been associated with several cases of hereditary PC deficiency (Broekmans et al 1983c, McGehee et al 1984, Samama et al 1984, Marlar 1985). To avoid this complication, it is recommended that heparin therapy be continued for 4–5 days after initiation of coumarin therapy and that minimal loading doses of coumarin be used in PC deficient patients.

One experimental approach to treatment of PC deficiency involves the use of anabolic steroid therapy. Stanazolol increases levels of both antithrombin III and PC in normal healthy subjects and patients undergoing elective surgery (Kluft et al 1984, Preston et al 1983). Postsurgical drop in PC levels was reduced in the latter group. Caution must be used in such therapy, however, since levels of several vitamin K-dependent factors were increased as well. The level of PC in heterozygous type I deficiency is increased to near normal levels during Stanazolol treatment (Broekmans et al 1987, Mannucci et al 1984), presumably through increased synthesis from the normal allele. No treatment of a PC homozygous deficient infant has been reported. No effect on PS antigen levels was observed (Broekmans et al 1987). Importantly, the effectiveness of such treatment in preventing thrombosis has not been determined. Similar work was also done using Danazol which also increased PC levels in heterozygous PC deficiency until drug withdrawal, after which the PC levels declined to their previous values (Gonzalez et al 1985). As described above, Danazol treatment of a type I/type II PC deficient double heterozygote led to increase only of the dysfunctional protein in circulation (Grippo et al 1987).

FUTURE PROSPECTS

A number of areas are currently the objects of intensive research. Among these is the use of genetic engineering technology for the development of clinical tests for deficiencies of PC or PS and for study of structure/function relationships in these proteins. Molecular biology studies have made great contributions in recent years in the study of hemophilia, and newer forms of such technology are constantly being developed and applied to study inherited diseases. In clinical situations, such studies may help to identify patients at risk for thrombosis and to provide new therapeutic agents.

The delineation of new modes of regulation of the components of the PC pathways continues. New PC inhibitors are being identified, and their interactions with a variety of plasma proteins intensively studied. New data are continually being generated about the genetic regulation of the various proteins of the PC pathways which may help in understanding the control of their plasma levels.

And finally, more information is becoming available about the nature of the extensive posttranslational modifications of these proteins, from ideas concerning the purpose of the β-hydroxylation of certain Asp and Asn residues of PC and PS to identification of the amino acid sequences that signal γ-carboxylation. Such data will prove invaluable in the process of understanding the regulation of thrombosis by APC and PS at a molecular level.

REFERENCES

Aznar J, Dasi A, España F, Estelles A 1986 Thrombosis Research 42: 313–322
Baker M E, French F S, Joseph D R 1987 Biochemistry Journal 243: 293–296
Barbui T, Finazzi G, Mussoni L et al 1984 Lancet 2: 819
Bauer K A, Kass B L, Beeler D L, Rosenberg R D 1984 Journal of Clinical Investigation 74: 2033–2041
Beckmann R J, Schmidt R J, Santerre R F, Plutzky J, Crabtree G R, Long G L 1985 Nucleic Acids Research 13: 5233–5247
Berrettini M, Griffin J H 1987 In: Contributions to fetal health (in press)
Bertina R M, Broekmans A W, van der Linden I K, Mertens K 1982 Thrombosis and Haemostasis 48: 1–5
Bertina R M, Broekmans A W, Krommenhoek-Es C, van Wijngaardin A 1984 Thrombosis and Haemostasis 51: 1–5
Boerger L M, Morris P C, Thurnau G R, Esmon C T, Comp P C 1987 Blood 69: 692–694
Branson H E, Katz J, Marble R, Griffin J H 1983 Lancet 2: 1165–1168
Briet E, Engesser L, Brommer E J P, Broekmans A W, Bertina R M 1987 Thrombosis and Haemostasis 58: 39a
Broekmans A W, van der Linden I K, Veltkamp J J, Bertina R M 1983a Thrombosis and Haemostasis 50: 350
Broekmans A W, Veltkamp J J, Bertina R M 1983b New England Journal of Medicine 309: 304–344
Broekmans A W, Bertina R M, Loeliger E A, Hofman V, Klingemann H G 1983c Thrombosis and Haemostasis 49: 251
Broekmans A W, Bertina R M, Reinalda-Poot J et al 1985a Thrombosis and Haemostasis 53: 273–277
Broekmans A W, Engesser L, Briet E, Brommer E J P, Bertina R M 1985b Thrombosis Research 54: 57a
Broekmans A W, Conard J, van Weyenberg R G, Horellou M H, Kluft C, Bertina R M 1987 Thrombosis and Haemostasis 57: 20–24
Burdick M D, Schaub R G 1986 Federation Proceedings 45: 1072
Caput D, Beutler B, Hartog K, Thayer R, Brown-Shimer S, Cerami A 1986 Proceedings of the National Academy of Science USA 83: 1670–1674
Cariou R, Tobelem G, Soria C, Caen J 1986 New England Journal of Medicine 314: 1193–1194
Colucci M, Stassen J M, Collen D 1984 Journal of Clinical Investigation 74: 200–204
Comp P C, Esmon C T 1979 Blood 54: 1272–1281
Comp P C, Esmon C T 1981 Journal of Clinical Investigation 68: 1221–1228
Comp P C, Esmon C T 1984 New England Journal of Medicine 311: 1525–1528
Comp P C, DeBault L E, Esmon N L, Esmon C T 1983 Blood 62: 299a
Comp P C, Nixon R R, Cooper R, Esmon C T 1984 Journal of Clinical Investigation 74: 2082–2088
Comp P C, Thurnau G R, Welsh J, Esmon C T 1986a Blood 68: 881–885
Comp P C, Doray D, Patton D, Esmon C T 1986b Blood 67b: 504–508
Cosio F G, Harker C, Batard M A, Brandt J T, Griffin J H 1985 Journal of Laboratory and Clinical Medicine 106: 218–222
D'Angelo A, Lockhart M S, Vigano-D'Angelo S, Taylor F B 1987 Blood 69: 231–237
Dahlback B 1986 Journal of Biological Chemistry 261: 12022–12027
Dahlback B, Stenflo J 1980 European Journal of Biochemistry 107: 331–335
Dahlback B, Stenflo J 1981 Proceedings of the National Academy of Science USA 78: 2512–2516
Dahlback B, Lundwall A, Stenflo J 1986 Proceedings of the National Academy of Science USA 83: 4199–4203
DiScipio R G, Davie E W 1979 Biochemistry 18: 899–904
Drakenberg T, Ferlund P, Roepstorff P, Stenflo J 1983 Proceedings of the National Academy of Science USA 80: 1802–1806
Esmon C T, Esmon N L, Harris K W 1982b Journal of Biological Chemistry 257: 7944–7947
Esmon N L, Owen W G, Esmon C T 1982a Journal of Biological Chemistry 257: 859–864
Esmon N L, DeBault L E, Esmon C T 1983a Journal of Biological Chemistry 258: 5548–5553
Esmon N L, Carroll R C, Esmon C T 1983b Journal of Biological Chemistry 258: 12238–12242
España F, Berrettini M, Griffin J H 1988 Manuscript submitted
Foster D, Davie E W 1984 Proceedings of the National Academy of Science USA 81: 4766–4770
Foster D C, Rudinski M A, Schach B G et al 1987 Biochemistry 26: 7003–7011
Francis R B, Thomas W 1984 Thrombosis and Haemostasis 52: 71–74
Freyssinet J M, Wiesel M L, Gauchy J, Boneu B, Cazenave J P 1986 Thrombosis and Haemostasis 55: 309–313

Fulcher C A, Gardiner J E, Griffin J H, Zimmerman T S 1984 Blood 63: 486–489

Galvin J B, Kurosawa S, Moore K, Esmon C T, Esmon N L 1987 Journal of Biological Chemistry 262: 2199–2205

Gardiner J E, Griffin J H 1983 In: Brown E B (ed) Progress in hematology XIII. Grune & Stratton, New York. p 265–278

Gardiner J E, Griffin J H 1985 In: A V Hoffbrand (ed) Recent advances in haematology IV. Churchill Livingstone, London. p 269–283

Gardiner J E, McGann M A, Berridge C W, Fulcher C A, Zimmerman T S, Griffin J H 1984 Circulation 70: 820

Geiger M, Heeb M J, Binder B R, Griffin J H 1988 FASEB Journal 2: 2263–2267

Gladson C L, Scharrar I, Hach V, Beck K H, Griffin J H 1988 Thrombosis and Haemostasis 59: 18–22

Gladson C L, Groncy P, Griffin J H 1987 Archives of Dermatology 123: 1701–1706

Gonzalez R, Alberca I, Sala N, Vicente V 1985 Thrombosis and Haemostasis 53: 320–322

Griffin J H, Evatt B, Zimmerman T S, Kleiss A J, Widerman C 1981 Journal of Clinical Investigation 68: 1370–1373

Griffin J H, Mosher D F, Zimmerman T S, Kleiss A J 1982 Blood 60: 261–264

Griffin J H, Bezead A, Evatt B, Mosher D 1983 Blood 62: 301a

Gruppo R A, Francis R B, Marlar R A, Leimer P, Silberstein E B 1985 Thrombosis and Haemostasis 54: 142a

Guinto E R, Esmon C T 1984 Journal of Biological Chemistry 259: 13986–13992

Harris K W, Esmon C T 1985 Journal of Biological Chemistry 260: 207–210

Heeb M J, España F, Geiger M, Collen D, Stump D C, Griffin J H 1987a Journal of Biological Chemistry 262: 15813–15816

Heeb M J, España F, Geiger M, Collen D, Stump D C, Griffin J H 1987b Thrombosis and Haemostasis 58: 277

Heeb M J, Mosher D F, Griffin J H 1987c Thrombosis and Haemostasis 58: 514

Heeb M J, España F, Griffin J H 1988 Manuscript submitted

Hoskins J, Norman D K, Beckmann R J, Long G L 1987 Proceedings of the National Academy of Science USA 84: 349–353

Ishii H, Majerus P W 1985 Journal of Clinical Investigation 76: 2178–2181

Jackman R W, Beeler D L, Van deWater L, Rosenberg R D 1986 Proceedings of the National Academy of Science USA 83: 8834–8838

Jackman R W, Beeler D L, Fritze L, Soff G, Rosenberg R D 1987 Proceedings of the National Academy of Science USA 84: 6425–6429

Kakkar S, Melissari E, Kakkar V V 1987 Thrombosis and Haemostasis 58: 410a

Kamiya T, Sugihara T, Ogata K 1986 Blood 67: 406–410

Kisiel W, Canfield W M, Ericsson L H, Davie E W 1977 Biochemistry 16: 5824–5831

Kisiel W 1979 Journal of Clinical Investigation 64: 761–769

Kluft C, Bertina R M, Preston F E, Malia R G, Blamey S L, Lowe G D O, Forbes C D 1984 Thrombosis Research 33: 297–304

Long G L, Belagje R M, McGillivray R T A 1984 Proceedings of the National Academy of Science USA 81: 5653–5656

Lundwall A, Dackowski W, Cohen E 1986 Proceedings of the National Academy of Science USA 83: 6716–6720

McGehee W G, Klotz T A, Epstein D J, Rapaport S I 1984 Annals of Internal Medicine 100: 59–60

Malm J, Bennhagen R, Holmberg L, Dahlback B 1987 Thrombosis and Haemostasis 58: 400

Mammen E F, Thomas W R, Seegers W H 1960 Thrombosis et Diathesis Haemorrhagica 5: 218

Manabe S I, Matsuda M 1985 Thrombosis Research 39: 333–341

Manco-Johnson M J, Marlar R A, Hathaway W 1985 Thrombosis and Haemostasis 54: 142

Mannucci P M, Vigano S 1982 Lancet 2: 463–467

Mannucci P M, Bottaso B, Sharon C, Tripodi A 1984 La Ricerca Clinica Laboratoria 14: 673–679

Mannucci P M, Tripodi A, Bertina R M 1986a Thrombosis and Haemostasis 55: 440

Mannucci P M, Valsecchi C, Bottasso B, D'Angelo A, Casati S, Ponticelli C 1986b Thrombosis and Haemostasis 55: 31–33

Marciniak E, Wilson H D, Marlar R A 1985 Blood 65: 15–20

Marlar R A 1985 Seminars in Thrombosis and Haemostasis 11: 387–392

Marlar R A, Endres-Brooks J E 1983 Thrombosis and Haemostasis 50: 351

Marlar R A, Kleiss A J, Griffin J H 1981 New York Academy of Sciences 370: 303–310

Marlar R A, Kleiss A J, Griffin J H 1982 Blood 59: 1067–1072

Marlar R A, Endres-Brooks J E, Miller C 1985 Blood 66: 59–63

Maruyama I, Salem H H, Majerus P W 1984 Journal of Clinical Investigation 74: 224–230

Maruyama I, Bell C E, Majerus P W 1985 Journal of Cell Biology 101: 363–371

Maruyama I, Majerus P W 1987 Blood 69: 1481–1484
Maruyama I, Majerus P W 1985 Journal of Biological Chemistry 260: 15432–15438
Melissari E, Scully M F, Paes T, Ellis V, Kakkar V V 1986 Thrombosis and Haemostasis 55: 54–57
Melissari E, Scully M F, Parker C, Nicolaide K H, Kakkar V V 1987 Thrombosis and Haemostasis 58: 407
Miletich J P, Broze G J 1986 Circulation 74: (II) 92
Miletich J P, Leykam J F, Broze G J 1983 Blood 63: 603a
Mitchell C A, Hau L, Salem H H 1986 Thrombosis and Haemostasis 56: 151–154
Moore K L, Andreoli S P, Esmon N L, Esmon C T, Bang N U 1987 Journal of Clinical Investigation 79: 124–130
Nawroth P P, Stern D M 1986 Journal of Experimental Medicine 163: 740–745
Nawroth P P, Handley D A, Esmon C T, Stern D M 1986 Proceedings of the National Academy of Science USA 83: 3460–3464
Nesheim M E, Canfield W M, Kisiel W, Mann K G 1982 Journal of Biological Chemistry 257: 1443–1447
Odegaard B, Mann K 1987 Journal of Biological Chemistry 262: 11233–11238
Ogura M, Takamatsu J, Tanabe T, Maruyama I, Saito H 1987 Blood 70: 357a
Owen W G, Esmon C T 1981 Journal of Biological Chemistry 256: 5532–5535
Plutzky J, Hoskins J A, Long G L, Crabtree G R 1986 Proceedings of the National Academy of Science USA 83: 546–550
Polgar J, Lerant I, Muzbek L, Machovich R 1986 Thrombosis Research 43: 585–890
Preissner K T, Delvos U, Muller-Berghaus G 1987 Biochemistry 26: 2521–2528
Preston F E, Malia R G, Greaves M, Kluft C, Bertina R M, Segal D S 1983 Lancet 2: 517–518
Romeo G, Hassan H J, Staempfli S et al 1987 Proceedings of the National Academy of Science USA 84: 2829–2832
Sakata Y, Currinden S, Lawrence D, Griffin J H, Loskutoff D J 1985 Proceedings of the National Academy of Science USA 82: 1121–1125
Sakata Y, Loskutoff D J, Gladson C L, Hekman C M, Griffin J H 1986 Blood 68: 1218–1223
Sala N, Oliver A, Estivill X, Moreno R, Felez J, Rutllant M L 1985 Thrombosis and Haemostasis 54: 900
Sala M, Borrell M, Bauer K A et al 1987 Thrombosis and Haemostasis 57: 183–186
Salem H H, Maruyama I, Ishii H, Majerus P W 1984 Journal of Biological Chemistry 259: 12246–12251
Samama M, Horellou M H, Soria J, Conard J, Nicholas G 1984 Thrombosis and Haemostasis 51: 132–133
Sas G, Blasko G, Petro I, Griffin J H 1985 Thrombosis and Haemostasis 54: 724
Schwarz H P, Muntean W 1987 Thrombosis and Haemostasis 58: 218
Schwarz H P, Fischer M, Hopmeier P, Batard M A, Griffin J H 1984 Blood 64: 1297–1300
Schwarz H P, Heeb M J, Wencel-Drake J D, Griffin J H 1985a Blood 66: 1452–1455
Schwarz H P, Heeb M J, Griffin J H 1985b Thrombosis and Haemostasis 54: 57
Schwarz H P, Heeb M J, Lämmle B, Berrettini M, Griffin J H 1986 Thrombosis and Haemostasis 56: 382–386
Seegers W H, McCoy L E, Groben H D, Sakuragawa N, Agrawal B B L 1972 Thrombosis Research 1: 443
Seligsohn U, Berger A, Abend M, Rubin L, Attias D, Zivelin A, Rapaport S I 1984 New England Journal of Medicine 310: 559–562
Sharon C, Tirindelli M C, Mannucci P M, Tripodi A, Mariani G 1986 Thrombosis Research 41: 483–488
Sills R H, Marlar R A, Montgomery R R, Deshpande G N, Humbert J R 1984 Journal of Pediatrics 105: 409–413
Soff G A, Marlar R A, Sica D, Quereshi G D, Evans H J 1983 Clinical Research 31: 875a
Soria J, Soria C, Samama M, Nicolas G, Kisiel W 1985 Thrombosis and Haemostasis 53: 293–296
Steiner S A, Amphlett G W, Castellino F J 1980 Biochemical Biophysical Research Communications 94: 340–347
Stenflo J 1976 Journal of Biological Chemistry 251: 355–363
Stenflo J, Lundwall A, Dahlback B 1987 Proceedings of the National Academy of Science USA 84: 368–372
Stump D C, Thienpont M, Collen D 1986 Journal of Biological Chemistry 261: 12759–12766
Suzuki K, Stenflo J, Dahlback B, Teodorsson B 1983a Journal of Biological Chemistry 258: 1914–1920
Suzuki K, Nishioka J, Hashimoto S 1983b Journal of Biological Chemistry 258: 163–168
Suzuki K, Nishioka J, Hashimoto S 1983c Journal of Biochemistry 94: 699–705
Suzuki K, Nishioka J, Kusumoto H, Hashimoto S 1984a Journal of Biochemistry 95: 187–195
Suzuki K, Nishioka J, Matsuda M, Maruyama H, Hashimoto S 1984b Journal of Biochemistry 96: 455–460
Suzuki K, Kusumoto H, Deyashiki Y et al 1987a EMBO Journal 6: 1891–1987
Suzuki K, Deyashiki Y, Nishioka J et al 1987b Journal of Biological Chemistry 262: 611–616
Taylor F B, Lockhart M S 1985 Thrombosis Research 37: 639–649
Taylor F B, Carroll R C, Gerrand J, Esmon C T, Radcliffe R D 1981 Federation Proceedings 40: 2092–2098
Tirindelli M C, Franchi F, Tripodi A, Mariani G, Mannucci P M 1986 Thrombosis Research 44: 893–897
Travis J, Salvesen G S 1983 Annual Review of Biochemistry 52: 655–710

van Hinsbergh V W M, Bertina R M, van Wijngaarden A, van Tilburg N H, Emeis J J, Haverkate F
    1985 Blood 65: 444–451
van der Meer F J M, van Tilburg N H, van der Linden I K, Briet E, Bertina R M 1987 Thrombosis
    and Haemostasis 58: 277
Vehar G A, Davie E W 1980 Biochemistry 19: 401–410
Vigano S, Mannucci P M, Solinas S, Bottasso D, Mariani G 1984 British Journal of Haematology
    57: 217–220
Vigano D'Angelo S, Comp P C, Esmon C T, D'Angelo A 1986 Journal of Clinical Investigation 77: 416–425
Walker F J 1980 Journal of Biological Chemistry 255: 5521–5524
Walker F J 1981 Journal of Biological Chemistry 256: 11128–11131
Walker F J 1984a Journal of Biological Chemistry 259: 10335–10339
Walker F J 1984b Seminars in Thrombosis and Hemostasis 10: 131–138
Walker F J 1986 Journal of Biological Chemistry 261: 10941–10944
Walker F J, Sexton P W, Esmon C T 1979 Biochimica et Biophysica Acta 571: 333–342
Wen D, Dittman W A, Ye R D, Deaver L L, Majerus P W, Sadler J E 1987 Biochemistry 26: 4350–4357

15. Acquired immunodeficiency syndrome

J. E. Groopman

INTRODUCTION

What began as an unusual disorder of unknown etiology apparently clustered in the male homosexual communities of New York and California 7 years ago is now understood to be a progressive immunosuppressive and neurodegenerative retroviral infection of pandemic proportions. A considerable body of information has been developed on the molecular biology, protein chemistry, and cell biology of the human immunodeficiency virus (HIV), the causative agents of AIDS (Barre-Sinoussi et al 1983, Popovic et al 1983). Furthermore, a second pathogenic human retrovirus, HIV-2, which is genomically related but clearly distinct from HIV-1, has been associated with AIDS in West Africa and more recently Europe (Couroce et al 1987, Hahn et al 1987). Information on the epidemiological, clinical, basic science, and therapeutic aspects of HIV has been generated at a rate possibly unparalleled for other human disorders. We will review the salient features of AIDS with particular emphasis on manifestations of importance to the hematologist. It is clear that knowledge about AIDS is essential for both the practicing physician and the resesarch biologist for this decade and likely the upcoming years.

BIOLOGY OF HIV

HIV (previously known as human T-lymphotropic virus type III, HTLV-III, lymphadenopathy associated virus, LAV, or AIDS related virus, ARV), has been studied extensively during the past 4 years. Like all retroviruses, HIV is an RNA virus and utilizes the enzyme reverse transcriptase to make a DNA copy of the viral RNA. Its outer lipid envelope is about 100 nanometers in diameter and the genomic RNA is contained within a characteristic dense cylindrical core. The genome of HIV (Fig. 15.1) contains genes that code for structural components of the virus including

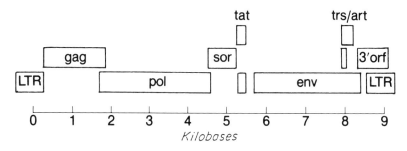

Fig. 15.1 HIV genome

the gag and env genes which encode core and envelope proteins respectively (Muesing et al 1985, Ratner et al 1985, Sanchez-Pescador et al 1985, Rabson & Martin 1985). A major envelope glycoprotein of HIV is 120 000 daltons and has recently been demonstrated to be essential for virus binding to its receptor, the CD4 protein (Allan et al 1985, Barin et al 1985, Dagleish et al 1984, McDougal et al 1986). The envelope gene is initially transcribed as a 160 kilodalton protein which subsequently forms the 41 000 dalton transmembrane segment and the 120 000 dalton external segment of the virus surface antigen. The major core protein encoded by the gag gene is 24 000 daltons. The pol gene encodes the viral reverse transcriptase. These genes, gag, pol, and env, are common to all retroviruses. At least four additional genes are found in HIV. Two of these, tat and trs/art are so-called 'multi-exon genes' which are formed by splicing together messenger RNAs that have been coded by the noncontiguous genome (Muesing et al 1986). These two genes, tat and trs/art, are thought to be important in regulating transcription of HIV (Sodroski et al 1986, Muesing et al 1986). Their role in regulation of translation of protein is somewhat controversial. Mutations occurring in either tat or trs/art genes will abrogate virus replication (Fisher et al 1986a). The sor gene is of unclear function and may act to anchor the membrane of the virus.

The 3'orf gene may function to reduce viral replication, acting in an opposite fashion to tat and trs/art (Fisher et al 1986b, Luciw et al 1987). Further work is necessary to better define the functional properties of the tat, trs/art, sor, and 3'orf genes. It is clear though that these genes are expressed during the life cycle of the virus in man since serum of HIV infected individuals contains antibodies to the protein products of these genes (Arya & Gallo 1986).

The genomic sequence and structure of HIV-2 is more similar to the pathogenic simian retrovirus SIV (also known as STLV-III) than to HIV-1. It does have the structural gag and env genes, the pol gene which encodes a reverse transcriptase, as well as a tat gene (Esteban et al 1987).

The receptor for HIV-1 has been identified as the CD4 protein (Dalgleish et al 1984, Klatzmann et al 1984, Maddon et al 1986). Laboratory studies of AIDS or ARC patients demonstrated depletion of CD4 helper lymphocytes in the peripheral blood with a striking inversion of the ratio of CD4 (helper) cells to CD8 (suppressor) cells (Seligmann et al 1987). The CD4 protein has also been identified on monocyte-macrophages, neuronal cells, and cell lines derived from colonic epithelium. The function of the lymphocyte CD4 protein is not known, but its close association with the major histocompatibility complex antigen type II (MHC II) present on antigen presenting cells during recognition of foreign antigen suggests that it is an important component in the immune response. It was observed that HIV replicated in vitro in CD4 positive lymphocytes and apparently not in other types of lymphocytes (Klatzmann et al 1984). These initial observations led to further work that defined the receptor for HIV on the surface of target cells as the CD4 molecule. HIV infection of CD4 positive cells could be blocked in vitro by monoclonal antibodies directed against specific epitopes (Leu3a, OKT4A) on the CD4 protein. In addition, immunoprecipitation of the CD4 protein during exposure of target cells to HIV resulted in coprecipitation of the major glycoprotein of HIV, gp120 (McDougal et al 1986). Transfection of human cells that do not normally express this CD4 protein on their surface with the CD4 gene makes them susceptible to HIV infection (Maddon et al 1986). Thus, the CD4 molecule appears to be necessary for HIV infection. Recently, soluble CD4 has been produced by truncating the transmembrane and cytoplasmic domains of the molecule (Smith et al 1987). The hydrophilic external portion of CD4 has been shown to bind with very high affinity $(Kd > 10^{-9} M)$ to gp120. Furthermore, soluble CD4 can completely block HIV infection of susceptible CD4 positive target cells. These in vitro observations suggest that therapeutic strategies may be derived through a better understanding of the interaction of HIV with its receptor.

Following this specific binding of HIV to the CD4 protein on the cell surface, the virus enters the cell and is uncoated. The mechanism of virus entry and uncoating is still not known. Following this step, the genomic RNA is transcribed by the viral reverse transcriptase into a DNA copy. This DNA copy then forms a circular structure and is integrated into the whole cellular DNA by a virally encoded enzyme, an integrase. Much of the HIV DNA is unintegrated and found in the cytoplasm, but the proportion that is integrated into the host cellular genome is termed a provirus (Shaw et al 1984).

The activation of HIV infected cells with antigen or exposure to other pathogens such as herpes viruses may be important in sustaining the replication cycle of HIV (Zagury et al 1986, Folks et al 1986). Following such activation, the viral genome is transcribed into RNA with subsequent synthesis of viral proteins, assembly of the proteins with the genomic viral RNA at the surface of the cell, and release of mature viral particles by budding (Rabson & Martin 1985). It is still unclear whether virus is transmitted via release of free virions, which is observed in vitro, or by cell to cell contact and fusion.

The mechanisms whereby HIV interferes with normal lymphocyte function is not clear. HIV is cytopathic to CD4 positive lymphocytes in vitro but not particularly cytopathic to monocyte-macrophages (Nicholson et al 1986, Gartner et al 1986, Salahuddin et al 1986). The life cycle and effects of the virus in these two different cell types is clearly quite different. It has been speculated that the persistence of HIV within the monocyte-macrophage, and the role of this cell in the circulation with egress into tissues, may be quite important as a mechanism for dissemination of HIV infection in man. Two major hypotheses have been proposed to account for the cytopathic effects of HIV: the significant amount of unintegrated viral DNA in the cytoplasm may be toxic; or following infection, cell fusion occurs by binding of the viral envelope glycoprotein gp120, expressed on the surface of infected cells, with the CD4 molecule expressed on uninfected cells (Zagury et al 1986, Lifson et al 1986). This binding of gp120 to the CD4 protein results in multinucleated giant cells and subsequently cell death. Although syncytia may be observed in vitro, they are generally not seen pathologically in vivo except in brain (Gartner et al 1986).

It is clear that HIV is a persistent infection in man because the retrovirus integrates into the target cell genome in a proviral form. Each time the cell replicates and divides, it carried the viral genome with it. Thus, it must be assumed that individuals infected with HIV are infected permanently and are potentially infectious to others. HIV is only transmissable through parenteral exposure, sexual contact (heterosexual or homosexual), exchange of body fluids, blood or blood products, or during pregnancy (Curran et al 1985). It is believed that most of the virus is in a latent form in the infected host, and as stated before, this latent form of the virus may be activated through exposure to exogenous stimuli such as alloantigens from blood or semen or by pathogens such as concurrent herpes virus infection (Folks et al 1986). It is also clear that the biology of the virus may differ according to the cell type infected. This difference in viral effects according to cell type probably results from both host cell factors as well as the interaction of the viral genes tat, trs/art, and/or 3'orf.

THE CLINICAL SPECTRUM OF HIV INFECTION IN ADULTS

Considerable progress has been made in developing a systematic characterization of the clinical findings associated with HIV infection. Classification schema have been developed by the Centers for Disease Control and the Walter Reed Army Institute of Research (Centers for Disease Control 1986, Redfield et al 1986). Both of these classification systems encompassed the spectrum of clinical manifestations ranging from asymptomatic infection with HIV to severe immunodeficiency manifest as opportunistic infections, neoplasms, and/or neurologic dysfunction. Initially, the only widely accepted and unambiguous definition was for the most severe manifestation of HIV infection, AIDS. AIDS has been defined as a disease at least moderately predictive of the defect of cell mediated immunity occurring in a person with no known cause with diminished resistance to that disease. Such diseases include *Pneumocystis carinii* pneumonia, other serious opportunistic infections, and/or Kaposi's sarcoma. Diagnoses are considered to fulfill the case definition only if based on sufficiently reliable methods such as culture, histology, etc. In adults with HIV seropositivity, additional diseases fulfilling the criteria of AIDS include disseminated histoplasmosis, Isosporiasis, bronchial or pulmonary candidiasis, and lymphoma.

In addition, several definitions for the less severe manifestations of HIV infection that may precede the development of AIDS have also been suggested. These are reviewed in Table 15.1.

Subsequent to the identification of HIV as the etiologic agent of AIDS, hierarchical classification systems for HIV infection related disorders have been developed. It is important to keep in mind that the full expression of HIV infection is not known, so that these systems may be changed. Most recently, the American Medical Association has developed a modified Centers for Disease Control classification of HIV infection (Ostrow et al 1987). This groups patients according to initial infection, chronic asymptomatic infection, persistent generalized lymphadenopathy, and other diseases including constitutional disease, neurologic disease, secondary infectious diseases, secondary cancers, and other conditions. This system appears to be the most complete one to date and most ammenable to clinical, basic science, and epidemiological studies.

EPIDEMIOLOGY OF HIV

There are currently 70 000 cases of frank AIDS reported in the United States, with an estimated 1–2 million HIV infected individuals (Curran et al 1985). It is believed that there are 3–10 million HIV infected individuals worldwide, with approximately 1 million infected in Western Europe and more than 2–4 million in Central Africa. The major risk groups for AIDS in the West include homosexual and bisexual men, intravenous drug abusers, both IV drug abusers and homosexual men, heterosexual contacts, recipients of blood products, and children born to infected mothers (Curran et al 1985). In the United States and Western Europe the major forms of transmission

Table 15.1 Modified CDC classification of HIV infection

Group I: Initial infection
Patients in this group may be designated as symptomatic seroconversion or asymptomatic seroconversion
Symptomatic infection may include a mononucleosis-like syndrome, aseptic meningitis, rash, musculo-skeletal complaints and hematologic abnormalities as well as other clinical and laboratory findings
Asymptomatic infection may occur with or without hematologic abnormalities

Group II: Chronic asymptomatic infection
Patients in this group may be designated as having a normal laboratory evaluation, specified laboratory abnormalities or laboratory evaluation pending or incomplete
Laboratory abnormalities associated with HIV infection include: anemia, leukopenia, lymphopenia, decreased T-helper lymphocyte count, thrombocytopenia, hypergammaglobulinemia and cutaneous anergy

Group III: Persistent generalized lymphadenopathy
Patients in this group may be designated on the basis of laboratory evaluation in the same manner as those in Group II

Group IV: Other diseases
(Medical evaluation must exclude the presence of other intercurrent illnesses that could explain the symptoms

Subgroup IV-A: Constitutional disease
Patients in this group may be designated as having fever for more than 1 month, involuntary weight loss greater than 10% of baseline body weight, diarrhea lasting more than 1 month, or any combination of these

Subgroup IV-B: Neurologic disease
Category 1: CNS disorders: Includes (a) dementia, (b) acute atypical meningitis (occurring after initial infection), and (c) myelopathy
Category 2: Peripheral NS disorders: Includes (a) painful sensory neuropathy and (b) inflammatory demyelinating polyneuropathy

Subgroup IV-C: Secondary infectious diseases
Category 1: Patients in this group may be designated as having one or more of the following: *Pneumocystis carinii* pneumonia, chronic cryptosporidiosis, toxoplasmosis, extra-intestinal strongyloidiasis, isosporiasis, candidiasis (esophageal, bronchial or pulmonary), cryptococcosis, disseminated histoplasmosis, mycobacterial infection with *M. avium* complex or *M. kansasii*, disseminated cytomegalovirus infection, chronic mucocutaneous or disseminated herpes simplex virus infection and progressive multifocal leukoencephalopathy.
Category 2: Patients in this group may be designated as having one or more of the following: oral hairy leukoplakia, multidermatomal herpes zoster, recurrent Salmonella bacteremia, nocardiosis, tuberculosis or oral candidiasis (thrush)

Subgroup IV-D: Secondary cancers
Patients in this group may be designated as having one or more of the following: Kaposi's sarcoma, non-Hodgkin's lymphoma (small, noncleaved lymphoma or immunoblastic sarcoma), or primary lymphoma of the brain

Subgroup IV-E: Other conditions
Includes patients with clinical findings or diseases, not classifiable above, which may be attributed to HIV infection and/or which may be indicative of a defect in cell-mediated immunity. Patients in this group may be designated on the basis of the types of clinical findings or diseases diagnosed, e.g. chronic lymphoid interstitial pneumonitis

appear to be homosexual contact, particularly receptive anal intercourse, or parenteral drug abuse. In regions of Central Africa and Haiti, where seroprevalence rates are 5% or greater among the general population, heterosexual transmission appears to be an important factor. It has been difficult to discern whether certain cultural practices such as scarification, female circumcision, or frequent injections with poorly sterilized needles may be important in the developing world in transmission of HIV.

Although all the major groups may manifest the opportunistic infections and/or neoplasms fulfilling the criteria for AIDS, there is an interesting disproportionate occurrence of Kaposi's sarcoma among homosexual verses heterosexual AIDS cases (Groopman et al 1987a). Kaposi's sarcoma will be diagnosed in up to 40% of homosexual men with AIDS at some time during their illness while it is recognized in only 5–10% of heterosexual cases of AIDS. This discrepancy has not yet been explained, but suggests that there is another transmissable agent, perhaps a virus, present in the homosexual community which is not present in the heterosexual community at risk for AIDS. Considerable effort has been made to identify a second transmissable agent, but to date this has not been successful. Although it has been speculated that recreational drugs such as amyl or butyl nitrite, or the cytomegalovirus, could be important in AIDS-related Kaposi's sarcoma, the data to support pathogenetic roles for these factors are unconvincing. It does appear though that the B-cell lymphomas associated with AIDS may be similar in molecular phenotype to the Burkitt's lymphoma in Africa, with evidence of Epstein-Barr virus genome integrated into the lymphoma DNA, over expression of the c-myc oncogene, and characteristic chromosomal rearrangements such as 8;14 or 8;22 translocations (Groopman et al 1986).

The risk that AIDS poses for the general population should not be underemphasized or overemphasized. It is clear that anyone can become infected with HIV given the appropriate exposure. Heterosexual transmission, particularly to women who have vaginal intercourse with HIV infected men, is a real threat. The transmission from female to male is believed to be much less efficient than from male to female, but documented cases have occurred. Because of the lack of data with respect to HIV infection among the general population, and the difficulty in generating such data through widespread testing even on an anonymous basis, it is prudent that sexually active heterosexuals as well as homosexuals be aware of AIDS and take the appropriate precautions such as the use of condoms to avoid infection.

HEMATOLOGICAL MANIFESTATIONS OF HIV

All hematopoietic elements are affected by HIV infection. The majority of patients with frank AIDS manifest anemia and granulocytopenia and about a third have thrombocytopenia (Spivak et al 1983, Zon et al 1987). These abnormalities may be attributable to concomitant infections, neoplasms, and/or myelosuppressive antibiotics or chemotherapy, or they may be a direct result of HIV infection. It is clear that decreased peripheral blood counts may also occur in the earlier clinical stages of HIV infection before overt AIDS, but at a lower frequency. Among asymptomatic HIV carriers, anemia, granulocytopenia, and thrombocytopenia were respectively found in 17%, 8%, and 13%. Thrombocytopenia may occur as an isolated hematological finding in this setting while anemia and granulocytopenia tend to occur simultaneously. These findings suggest that the pathophysiological mechanisms of thrombocytopenia in HIV infection may differ from the mechanism of anemia and granulocytopenia.

Bone marrow abnormalities on aspirate and biopsy have been observed in a significant number of AIDS patients (Spivak et al 1983, 1984). Again, confounding clinical variables such as coexistent infections or myelotoxic therapy may be operative in many of these cases. Nonetheless, hematopathological findings in HIV infection without such iatrogenic or other infectious complications include hypercellularity, plasmacytosis, lymphoid aggregates, and prominent dysplasia. The bone marrow generally contains adequate megakaryocytes in patients with thrombocytopenia. The anemia and granulocytopenia often occur with prominent dysplastic changes in the bone marrow and appear to represent ineffective hematopoiesis.

Several studies support an immune mediated mechanism for thrombocytopenia (Walsh et al 1985, McGrath et al 1986, Stricker et al 1985). Circulating immune complexes are frequent in HIV infected individuals, with elution of immunoglobulins from the platelet surface in the majority of cases. A controversy exists as to a nonspecific verses a specific immune mediated suppression. Stricker and colleagues have identified a 25 000 dalton platelet-associated antigen which is recognized by antibodies found in HIV infected persons that did not bind to other blood cells but did react with a similar antigen associated with cultured herpes simplex virus types 1 and 2 and human fibroblasts. The presence of this antiplatelet antibody in serum did not uniformly lead to thrombocytopenia. Evidence for immune complexes on the surface of platelets as opposed to a specific antiplatelet antibody has also been developed. An additional mechanism which may be operative in determining the circulating platelet count in HIV infected individuals is the clearance of circulating immune complexes in AIDS patients. Defective clearance of immune complexes attached to the C3b receptor of erythrocytes has been shown in the progression from asymptomatic HIV infection to development of overt AIDS (Inada et al 1986). Fc receptor mediated clearance has also been found to be defective in AIDS (Bender et al 1984). Thus, one might postulate that abnormal receptor clearance could mediate normalization of the platelet count in the presence of an antiplatelet antibody or nonspecific complexes binding to the Fc receptor of the platelet.

Treatment of thrombocytopenia associated with HIV infection is also controversial. Some patients who do not manifest frank bleeding or a marked predisposition to hemorrhage (such as petechiae and spontaneous ecchymoses) may be observed with occasional normalization of the platelet count without treatment. Some groups have used corticosteroids but others are reluctant to treat with potentially immunosuppressive agents that might accelerate the development of frank AIDS or predispose to certain opportunistic infections such as cryptococcal meningitis or *Pneumocystis carinii* pneumonia. Other investigators have advocated use of agents such as Danazol, antiRh (D), Vincristine, or high dose intravenous gammaglobulin. We have had considerable success in management with high dose intravenous gammaglobulin, but similar to the situation in classical immune thrombocytopenia, the benefit in terms of elevation of the platelet count is generally not sustained. Splenectomy is an important and generally effective modality of treatment for patients with HIV related thrombocytopenia who manifest severe thrombocytopenia and/or clinical episodes of bleeding.

The pathogenesis of anemia and granulocytopenia in HIV infected patients appears to result from ineffective hematopoiesis. We have recently studied in vitro proliferation of myeloid and erythroid progenitors in the presence of colony stimulating factors and erythropoietin (Donahue et al 1987). Our studies revealed normal numbers and normal response of both myeloid and erythroid progenitors to recombinant granulocyte macrophage stimulating factor and recombinant human erythropoietin, but suppression of such progenitor proliferation in the presence of anti-HIV antibodies. More specifically, progenitor proliferation could be inhibited using polyclonal animal sera which had been raised to recombinant envelope gp120. Other investigators who may have studied patients on myelosuppressive therapy or with co-existent myelosuppressive infections have found decreased numbers of myeloid progenitors (Leiderman et al 1987). These studies used conditioned medium as a source of colony stimulating factor and not purified hormone. Nonetheless, they are of interest because a putative glycoprotein of 84 000 dalton molecular weight was identified as being a suppressive factor released by cultured bone marrow mononuclear cells from HIV infected individuals. Further studies are required to characterize this factor.

Recombinant human granulocyte macrophage colony stimulating factor has been administered in a phase I study to severely leukopenic patients with AIDS (Groopman et al 1987). This study demonstrated an exquisite sensitivity of these patients to the myeloid hormone, with normalization of circulating white blood cell count in all patients. The cell types recruited were mainly granulocytes and bands as well as eosinophils with a variable increase in monocytes and lymphocytes. No discernible effect was observed on the circulating platelet count or hemoglobin. Thus, if ineffective hematopoiesis is a mechanism of granulocytopenia in HIV infection, it apparently can be overcome through administration of recombinant granulocyte-macrophage colony stimulating factor.

In addition to the circulating cytopenias seen in HIV infection, coagulation abnormalities have been observed in some patients. Antiphospholipid antibodies have been observed in a significant number of patients with AIDS or ARC (Cohen et al 1986, Canosa et al 1987). Their presence has been associated with other disease conditions such as systemic lupus erythematosis with thrombocytopenia, arterial and venous thrombosis, and recurrent abortions. The family of antiphospholipid antibodies include lupus anticoagulant, anticardiolipin antibodies, and Venereal Disease Research Laboratory tests (VDRL) for syphilis. The lupus anticoagulant is an IgG or IgM immunoglobulin which is capable of prolonging the lipid dependent coagulation tests. The lupus anticoagulant antibody may be directed against the phospholipid components of the prothrombin activator complex and/or against the phospholipid in the platelet membrane. Of particular note for the astute clinician caring for a patient population of homosexual men or intravenous drug abusers, the presence of the lupus anticoagulant correlates with false positive serology for syphilis and may lead to that diagnosis inappropriately. Bloom et al (1984, 1986) first reported the presence of a prolonged partial thromboplastin time in four homosexual patients with AIDS that appear to be due to a lupus anticoagulant. One of these patients had a documented deep venous thrombosis and pulmonary embolism. Other investigators have subsequently reported the presence of a plasma anticoagulant in HIV infected individuals. We recently studied the level of anticardiolipid antibodies in 73 homosexual men using an enzyme linked immunosorbent antigen (Canosa et al 1987). High levels of IgG anticardiolipid antibodies were present in 23 of 28 patients with AIDS, 12 of 14 patients with ARC, and 5 of 10 HIV seropositive asymptomatic homosexuals and none of 13 asymptomatic HIV negative health homosexuals. Elevated levels of IgM anticardiolipin antibodies were detected only in 4 patients with AIDS. There were no thrombotic episodes detected in these patients with high anticardiolipin antibodies. Further study is required to better define the prevalence of such antibodies and the mechanism for their appearance in HIV infected individuals.

Similar to antibodies demonstrated against platelets and phospholipids, antibodies directed against the red cell membrane have been detected in HIV infected subjects. In a retrospective review of 55 patients from the transfusion service at San Francisco General Hospital, a direct antiglobulin (Coombs) test was positive in 10 patients (Toy et al 1985). This compared to 0.6% of the general hospital population. Of the 10 patients with the positive direct antiglobulin test, erythrocytes were coated with IgG and complement in 4, IgG in 4, and with complement alone in 2. The antibody screen was positive for an antiPl in 1 patient only. No patient had significant hemolysis. Similar studies from other groups have demonstrated a slightly elevated prevalence of positive direct antiglobulin tests as well (McGinnis et al 1986). A selection bias is present in these studies because the patients evaluated were those who required blood typing or transfusion. The frequency of red cell antibodies detected in unselected HIV infected individuals is thus probably much lower than that reported. Despite the production of such antibodies in some patients with HIV infection, the mechanism of anemia does not appear to be hemolytic. The antibodies may relate to the hyper-gammaglobulinemia seen in patients with HIV infection. Nonspecific immune complexes may attach to the erythrocytes yielding a positive direct antiglobulin test. Alternatively, the antibody may be directed against a specific determinant on the red cell membrane, such as the phospholipid. Furthermore, Inada et al (1986) has shown deposition of circulating immune complexes on erythrocytes via the C3b receptor.

Antineutrophil antibodies have also been detected in patients with HIV infection (Outwater & McCutchen 1985). Their presence may not correlate with peripheral granulocytopenia. It is of interest that we have treated one patient with severe neutro-penia and positive antigranulocyte antibodies with high doses of intravenous gamma-globulin. This patient showed a striking increase in his neutrophil count following gammaglobulin therapy. This later declined and upon retreatment with intravenous gammaglobulin, rose again. Thus, in some patients antigranulocyte antibodies may be an important mechanism for granulocytopenia. Antilymphocyte antibodies have also been described in patients with AIDS in homosexual men with lymphadenopathy. Their significance with respect to loss of circulating lymphocyte populations is still unclear.

BLOOD PRODUCTS AND HIV

In 1982 it became clear that patients with hemophilia with no sexual risk factors for AIDS had developed the disease (Levine 1985). This provided the first evidence that AIDS could be transmitted by blood products. Since that time, detailed epidemio-logic, serologic and virologic studies have clearly established transmission of HIV by a variety of blood products. Over the past 4 years screening of blood donors for HIV antibody with an accurate ELISA assay has been instituted, so that the current risk of contamination of a blood product with HIV is estimated to be 1 in 200 000 to 1 in a million (Esteban et al 1986).

The percentage of AIDS cases in the United States in which blood transfusion was the only risk factor has remained relatively constant over the last 4 years, compris-ing 1.5–2% of the total cases in adults (Curran et al 1985). Among women with AIDS, exposure to blood products is a primary risk factor in 10% of cases. Blood transfusion is implicated in about 13% of pediatric AIDS cases. Nine per cent of all transfusion associated AIDS cases have occurred in children, although children represent less than 2% of transfusion recipients. This suggests that clinical progression from HIV infection to frank AIDS may be more rapid in a child who is infected via transfusion compared to an adult.

There are approximately 20 000 individuals in the United States with hemophilia and about one-half of these require infusion of clotting concentrates once a week. Although about 1% of AIDS cases occur in hemophiliacs, and about 6% of pediatric AIDS cases have hemophilia, it is clear from surveillance studies in these populations that between 50 and 90% of hemophiliacs have antibody to HIV (Levine 1985). Nonetheless, only 2% of these HIV seropositive individuals have developed frank AIDS, which suggests that the latent period is unusually long in this population or that some protective factor exists.

Prospective studies of hemophiliacs who received the recently developed heat treated factor concentrates suggest that HIV infection in hemophiliacs should be extremely uncommon in the future (Ragni et al 1987). Because commercial clotting factor concentrates are prepared from pools of plasma from several thousand different donors, they have frequently been associated with transmissable pathogens such as hepatitis and more recently HIV. Bear in mind though that, most single donor blood components, such as platelets, plasma, and red cells even when frozen and washed may also transmit HIV as well as hepatitis virus. There is strong evidence that albumin and immunoglobulin preparations which do not transmit hepatitis also do not transmit HIV.

Studies from the Centers for Disease Control have modelled the incubation period for transfusion associated AIDS with a mean of 20–30 months in children and 30–40 months in adults (range of 4–90 months in both groups) (Curran et al 1985, Berkman & Groopman 1988). Again, the reason for this age difference is not known, but neonates may be highly susceptible to HIV or the incubation period may be dose related with a proportionally larger inoculum of virus that contaminates a single unit delivered to a lower weight infant or child. These models are relatively crude and some investigators believe that the incubation period may actually be 5–15 years in adults.

Although the interval from transfusion of a contaminated unit to the development of clinical AIDS may be quite long, the interval to development of antibody to HIV is short. An experimental model of antibody seroconversion has been developed in the chimpanzee whereby detectable antibody to HIV is evident between 3 and 12 weeks after inoculation (Nara et al 1987). In several anecdotal situations such as cardiac surgery patients prospectively followed after receipt of anti-HIV positive blood, the seroconversion interval was 6–8 weeks (Marlink et al 1986). It appears though that the risk of seroconverting to HIV, and thus being infected with the virus, following receipt of a blood product from an HIV seropositive donor is 90–100% (Peterman et al 1985).

The clinical manifestations of HIV infection in patients who contracted the virus due to transfusion of blood products is similar in most regards to that of the other risk groups. The majority of individuals who seroconvert are entirely asymptomatic; some do develop an acute mononucleosis-like illness with pharyngitis, fever, generalized lymphadenopathy, headache, malaise, and an evenescent rash (Ho et al 1986). It appears that Kaposi's sarcoma and/or lymphoma are less common in transfusion-associated AIDS compared to homosexual men with AIDS.

Blood donors throughout the United States and Western Europe are currently tested for antibodies to HIV using an enzyme immunoabsorbent assay (ELISA) with antigens purified from disrupted whole virus. The majority of inaccurate tests appear to be false-positives, with a very low rate of false-negatives (Petricciani 1985). A confirmatory test utilizing an electrophoretic technique, the Western blot, detects antibodies to viral antigens of specific molecular weights (Groopman et al 1986b). A positive Western blot is generally taken as demonstrating antibodies to the core (p24) and envelope (gp41 and/or gp120) antigens. The American Red Cross has reported that over 5 million units were screened with 90% of the repeatedly reactive ELISA tests being false-positives. The false-negative population appears to be that of individuals who are in the process of seroconverting; they do not have demonstrable antibody but may have circulating antigen detectable by a new assay for the p24 core protein (Goudsmit et al 1987). It is currently debated whether all blood donors should be tested for viral antigen in addition to antibody, with estimates of detection of such donors being 1 in 250 000 to 1 in 1 million. More important is the need to test for HIV-2, which as stated previously is appearing in Western Europe. It is likely that ELISA assays will be formatted to detect antibody to both HIV-1 and HIV-2 in the near future (Couroce 1987).

The optimal interventions to prevent transfusion associated AIDS now include exclusion of potential donors with high risk behavior through a questionnaire administered at the time of donation; laboratory screening techniques for anti-HIV antibody; inactivation of HIV in the blood product; and autologous transfusion in cases of elective surgery. These measures have considerably altered the risk of transmitting HIV via blood products, and will ultimately entirely eliminate any risk as the screening assays are improved over their currently excellent performance.

VACCINE AND THERAPEUTIC DEVELOPMENTS

To date, attempts to develop a vaccine to protect against HIV infection have failed in the chimpanzee model. A number of approaches have been attempted including subunit vaccine based on inactivated native virus, recombinant envelope protein, or recombinant constructions of the envelope inserted into the vaccinia virus (Putney et al 1986, Zarling et al 1986, Lasky et al 1986). It is not clear at this time whether the failure to protect the chimpanzee is related to a high inoculum of virus used as the challenge, relatively weak humoral and/or cellular immune responses of the animal, or something fundamental to the biology of HIV. Despite these failures in the chimpanzee, several phase I studies in man have begun to assess the safety and immunogenicity of a subunit envelope glycoprotein vaccine or a vaccinia based construction. The results of these studies have not yet been obtained.

Strides have been made in identifying therapeutic agents to treat AIDS (Yarchoan & Broder 1987). Although there is no 'cure' for AIDS at this time, an antiviral nucleoside derivative, 3'3'-azidothymidine (AZT) has been shown in a randomized placebo controlled trial to both reduce the incidence of opportunistic infections and reduce mortality in patients with AIDS or advanced ARC (Fischl et al 1987, Richman et al 1987). AZT is a relatively myelotoxic drug resulting in significant anemia and dose limiting leukopenia. Its role in the therapy of less symptomatic HIV infected individuals is not yet defined. It is likely that the optimal therapy of HIV infection will include a combination or multiagent approach with drugs like AZT in addition to myeloprotective agents such as GM-CSF and perhaps immunomodulatory drugs (Groopman et al 1987b). It is clear that the upcoming years will be one of ongoing clinical trials of reverse transcriptase inhibitors such as AZT in combination with some of these other agents.

CONCLUSION

Pathogenic human retroviruses have emerged in the last decade with major importance for world health. Two distinct lymphotropic retroviruses, HIV-1 and HIV-2, have been identified and are associated with clinical AIDS. Several million individuals have been infected with these viruses in the United States, Western Europe and Africa, resulting in a pandemic with significant impact on health care resources. The hematologist should be aware of the basic biology and clinical aspects of HIV, since many of its clinical manifestations are hematological and therapy with antiviral agents to date has resulted in dose-limiting myelotoxicity. The optimal approach to AIDS, and a better understanding of its basic science and clinical scope, will necessitate a close relationship, with communication and cooperation, between the bedside physician and the laboratory researcher. Most importantly, an open mind should be kept in terms of the likelihood that all of the dimensions of AIDS, and certainly much of the biology of these pathogenic retroviruses, is yet to be described.

REFERENCES

Abrams D I, Chinn E K, Lewis B J, Volberding P A, Conant M A, Townsend R M 1984 Am J Clin Pathol 81 (1): 13
Allan J S, Coligan J E, Barin F et al 1985 Science (Wash DC) 228: 1091
Anderson K C, Gorgone B A, Marlink R G et al 1986 Ann Intern Med 105: 519–527
Arya S K, Gallo R C 1986 Proc Natl Acad Sci USA 83: 2209–2213
Barin F, McLane M F, Allan J S, Lee T H, Essex M 1985 Science 228: 1094–1096
Barre-Sinoussi F, Chermann J C, Rey F 1983 Science (Wash DC). 220: 868–871
Bender B S, Quinn T C, Lawley T J et al 1984 Clin Res 32: 511a
Berkman S, Groopman J 1988 Transfusion Med Reviews (in press)
Bloom E J, Abrams D I, Rodgers G M 1984 Blood 64 (1): 93a
Bloom E J, Abrams D I, Rodgers G 1986 JAMA 256 (4): 491–493
Bowen D L, Lane H C, Fauci A S 1985 Ann Intern Med 103: 704–709
Brettler D B, Brewster F, Levine P H et al 1987 Blood 70: 276–281
Canoso R T, Zon L I, Groopman J E 1987 Brit Journ Haematol 65: 495–498
Centers for Disease Control, US Department of Health and Human Services 1986 Ann of Intern Med 105: 234–236
Coffin J M 1986 Cell 46: 1–4
Cohen A J, Phillips T M, Kessler C M 1986 Ann Int Med 104: 175–7
Cooper D A, Gold J, Maclean P et al 1985 Lancet 1: 537–540
Couroce A M 1987 Lancet i: 1151
Curran J W, Lawrence D N, Jaffe H et al 1984 New Engl J Med 310: 69–75
Curran J, Morgan W, Hardy A, Jaffe H, Darrow W, Dowdle W R 1985 Science 229: 1352–1357
Dalgleish A G, Beverley P C L, Clapham P R et al 1984 Nature 312: 763–7
Donahue R E, Johnson M M, Zon L I, Groopman J E 1987 Nature 326: 200–203
Esteban, Emerman M, Guyader M et al 1987 EMBO 6: 3755–3760
Fauci A S, Masur H, Gelmann E P, Markham P D, Hann B H, Lane H D 1985 Ann Intern Med 102: 800
Fisher A G, Feinberg M B, Josephs S F et al 1986a Nature 320: 367–371
Fisher A G, Ratner L, Mitsuya H et al 1986b Science 233: 655–659
Fischl M A, Richman D D, Brieco M H et al 1987 New Engl J Med 317 (4): 185–191
Folks T M, Powell D, Lightfoote M et al 1986 J Exp Med 164: 280–290
Gallo'R, Salahuddin S, Popovic M et al 1984 Science 224: 200–203
Gartner S, Markovits P, Markovits D M, Kaplan M H, Gallo R C, Popovic M 1986 Science 233: 215–219
Gold J E, Haubenstock A, Zalusky R 1986 N Engl J Med 314 (19): 1252
Goudsmit J, de Wolf F, Paul D A et al 1986 Lancet ii:177–180
Groopman J E 1987 Semin Oncol 14: 1–6

Groopman J E, Sullivan J L, Mulder C et al 1986a Blood 67: 612–615
Groopman J E, Chen F W, Hope J A et al 1986b J Inf Dis 153: 736–742
Groopman J E, Mitsuyasu R T, DeLeo M J, Oette D, Golde D W 1987 N Engl J Med 317: 593–598
Hahn B H, Kong L I, Lee S W et al 1987 Nature 330: 184–186
Ho D D, Sarngadharan M G, Resnick L, Dimarzo-Veronese F, Rota T R, Hirsch M S 1985 Ann Intern Med 103 (6pt 1): 880–883
Inada Y, Lange M, McKinley G F et al 1986 AIDS Res 2: 235–238
Klatzmann D, Champagne E, Chamaret S et al 1984 Nature 312: 767–768
Kroegel C, Hess G, Meyer zum Buschenfelde K H 1987 Lancet i: 1150
Lasky L A, Groopman J E, Fennie C W et al 1986 Science 233: 209–212
Leiderman I Z, Greenberg M L, Adelsberg B R, Siegal F P 1987 Blood 70: 1267–1272
Levine P H 1985 Ann Int Med 103: 723–726
Levy J A, Hoffman A D, Kramer S M et al 1984 Science 225: 840–842
Levy J, Cheng-Mayer C, Dina D, Luciw P 1986 Science 232: 998–1001
Lifson J, Coutre S, Huang E, Engleman E 1986 J Exp Med 164: 2101–2106
Luciw P A, Cheng-Mayer C, Levy J A 1987 Proc Natl Acad Sci USA 84: 1434–1438
McDougal J S, Kennedy M S, Sligh J M et al 1986 Science 231: 382–385
McGinnis M H, Macher A M, Rook A H, Alter H J 1986 Transfusion 26: 405–407
McGrath K M, Spelman D, Barnett M, Kellner S 1986 Am J Hematol 23 (3): 239
Maddon P J, Littman D R, Godfrey M et al 1985 Cell 42: 93–104
Maddon P J, Dalgleish A G, McDougal J S et al 1986 Cell 47: 333–348
Marlink R G, Allan J S, McLane M F et al 1986 N Engl J Med 315: 1549
Martin P W, Burger D R, Caouette S et al 1986 N Engl J Med 314: 1577–1578
Mintzer D M, Real F X, Jovino L, Krown S E 1985 Ann Intern Med 102 (2): 200
Muesing M, Smith D, Cabradilla C et al 1985 Nature 313: 450–458
Muesing M A, Smith D H, Capon D M 1986 Cell 48: 691–701
Nicholson J K, Cross G D, Callaway C S, McDougal J S 1986 J Immunol 137 (1): 323
Ostrow D G, Solomon S L, Mayer K H, Haverkos H 1987 Amer Med Assoc, Chicago, IL
Outwater E, McCutchean J A 1985 Clin Res 33: 413a
Peterman T A, Jaffe H W, Feorino P M et al 1985 JAMA 254: 2913–2917
Popovic M, Sarngadharan M G, Read E, Gallo R C 1984 Science 224: 497–500
Rabson A B, Martin M A 1985 Cell 40: 477–480
Ragni M V, Winkelstein A, Kingsley L, Spero J A, Lewis J H 1987 Blood 70 (3): 786–790
Ratner L, Haseltine W, Patarca R et al 1985 Nature 313: 277–284
Redfield R R, Wright D C, Traumont E C 1986 N Engl J Med 314: 131–132
Richman D D, Fischl M A, Grieco M H et al 1987 N Engl J Med 317: 194–197
Salahuddin S Z, Rose R M, Groopman J E, Markham P D, Gallo R C 1986 Blood 68 (1): 281–284
Sanchez-Pescador R, Power M, Barr P et al 1985 Science 227: 484–492
Seligmann M, Chess L, Fahey J L et al 1984 N Engl J Med 20: 1286–1292
Seligmann M, Pinching A J, Rosen F S et al 1987 Ann Int Med 107: 234–242
Shaw G M, Hahn B H, Arya S K et al 1984 Science 226: 1165–1171
Smith D H, Byrn R, Gregory T et al 1987 Science (in press)
Sodroski J, Goh W C, Rosen C et al 1986 Nature 321: 412–417
Spivak J L, Bender B S, Quinn T C 1984 Am J Med 77 (2): 224
Spivak J L, Selonick S E, Quinn T C 1983 JAMA 250 (22): 3084
Stricker R B, Abrams D I, Corash L, Shuman M A 1985 N Engl J Med 313 (22): 1375
Toy P T, Reid M E, Burns M 1985 Am J Hematol 19 (2): 145–148
Treacy M, Lai, L, Costello C, Clark A 1987 Brit J Haematol 65: 289
Tucker J, Ludlam C A, Craig A et al 1985 New Engl J Med 314: 1115
Wall R A, Denning D W, Amos A 1987 Lancet i: 566
Walsh C M, Nardi M A, Karpatkin S 1984 N Engl J Med 311 (10): 635
Walsh C, Krigel R, Lennette E, Karpatkin S 1985 Ann Intern Med 103: 542–546
Ward J W, Deppe Da, Samson S et al 1987 Ann Intern Med 106: 61–62
Yarchoan R, Broder S 1987 N Engl J Med 316: 557–564
Zabury D, Bernard J, Leonard R et al 1986 Science 231: 850–853
Zarling J, Morton W, Moran T et al 1986 Nature 323: 344–346
Zon L I, Arkin C, Groopman J E 1987 Brit J Haematol 66: 251–256

16. Plasma cell disorders: recent advances in the biology and treatment

B. G. M. Durie

INTRODUCTION

The plasma cell disorders represent a collection of disease states, in which there is clonal expansion of the plasma cell population, which is either (a) non-malignant (e.g. monoclonal gammopathy of undetermined significance, primary systemic amyloidosis); or (b) malignant, resulting in such disorders as multiple myeloma and Waldenstrom's macroglobulinemia. Although the plasma cell disorders have similarities to other B cell states such as hairy cell leukemia, chronic lymphocyte leukemias and non-Hodgkin's lymphomas, the disorders involving the terminally differentiated plasma cell, are discretely different. The aetiology, epidemiology, pathogenesis and effects of treatment show patterns which are distinctive and characteristic of the plasma cell disorders.

Within the past five years, much new information has become available concerning the biology of the plasma cell. The molecular genetics of the immunoglobulin genes has been further elucidated (Tonegawa 1983, Arnold et al 1983, Yancopaulas & Alt 1986), as has the cellular immunology of T cells, B cells, plasma cells, and associated monocytes and macrophages (Gordon & Guy 1987, O'Garra et al 1988, Farham 1988). With the availability of recombinant DNA technology many important lymphokines and other cytokines have been well characterized and made available for in vitro and clinical testing (Kawano et al 1988, Tosato et al 1987, Kehrl et al 1987). It has thus become possible to dissect the complex interactions in the milieu of the bone marrow where the clonal expansion of plasma cells occurs. New knowledge about the role of the bone cells (osteoclasts and osteoblasts), and bone marrow myeloid cells has also been gathered (Hahn 1986, Garrett et al 1987).

In this chapter the impact of the new information upon the evaluation and treatment of patients with plasma cell disorders will be detailed. It should be noted that computer, medline searches for manuscripts dealing with plasma cell disorders, including multiple myeloma, plasmacytomas, amyloidosis, and related malignant and benign conditions, reveal in excess of 1000 manuscripts published for each calendar year. Therefore comments made and references used as a part of this chapter, reflect both the difficulty in reviewing this amount of data and the annotated perspective of the author. As yet advances in understanding the biology have not had a major effect upon treatment, or treatment outcome. However, now, for perhaps the first time, there are many new ideas about better approaches to management which give promise for improvements in the near future (Buzaid & Durie 1988).

Aetiology, epidemiology and pathogenesis

The exact cause or causes of human multiple myeloma are unknown. There are many reasons for this, including the fact that the disease is usually not familial and that it usually does not have an obvious environmental cause. In addition, extensive testing has failed to reveal a uniform specificity for the monoclonal protein used as a hallmark of this disease in 99% of patients. This latter point is perhaps the key question. Initial investigators sought to identify the foreign antigen specificity of myeloma monoclonal proteins. The surprising finding was that myeloma proteins almost never have a clear-cut specificity for foreign antigen (Pillot et al 1976). The simple conclusion was therefore that foreign antigen was not an immediate trigger for multiple myeloma and related plasma cell disorders. However, a more complete understanding of the mechanisms of interaction between foreign antigens, and B cells, T cells and macrophages, which has been accrued within the last few years, leads to the conclusion that the apparent lack of a relationship with a foreign antigen may be misleading (Cooke 1986).

A major breakthrough in understanding has been the observation that monoclonal proteins can have auto-reactivity, or are in fact antibodies against auto-antibodies (anti(anti) idiotypes) (Zouali et al 1984, Shoenfeld et al 1986, Davidson et al 1987). A preliminary assessment is therefore that myeloma cells may arise from B cells within the idiotypic (anti) idiotypic network of Jerne (1987). An important property of this network is that beyond level 3 in the hierarchy, the anti-idiotypic antibodies produced may lack specificity for the original stimulating antigen be it foreign or autologous (Raychaudhuri et al 1987). Although it is no more than a hypothesis at this point, the data are sufficient to consider that myeloma may rise from B cells within this hierarchal network. This is important because it allows one both to classify the types of defects which could give rise to expansion of monoclones and also lead to the development of therapeutic strategies which might inhibit the expansion of such monoclonal populations.

The general types of molecular and cellular defects which could give rise to myeloma, are summarized in Table 16.1. Considerable data, particularly from mouse plasma-

Table 16.1   Pathogenesis of myeloma: types of potentially causative defect

A	B
Inherited	Immunoglobulin gene defect
Acquired	Other gene regulatory defect
	Idiotype specific T cell deficiency
	Specific monocyte/macrophage abnormality
	Other associated abnormalities e.g. fibroblasts, myeloid stem cells, bone cells (osteoclast, osteoblast)

cytomas, indicate a variety of defects in immunoglobulin gene rearrangement in malignant plasma cells. Obviously from a theoretical standpoint, there is the potential for mutational abnormality in the variable and/or constant structural domains as well as defects in the promoter, leader, enhancer and switch regions (Yancopoulas & Alt 1986). Examples of molecular abnormalities noted include: isotope switching by DNA deletion in B malignancies (Gorzillo et al 1987); a mutation in the 3' flanking region, resulting in decreased transcription of alpha heavy chain (Gregor & Morrison 1986); mutations which stabilize myc transcripts and enhance transcription in two mouse plasmacytomas (Bauer et al 1986), and the observation of rapid induction of plasmacytomas in mice by Pristane when Avian v-myc and a defective raf oncogene have been inserted (Potter et al 1986). Another observation of interest was the transcription of unrearranged immunoglobulin lambda variable region in a kappa producing myeloma (Picard & Schaffer 1984). Just which molecular defect or defects are crucial in the majority of myelomas remain to be determined. However, it is likely that in addition to molecular changes within the plasma cells, defects in T cells and/or monocytes or macrophages are also important. For example the presence of peritoneal macrophages enhances myeloma induction in BALB/C mice (Potter 1973). Such defects may be inherited or acquired, and may be related to the pathogenesis of myeloma in individual patients. It is of particular interest that although small amounts of interleukin-6 (IL-6) are produced by plasma cells, IL-6 is produced predominantly by macrophages and fibroblasts (Tosato et al 1987). Any defect leading to enhanced production of IL-6 could increase plasma cell growth and differentiation.

SPECIFIC AETIOLOGIC FACTORS IN MYELOMA

In most patients, the specific factors resulting in the molecular and/or cellular defects causing multiple myeloma are never determined. In a few instances, there is a familial tendency or a striking environmental factor such as radiation exposure or perhaps Aleutian mink disease exposure (Shoenfeld et al 1982, Blattner 1980, Blattner 1981). However, these cases are rare, and in most instances the cause is unknown. Nonetheless, there are a number of new observations which relate to possible aetiology and pathogenesis. First of all, two case control studies have evaluated the potential role of chronic immunologic stimulation (Linet et al 1987, Cohen et al 1987). No statistically significant associations were found between multiple myeloma and prior history of medical conditions believed to cause prolonged stimulation of the immune system, other immune disorders, allergy related disorders or lymphoid tissue surgery. It must be emphasized that although these studies seem to make it unlikely that broad antigenic stimulation, to which many individuals are exposed, is aetiologic in myeloma, they do not exclude the possibility that antigenic stimulation by a critical antigen in a given individual could trigger an anomalous immune response. Numerous studies have indicated associations between myeloma and several occupations and types of environmental exposure (Alberts & Lanier 1987, Nandakumar et al 1986, Gallagher et al 1983, Cuzick et al 1983, Guidotti et al 1982, Leech et al 1983, Kyle & Greip 1983, Sharpira & Carter 1986, Bourguet et al 1987, Pearce et al 1985, Leech et al 1985, Turesson et al 1984). The occupations showing highest risk have included farming, woodworking, leather work, commercial painting industries and cosmetology (in women). Specific exposures correlated with an increased risk of myeloma include pesticides, plastics, rubber, petroleum products and asbestos. Further case control and epidemiologic studies are necessary to further clarify specific causative factors. Other important points are that myeloma is more common in blacks and also increases in frequency with age (Blattner 1980, Blattner et al 1981). This latter aspect has been associated with the loss of immune regulatory functions which occurs with age. However, this may or may not be the critical factor. Evaluation of specific immunologic, and molecular defects observed in patients with the potential effects of various environmental hazards should prove to be especially revealing.

MONOCLONAL GAMMOPATHY OF UNDETERMINED SIGNIFICANCE (MGUS) AND SMOLDERING MYELOMA

The general categories of disorders classified as MGUS (Kyle 1987), smoldering myeloma (Kyle & Griepp 1980), and related diseases include: true (idiopathic) MGUS; non-myelomatous B cell malignancies, with associated monoclonal proteins (CLL, lymphomas, and hairy cell leukemia), and also monoclonal protein abnormality associated with miscellaneous hematologic disorders, such as pernicious anemia, pure red cell aplasia, or other diseases such as connective tissue diseases, neurologic diseases, and disease conditions in which there is specific symptomatic antibody activity associated with the monoclonal gammopathies, such as coagulation factor activity, calcium binding, or nephrotoxicity (e.g. Fanconi's syndrome) (Kyle & Griepp 1982). Primary systemic amyloidosis which occurs in the absence of overt multiple myeloma, is also a special category of monoclonal gammopathy.

Diagnosis of MGUS

MGUS per se refers to a group of conditions in which a monoclonal protein is found in the serum and/or the urine, in the absence of a clear cut causative disease state (Kyle 1987). Perhaps the best way to consider MGUS is as a pre-myelomatous condition. Approximately 30% of patients develop myeloma or a related condition after 10 years. Major interest has focused upon the methods, to distinguish between MGUS and early multiple myeloma. Obviously, this is an important clinical point.

Several studies have indicated that the plasma cell labeling index is a reliable diagnostic test to distinguish between MGUS and smoldering myeloma on the one hand, and active multiple myeloma, on the other hand, particularly when differentiation is difficult, using standard clinical criteria (Durie et al 1980, Latreille et al 1982, Greipp & Kyle 1983, Boccardoro et al 1984). Of particular interest, is the description of a new 2-color immunofluorescence slide procedure that uses antibodies, 5-bromo-2-deoxyuridine (BU-1) and cytoplasmic immunoglobulin to label plasma cells from patients with monoclonal gammopathies (Greipp et al 1987, Durie 1987b). This BU-1 method for S phase measurement, has several advantages over traditional tritiated thymidine labeling, including availability to the practicing physician, the ease and speed of performance, and the lower cost. A particular advantage is the ability to have results within four hours of bone marrow processing. An additional important point, which may prove to have clinical relevance, is the evaluation of the labeling indices of peripheral blood B cells, which have the same cytoplasmic chain isotype, as the monoclonal protein (Witzig et al 1988). Testing of blood samples (which are obviously easier to obtain than bone marrow), has shown that peripheral B cell labeling indices can be used as a measure of disease activity in patients with monoclonal gammopathies. In a recent study (confirming prior observations (Durie 1986)), significantly higher labeling indices in peripheral blood B cells were noted in patients with relapsing disease or in patients who relapsed within six months of the study.

Both MGUS and smoldering myeloma (see definitions in Tables 16.2 and 16.3), are usually asymptomatic and require no treatment. However, since 30% of the

Table 16.2   Criteria for monoclonal gammopathy of undetermined significant (MGUS), indolent myeloma and smoldering myeloma (stage I or IIA)

MGUS
1. Monoclonal gammopathy
2. M component level
    a. IgG ≤3.5 g/dl
    b. IgA ≤2.0 g/dl
    c. BJ ≤1.0 g/24 h
3. Bone marrow plasma cells <10%
4. No bone lesions
5. No symptoms

Indolent myeloma: criteria as for myeloma (Table 3) with the following limitations:
1. No bone lesions or only limited bone lesions (≤3 lytic lesions); no compression fractures
2. M component levels
    a. IgG <7 g/dl
    b. IgA <5 g dl
3. No symptoms or associated disease features
    a. Performance status >70%*
    b. Hemoglobin >10 g/dl
    c. Serum calcium: normal
    d. Serum creatinine <2.0 mg/dl
    e. No infections

Smoldering myeloma: criteria as for indolent myeloma with additional constraints:
1. There must be no demonstrable bone lesions
2. Bone marrow plasma cell ≥10% ≤30%

* Karnofsky scale

Table 16.3   Criteria for diagnosis of multiple myeloma

Major criteria
  I. Plasmacytoma on tissue biopsy
 II. Bone marrow plasmacytosis with >30% plasma cells
III. Monoclonal globulin spike on serum electrophoresis exceeding 3.5 g/dl for IgG peaks or 2.0 g for IgA peaks, ≥1.0 g/24 h of κ or λ light chain excretion on urine electrophoresis in the absence of amyloidosis

Minor criteria
a. Bone marrow plasmacytosis with 10% to 30% plasma cells
b. Monoclonal globulin spike present, but less than the levels defined above
c. Lytic bone lesions.
d. Normal IgM <50 mg, IgA <100 mg, or IgG <600 mg/dl

  Diagnosis will be confirmed when any of the following features are documented in symptomatic patients with clearly progressive disease.
  The diagnosis of myeloma requires a minimum of one major + one minor criterion of three minor criteria that must include a + b.
1. I + b, I + c, I + d (I + a not sufficient)
2. II + b, II + c, II + d
3. III + a, III + c, III + d
4. a + b + c, a + b + d

patients eventually develop multiple myeloma, there is interest in what causes this transition in some patients, but not others. The focus is the intrinsic biology of the plasma cells and the potential regulatory mechanisms involved. Obviously if inhibition of mutational change in the plasma cells and/or enhanced immunosurveillance of the idiotypic clone could be accomplished, this would be a major achievement.

PRETREATMENT EVALUATION OF MULTIPLE MYELOMA: PROGNOSTIC FACTOR ANALYSIS AND STAGING

For many years it has been recognized that patients with multiple myeloma can have a very variable clinical course, with an anticipated survival duration from a few weeks to in excess of 10 years (Durie 1986). Several clinical staging systems have been developed with patients classified into good and poor risk groups (Bataille et al 1986). In general these classification systems have worked well both for individual counselling, for large single institutions, and cooperative group studies. However, in recent years there has been a proliferation of modified staging systems and proposals to introduce new systems of classification. This has made it more difficult to routinely classify patients and compare results of the published data.

The use of serum β_2 microglobulin

There is now a need to simplify and standardize prognostic factor classification and staging. It is therefore of some importance that a large number of studies from several countries, have documented the utility of pretreatment serum β_2 microglobulin, as a powerful, reliable, pretreatment prognostic factor in patients with multiple myeloma (Bataille et al 1982, 1983, 1984, 1986, Brenning et al 1986, Child & Kushwaha 1984, Child et al 1983, Cuzick et al 1985, Garewal et al 1984, Norfold 1979). There are several advantages in using serum β_2 microglobulin. Firstly, methods of measurement can be standardized and cross tested. Pretreatment serum samples can be sent to a central laboratory for testing. Subjective evaluations such as assessment of performance status, bone pain and involvement on skeletal X-rays, can be avoided. Although serum β_2 microglobulin is a very powerful, single prognostic factor, several combinations of factors have been proposed, including the combination of serum β_2 microglobulin and serum albumin. This type of classification is shown in Table 16.4. In

Table 16.4   New staging system: stratification of myeloma patients according to serum β2M and serum albumin level

Stratification stage	No. of patients*	Number alive (%)	Median survival** (months)
I. Low risk Sβ2M <6 µg/ml, and SA >3.0 g/dl	81	63 (78)	55
II. Intermediate Sβ2M ≥6 µg/ml, but SA >3.0 g/dl	46	19 (41)	19
III. Poor risk SA ≤3.0 g/dl	18	6 (33)	4

an analysis of previously untreated patients, the combination of serum albumin, with serum β_2 microglobulin allowed excellent separation of patients into good, intermediate and poor risk categories (Bataille et al 1986). Obviously this is only one of several types of classifications which are possible, depending upon the goals of the staging system.

As attempts are made to select different treatment for patients in different prognostic categories, slightly different group separations are required. For example, patients with poor risk myeloma under age 40 can be considered candidates for high-dose chemotherapy plus bone marrow transplantation. Conversely, patients with good risk myeloma over the age of 65, can be considered for much simpler approaches to therapy including for example glucocorticoids. Serum β_2 microglobulin levels combined with age, serum albumin or other factors can therefore offer the possibility of both well standardized and flexible approaches to prognostic factor classification and staging.

Other prognostic evaluation in multiple myeloma

Although serum β_2 microglobulin is very useful, there are other considerations, for example the bone marrow histology, the cellular morphology of bone marrow plasma cells and many other laboratory and clinical features have been shown to have prognostic importance (Bartl et al 1982, Fritz et al 1984, Griepp et al 1985). For particular institutions, and combined with new protocols for treatment evaluation, such parameters may be usefully employed, particularly to identify very high-risk multiple myeloma, or exclude from study patients who have gammopathies not requiring therapy. In recent years, the use of computerized tomography and magnetic resonance imaging, has proved especially useful in evaluating patients with multiple myeloma, to document the presence or absence of bone disease, and to evaluate the extent and distribution of bone disease (Fruehwald et al 1988, Ludwig et al 1987, Schreiman et al 1985, Solomon et al 1984). Magnetic resonance imaging is especially useful in detecting myeloma associated focal bone lesions, as well as soft tissue disease adjacent to the spine.

Ideally the best classification (as a basis for treatment) would include measurement of intrinsic drug sensitivity (Durie et al 1983). Although colony assay and other systems have been used to determine in vitro drug sensitivity, unfortunately it has not proved possible to routinely apply this approach. However, recent investigations of parameters such as CALLA positivity (Durie & Grogan 1985), serum LDH levels (Barlogie et al 1988) and the measurement of P-glycoprotein (Durie & Dalton 1988), suggest it may be possible to identify patients most likely to be resistant to standard approaches both at diagnosis and subsequently.

TREATMENT SELECTION IN MULTIPLE MYELOMA

If multiple myeloma is confirmed by the presence of at least the minimal criteria for diagnosis of multiple myeloma (Durie 1986), as outlined in Table 16.3, the next step is to select the induction regimen, and proceed with therapy. For the first time in many years, there have been several promising reports of new approaches to treatment in multiple myeloma both for patients with previously untreated disease (Durie et al 1986b), as well as for patients at later stages (Buzaid & Durie 1988).

Induction therapy

As far as induction approaches, there is an accumulation of evidence indicating that combination chemotherapy imparts some survival benefit in multiple myeloma. Unfortunately the impact on survival is not of major proportion (e.g. survival of 20% at 8 years with combination therapy versus 10%, with simpler regimens). Also no patient subset appears to be cured. Nonetheless, the benefit is real. The evidence consists of a few studies that show definite survival benefit which is statistically significant with combination approaches v. simpler regimens (Harley et al 1979, Salmon et al 1983, Durie et al 1986b, MacLennan et al 1987), as well as a larger number of other studies, essentially all of which show either the equivalent results with combination approaches or slightly better results with the combination approach (Woodruff 1981, Sporn & McIntyre 1986). Considering all the published data in total, one has to conclude, that combination therapy is at least as good as, and in many instances slightly or significantly better than, simpler treatment. Conversely, there are many reports of very poor survival with single agent regimens.

Table 16.5   Comparison of SWOG studies 7927/28 and 7704/05 (Durie et al 1986b)

Protocol	Treatment	Median survival (months)	P values	No. of patients
SWOG 7927/28	VMCP-VBAP	48	0.008	200
	VCP	29		
SWOG 7704/05	Combination chemotherapy induction	42	0.021	275
		23		
	MP			

Total number of patients in 7927 plus 7704 studies was >700. In exact comparison of VMCP/VBAP alone, versus VCP 200 patients were involved. (Durie et al 1986b. Reproduced with permission from Journal of Clinical Oncology)

Two Southwest Oncology Group studies have shown clear survival benefit for combination therapy (Durie et al 1986b, Salmon et al 1983). The results are summarized in Table 16.5. The combined results in a total of >700 patients show that the VMCP/VBAP (or a similar regimen) was significantly superior to melphalan/prednisone or vincristine/cytoxan/prednisone. This survival benefit was seen in patients with stage I, II and III disease. The most substantial survival benefit was in patients with stage IIIA disease. The longer term follow up of the 1979 study (SWOG 79/2728) shows that the survival benefit is sustained out to the 8 year time point with 30% v. 15% of patients being alive at 6 years; 20% v. 10% of patients being alive at 8 years (Table 16.6). Although this is not a dramatic survival benefit, it is a significant and sustained survival benefit with the VMCP/VBAP regimen, which is extremely well tolerated, and does not impart significant additional morbidity.

Table 16.6   Long-term survival on SWOG study 7704/05 (Durie et al 1986b)

| | Percentage survival | |
	6 years	8 years
VMCP/VBAP*	15	10
MP	30	20

* See Durie et al 1986b

The largest study to support this observation, has yet to be reported in full (MacLennan et al 1988), but was presented in a preliminary fashion at the recent Blenheim Palace meeting on multiple myeloma. At this meeting, the preliminary results of a recent MRC study were outlined, indicating a survival benefit for the ABCM regimen over melphalan/prednisone ($P < 0.004$ for difference). The ABCM regimen which incorporates the drugs used in the VMCP/VBAP regimen (excluding the vincristine), produced results almost identical to those which have been achieved with the VMCP/VBAP regimen.

It is important to discuss why all the other studies which have attempted to assess the benefit for combination approaches have not shown significant survival improvement. Firstly, some reported studies involved very small numbers of patients and can only be construed as preliminary. In most instances, however, this is clearly not the case, and there are other explanations. Although analysis of all published data is controversial, three major points are evident:

1. The incorporation of adriamycin along with alkylating agents as an integral part of the treatment regimen seems to be critical (e.g. as VCMP/VBAP or ABCM). Studies without this feature show lesser benefit;
2. Although patients are classified in terms of routine staging and a variety of other parameters, unfortunately all of the features which can influence the treatment outcome have not been controlled for in many published studies, including serum β_2 microglobulin, age, serum albumin and several other prognostic factors. It is clear from very recent analyses (MacLennan et al 1986), that significant variations in these parameters could account for major differences in survival outcome;
3. The third important point is that glucocorticoids are a critical component in therapy. A recent dose intensity analysis showed that the dose of prednisone administered, clearly influenced survival duration (Belch et al 1987). A number of combination regimens with good survival outcome (e.g. with M_2 protocol) have included $\geqslant 14$ days of prednisone along with alkylating agents and other drugs. Several reports have suggested a role of glucocorticoids in the treatment of multiple myeloma for over 20 years (Buzaid & Durie 1988). The exact response rates and impact upon survival duration have been remarkably poorly evaluated. However, recent studies have documented substantial responses, even in patients with refractory disease (Buzaid & Durie 1988). In fact, high dose or alternate day glucocorticoids may represent the single most efficacious approach, in refractory disease. The overall response rate in the various studies is approximately 40% in previously treated patients (Alexanian et al 1986, Perren et al 1986). If anything, response is more likely in refractory patients, rather than patients who have been initially sensitive to standard chemotherapy regimens. This may relate to the cellular biology of the drug resistant cells. Recent studies using the 8226 doxorubicin resistant sublines, have indicated remarkable sensitivity to glucocorticoids, alpha interferon and tumor neurosis factors, as well as a variety of other biologic agents (Croghan et al 1988). Steroids must therefore be considered as a more integral part of induction regimens.

The VAD regimen

One of most important new approaches in myeloma therapy in recent years has been the introduction of the VAD, 4 day infusion chemotherapy schedule (Barlogie et al 1984, Monconduit et al 1986a,b, Sheehan et al 1986). In patients with relapsing disease, response rates have ranged from 38% to 73%. In patients with resistant disease, the response rates range from 32% to 50%. There are several important features of the VAD regimen, beyond the fact that it does have significant activity in patients with multiple myeloma. Firstly, it represents a relatively expensive approach which requires placement of a central catheter and very close follow up and monitoring. The need for a central catheter results in significant additional risks including both clotting problems at the site of the venous insertion, as well as the risk of infection. The risk of infection is particularly important in view of the overall toxicity observed with the VAD regimen. The intensive steroid program accentuates the risk of infection. In the Barlogie et al series, 11 of 29 patients, had episodes of fever (nine of which required hospitalization). An infectious agent was identified in eight patients, four cases of pneumonia, two cases of Gram-positive bacteremia (probably catheter related), and two cases of Gram-negative sepsis. Four patients had viral infections, including herpetic esophagitis, herpes zoster infection, and cytomegalovirus infection with hepatitis. Similar toxicity has been observed by other investigators. Infectious complications as well as other steroid related complications have necessitated reduction in steroid dosages in many patients, and the addition of prophylactic antibiotics, as a standard approach. Several modified VAD regimens have been utilized with some incorporating potentially less toxic steroid schedules.

A recent innovation involving the VAD regimen (and similar regimens), has been the addition of verapamil (Durie & Dalton 1988, Gore et al 1988), in an effort to overcome resistance to adriamycin and vincristine. This is based on in vitro and preliminary clinical data, indicating efficacy for this approach (Durie & Dalton 1988). The general concept is that verapamil (a calcium channel blocker) binds to P-glycoprotein in the cell wall of the drug resistant myeloma cells and interferes with the active efflux of adriamycin and vincristine from drug resistant cells. This active efflux in drug resistant cells is the process associated with decreased DNA effects, and decreased efficacy of these drugs. Obviously, it may prove possible to identify more potent calcium channel blocking or related compounds which can more effectively interfere with this drug resistance mechanism. However, in the interim, preliminary results with verapamil are encouraging and further studies are ongoing.

High dose chemotherapy with and without transplantation

A major new area of investigation has been the use of high dose chemotherapy alone, or with autologous or allogeneic bone marrow transplantation (Buzaid & Durie 1988). Overall results have recently been reviewed (Buzaid & Durie 1988). In summary, it is clear that high dose chemotherapy regimens, such as high dose melphalan, have very high objective response rates in previously treated as well as refractory patients with multiple myeloma (McElwain & Powles 1983, Kantarjian et al 1984, Lenhard et al 1984, Barlogie et al 1986, Selby et al 1987). The major disappointment is that although even apparent complete responses have been observed, relapse supervenes in most if not all of the patients treated in this fashion. The major hope is that additional manoeuvres such as the purging of autologous bone marrow, the addition of total body irradiation (TBI) to high dose melphalan or the use of another alkylator, and/or other high dose chemotherapy or preparative regimens, may make an impact and convert the complete responses into sustained complete remissions.

Besides the initial very important observations with high dose melphalan alone (McElwain & Powles 1983, Selby et al 1987), the two most noteworthy recent studies are results with the high dose melphalan plus TBI with autologous marrow rescue and the results of the European (allogeneic) bone marrow transplant study group

(Barlogie et al 1987, Gahrton et al 1987). Barlogie et al recently reported that when total body irradiation was combined with high dose melphalan and autologous bone marrow transplantation the response rate increased and lasted longer. Of seven patients treated who failed standard alkylating agent regimens and VAD chemotherapy, six achieved a response (defined as >75% decrease in the M component), with a median response duration of 15 months. Five patients remain alive and well without further therapy from 2–21 months later. However, the use of autologous bone marrow transplantation carries two major problems. Firstly, multiple myeloma is difficult to eradicate from bone marrow, even with the high dose chemotherapy and radiation. Secondly, to date, bone marrow purging in this disease has not been completely successful. Newer purging techniques may prove to be better.

The initial results with allogeneic bone marrow transplantation are as yet preliminary, but are extremely interesting (Osserman et al 1982, Gahrton et al 1987, Ozer et al, in press). The special problems with the allogeneic transplant patients include graft v. host disease, plus the severe age restrictions which apply with patients with multiple myeloma, a disease predominantly of the elderly. Nevertheless, from the European Cooperative Group for bone marrow transplantation results, it is clear that sustained remissions can be achieved even in patients with previously refractory disease. Whether any of these will be converted into long-term remission or cures, remains to be seen. It is disappointing that late relapses have been noted in the longest survivors. But so far, relapsing patients have apparently not required retreatment. The experience represents an important step forward in the attempt to develop potentially curative therapy for a subset of patients with multiple myeloma.

Interferon treatment in multiple myeloma
Within the last five years, many studies have evaluated the role of interferons in multiple myeloma (Cooper & Welander 1986, Costanzi et al 1985, Mandelli et al 1987, Oken et al 1988, Quesada et al 1986). Although the response rate of only approximately 20% in previously treated patients was less than hoped for, more recent results with combined interferon plus chemotherapy for induction, and using alpha 2b interferon as a maintenance therapy for patients following chemotherapy induction, are really very promising. With short initial follow up, reports so far document increased response rates and prolonged remissions, without a clear translation into prolongation of survival duration. Early results in the Italian Cooperative Group study, utilizing alpha 2b interferon v. zero in maintenance are particularly encouraging. Further follow up in this study, plus two other ongoing studies by the National Cancer Institute of Canada, and the Southwest Oncology Group, will provide more complete information as to the benefit of interferon maintenance in myeloma.

GENETICS OF MULTIPLE MYELOMA

Until recently very little was known about the frequency and types of chromosomal abnormalities in multiple myeloma. However, three human studies have just been published which give a good perspective of the major changes (Dewald et al 1984, Gould et al 1988, Lewis & MacKenzie 1984). The studies all emphasize that the cytogenetic abnormalities in multiple myeloma are non-random. In the study from the Mayo Clinic (Dewald et al 1984), a chromosomally abnormal clone was found in 18% of the patients with newly diagnosed myeloma, in 63% of patients with aggressive disease and in 40% of the patients with plasma cell leukemia. Survival in the newly diagnosed patients was significantly shorter for those with abnormal chromosomes who had a median survival of approximately six months. In this study, the most common abnormal chromosomes were chromosomes 1, 11 and 14. In this series, the single most common anomaly was an 11;14 translocation. Among patients who subsequently developed preleukemia, or acute non-lymphocytic leukemia, the most commonly observed abnormalities involved chromosome number 7. The other studies also emphasize abnormalities of chromosomes 1, 11 and 14, but also noted abnormalities of chromosome 3, 5, 7, 8, 9, 13, 15 and 16. In one of the other studies, 46% of 115 evaluable patients had an abnormal karyotype, plus there was an association between t(8;14) (q24;q32) and IgA protein isotype (Gould et al 1988). Although clonal evolution does occur in myeloma, the changes found in later disease are usually also observable in early disease. The many differences in cytogenetic abnormalities as compared to Hodgkin's disease, non-Hodgkin's lymphomas, and other related lymphoproliferative diseases have been emphasized.

In addition to the information gained from direct clinical specimens; there has been considerable new information from multiple myeloma cell lines, including molecular studies carried out in both the human and mouse systems (Barletta et al 1987, Durie et al 1985, 1986a, Gazdar et al 1986, Grace et al 1982, Grogan et al 1987, Jernberg et al 1987, Koeppler et al 1987, Korsmeyer & Walkmann 1984, Lokhourst et al 1987, Potter et al 1987, Przepiorka et al 1984). In one study, chromosomal analysis from bilateral malignant pleural effusions (from a patient with very fulminant multiple myeloma) demonstrated in vivo karyotypic heterogeneity, with the evolution of new subclones. In another established culture, it was possible to evaluate rearranged cellular myc proto-oncogene. In two other studies, the human calcitonin gene was located to the short arm of chromosome number 11, and in another three permanent leukemia cell lines were established which actually produced calcitonin (Koeppler et al 1987, Przepiorka et al 1984).

Two studies have recently addressed what might be the nature of the major stem cell, or proliferative cell, in patients with multiple myeloma (Grogan et al 1987, Lokhourst et al 1987). In one study, cells with a novel pre-B phenotype appeared to be the major proliferative and stem cell compartment. In the other study so called 'spot' cells (areas of focal immunoglobulins) were identified as a potential major growth subpopulation. Other studies have emphasized the potential for oncogene abnormalities, particularly as associated with immunoglobulin gene rearrangement. A very recent observation has also raised the possibility that abnormalities of chromosome 6, which occur in myeloma may be associated with increased TNFβ secretion and associated osteoclast activation and bone disease (Durie et al 1986a). This will be discussed under bone disease.

THE IMMUNOBIOLOGY OF MULTIPLE MYELOMA

Studies of various immunologic parameters in patients with multiple myeloma continue to be very popular. Major areas of interest have been the immunoregulation of the myeloma clone or clones, potential defects in the associated T cell subsets, and the mechanisms of effects on the normal B cell clones with the resultant hypogammaglobulinemia (Mellsted et al 1984, Pilarski et al 1984, 1985a,b, Wearne et al 1985a,b, 1987). The published data are rather conflicting. Nonetheless, it is clear that B cells which are part of the myeloma clone do occur in the peripheral blood and that they have a variety of abnormal features. As mentioned above, the labeling index of circulating B cells correlates with disease activity and the presence of CALLA positive B lymphocytes in the peripheral blood, correlates highly with a *lack* of light chain isotype suppression (LCIS), which is characteristic of progressive myeloma. Several studies have evaluated the frequency and significance of LCIS, which has been noted to be a characteristic feature of stable disease, both pretreatment and in the plateau phase, post-therapy. These findings provide strong evidence for immunoregulation in multiple myeloma, the details of which require further exploration.

Other studies have also expanded the knowledge of the immune phenotype of the malignant plasma cell. Although plasma cells lack surface idiotype bearing immunoglobulin molecules, they can express or be induced to express a variety of the antigens, including myelomonocytic and T cell antigens (Durie et al 1988, Epstein et al 1988, Grogan et al 1988, Rossi et al 1988, Spier et al 1988). The aberrant expressions of antigens, such as CALLA, myelomonocytic antigens, and T cell antigens is in general, a very poor prognostic factor. However, in a very recent study, the expression of CALLA in bone marrow cells in myeloma, was found to correlate with responsiveness to very aggressive therapy, such as VAD. It may turn out that, as with other types of malignancy, the most aggressive subtype, may also turn out to be the one most likely to respond with very aggressive therapy. Further long term studies with correlation to treatment outcome are required.

Bone disease in myeloma

The most characteristic feature of multiple myeloma, which distinguishes it from other B cell malignancies, is the bone involvement which manifests as discrete multiple lytic bone lesions, although there is sometimes a diffuse osteoporotic pattern (Mundy & Bertolini 1986). Several recent studies have evaluated the mechanisms which result in bone destruction in multiple myeloma (Mundy & Bertolini 1986). The major conclusion is that the bone disease results from a combination of both osteoclast activation and inhibition of osteoblast function. The latter inhibition of osteoblast function, which is particularly important in the production of the punched out lytic lesions, is poorly understood. However, there is new exciting information about mechanisms which can activate the osteoclast. Several substances are known to be capable of activating the human osteoclast (Mundy & Bertolini 1986), including TNFβ (lymphotoxin), TNFα, interleukin 1, and probably interleukin 6. In a recent study it was shown that in myeloma cell supernatants (specifically supernatants from myeloma cells from patients with very aggressive myeloma bone disease), the production of TNFβ, or lymphotoxin, correlated with the activation of osteoclast function (Garrett et al 1987). Increased production of lymphotoxin (or a related lymphokine or lymphokines) is therefore important in some patients with aggressive bone disease. An additional ancillary observation is that the gene for TNFβ, is located on chromosome number 6.

Chromosomal abnormalities involving chromosome number 6 have been observed in a significant percentage of patients with multiple myeloma, in association myeloma, in association with very aggressive bone disease (Durie et al 1986a). Obviously these various preliminary observations represent only the start of investigations which may further elucidate the very complex biology of bone disease in multiple myeloma.

One of the goals of investigating the biology of bone disease in multiple myeloma is to develop better treatment for bone disease and hypercalcemia (Bataille et al 1981, Binstock & Mundy 1980, Ryzen et al 1985, Witte et al 1987). Several studies have addressed this issue, including the use of calcitonin, glucocorticoids and diphosphonates. Although calcitonin, particularly when combined with glucocorticoids, can be very effective treatment for hypercalcemia, it is not effective in all patients or the effect may be short lived. The effects of intravenous diphosphonates are therefore of particular interest. Clodronate is the most promising agent which is currently commercially available in Europe, but not in the United States (Witte et al 1987). Editronate is available in the US as an alternative (Ryzen et al 1985).

OTHER SPECIAL FEATURES OF MULTIPLE MYELOMA

Multiple myeloma is a disease which has a variety of special features in addition to the bone disease, including the unusual predilection for infection, neurologic complications and a tendency for both plasma cell leukemia and extramedullary disease in some instances (Durie 1987a). An additional special aspect is primary systemic amyloidosis which may or may not be associated with frank multiple myeloma. These various areas are dealt with in the following sections.

Infections in multiple myeloma

Little has been added to the traditional knowledge of infections as they occur with patients with multiple myeloma (Durie 1987a). Recent observations relate primarily to the infections which occur in patients who have been aggressively treated and/or are doing poorly (Espersen et al 1984). Infections which occur in patients who are neutropenic for other reasons have been observed, including both Gram-negative and Gram-positive infections. The presence of associated renal impairment is a particular risk factor. In patients receiving corticosteroids, there is a significant risk of both fungal and viral infections, as seen in other situations (Barlogie et al 1984, Monconduit 1986a,b, Sheehan et al 1986). Patients with multiple myeloma receiving bone marrow transplantation are particularly susceptible to infectious complications (Barlogie et al 1986, 1987, Gahrton et al 1987, Kantarjian et al 1984, Lenhard et al 1984, McElwain & Powles 1983, Osserman et al 1982, Selby et al 1987, Ozer et al 1988).

With the recent observations that high dose i.v. gammaglobulin may decrease infections early in the disease course in patients with chronic lymphocytic leukemia, there is renewed interest in this aspect for patients with multiple myeloma. Several studies have either been initiated or are planned in this area. The lack of efficacy of pneumococcal vaccination has again been noted (Birgens et al 1983).

Renal disease in myeloma

Renal complications are common in patients with multiple myeloma and are due to a variety of mechanisms, including direct plasma cell infiltration, the deposition of monoclonal components of different sizes and types, deposition of immune complexes, and functional renal disorders for which there is no clear cut anatomic lesion in the renal parenchyma (Durie 1987a). A recent review highlighted several of the important elements of renal dysfunction in myeloma (Rota et al 1987). In a series of 34 patients, renal failure proved to be totally reversible in seven patients, and partially reversible in nine, although improvement in renal function was often very slow, taking in excess of three months. Patients with reversible renal failure clearly had improved survival duration. Considering the triggering events (though the importance of dehydration and hypercalcemia were reaffirmed), the role of non-steroidal anti-inflammatory agents, as an important precipitating factor in renal failure was noted (Rota et al 1987). Indomethacin induced renal failure, has previously been reported (Paladini & Tonazzi 1982). Another important point was the correlation between the renal biopsy findings and the potential for complete recovery, which was observed only in the absence of global tubular atrophy and interstitial damage. The presence of cast induced tubular obstruction did not influence the outcome. There was no particular relationship between the iso-electric points of the light chains and the outcome. Because a subset of patients can clearly do well, there is justification for aggressive management in such patients, including dialysis and chemotherapy treatment. In addition, the acute reduction of serum and urine light chain concentrations with plasmapheresis can certainly be considered. Although several small studies have documented benefit from plasmapheresis, a large randomized study is necessary to show the true effects of plasmapheresis used in this setting. Because of the volume and other hemodynamic effects from plasmapheresis, caution must be observed to avoid further acute renal insult.

Three other brief reports document long-term survival in patients with multiple myeloma and renal failure (Briefel et al 1983, Barton & Vaziri 1984, Boyce et al 1984), using dialysis alone, and in one patient treated with renal transplantation. In the latter instance, a 41-year-old man received a cadaver kidney which functioned well for three-and-a-half years, following transplantation, while the myeloma was in a chemotherapy induced remission. It was clear in this instance and in other selected cases, cadaveric renal transplantation can be a useful option for patients with multiple myeloma.

Neurologic complications in myeloma
Reports have confirmed the fact that neurologic involvement in multiple myeloma is relatively common, and that there can indeed be rather complex effects on both the peripheral and central nervous system which are usually difficult to treat (Durie 1987a). The peripheral neuropathies of different types which occur, can be quite debilitating and especially refractory to conventional therapeutic approaches. Involvement of the central nervous system is usually an extremely poor prognostic sign. In the pathogenesis of neurologic dysfunction in patients with monoclonal gammopathies, the direct specificity of monoclonal proteins for nerve tissue has been reaffirmed. The potential for sequence homology between viral and/or bacterial proteins and nerve tissue, is of particular interest (Oldstone, 1987). The end result of this phenomenon is that antibody produced against the virus or bacterial infection can cross-react with nerve tissue. This phenomenon is clearly a component of some types of neurologic dysfunction in patients with monoclonal protein. In both benign monoclonal gammopathies, as well as overt multiple myeloma, similar types of peripheral neuropathy, have been reported (Noring et al 1982).

Extramedullary plasmacytomas

Extramedullary plasmacytomas have been increasingly recognized in recent years. There has been a major increase in reports detailing involvement by extramedullary plasmactomas in virtually every location throughout the body, ranging from reports of a solitary plasmacytoma of the foot (Newcott 1987) to multiple plasmacytomas with hemorrhage in the brain (Husain et al 1987). Almost any organ can sometimes be involved. The major site of extramedullary plasmacytomas remains the head and neck area (Kapadia et al 1982), particularly in the oral pharynx and in the upper airway system. In this location, as in other sites (Bataille 1982, Bataille & Sany 1981, Foucar et al 1983, Greenberg et al 1987, Knowling et al 1983, Loh 1984, Sidani et al 1983, Wiltshaw 1987), local extramedullary plasmacytomas tend to remain localized and surgical resection followed by local radiation represent the standard approach to treatment. Most extramedullary plasmacytomas are locally curable with a combination of surgery plus radiation, in a range of 3000–5000 rads. Since the typical pattern of spread is first to the regional lymph nodes, comprehensive radiation to the related lymph node systems is usually recommended, particularly in the head and neck areas (Knowling et al 1983). Although the majority of plasmacytomas are radiosensitive, some are remarkably radiation resistant and progress despite even higher doses of radiation and chemotherapeutic approaches. However, in sensitive patients, there can be a remarkable lack of disease progression in patients who receive adequate local therapy at the time of first evaluation. 70% of patients with extramedullary plasmacytomas of this type remaining alive and progression free at 10 years (Knowling et al 1983). In one study, the median survival for initially localized extramedullary plasmacytomas was over 100 months.

For patients with more widespread plasmacytomas, there are several important points to keep in mind. Firstly, the drug sensitivity pattern is quite different to that normally observed in traditional multiple myeloma (Wiltshaw 1987). Complete regressions with even single agent chemotherapy have been reported. In one study 12 of 20 patients (60%) with disseminated disease, had significant bone healing in response to chemotherapy. Failure with one chemotherapy agent was followed by significant and prolonged response with alternate back up treatment. This potential for excellent and sustained benefit from systemic therapy must be pursued aggressively, particularly in young patients. This is especially true in view of the normally well-preserved marrow reserves, and the normal renal function in these patients. It is reasonable to anticipate that high-dose chemotherapy with bone marrow transplantation or GM-CSF rescue could be a curative approach in a major subset of this category of patient.

Plasma cell leukemia

Plasma cell leukemia is an important subcategory of plasma disorder, very similar to multiple myeloma, but discreetly different (Kosmo & Gale 1987). The major characteristic feature is the increased number of plasma cells in the peripheral blood and the extensive organ infiltration which occurs. Plasma cell leukemia is defined as a malignant proliferation of plasma cells involving the blood stream with >20% of the differential white blood cell count, consisting of plasma cells, with an absolute plasma cell count of $>2 \times 10^9/l$. The various details of this entity have recently been reviewed (Kosmo & Gale 1987). Suffice it to say, that this generally represents a very poor prognosis subset of patients. Of interest, some patients responding to treatment can do so with relatively simple approaches, including single agent melphalan. Of interest, a sustained remission was recently reported in a patient treated with high doses of melphalan (Montecucco et al 1986). Conversely, the majority of patients are refractory to treatment, even with aggressive combination approaches. Further studies are needed to address the optimal approach to therapy for this group of patients.

Non-secretory myeloma

Non-secretory myeloma is an important subset because it is a type which is often difficult to diagnose because of the lack of a serum or urine monoclonal protein marker (Dreicer & Alexanian 1982, Smith et al 1986, Durie 1987a, Rubio-Felix et al 1987). Although many early reports of patients with this entity noted very advanced bone disease and other features of myeloma at the time of presentation (because of suspected delay in making the diagnosis), nonetheless, most reports document a survival similar to that observed with secretory myeloma of a similar stage. In contrast, two recent reports indicate that non-secretory myeloma may actually be a good prognosis subgroup. In one report from the MD Anderson Hospital, 29 consecutive patients with non-secretory myeloma are reported as a subset of 615 consecutive records reviewed (Dreicer & Alexanian, 1982). In this instance, the 29 patients (4.7%) with non-secretory myeloma frequently presented with low pre-treatment tumor mass (69% v. 24% for the average myeloma case). This earlier disease stage seemed to contribute a somewhat better than average median survival duration of 39 months in these non-secretory patients. In a report of 13 cases from the University Hospital in Manchester, England, involving a series of 172 consecutive multiple myeloma cases, a significantly longer survival was again noted with a median of 46 months in patients with non-secretory myeloma, v. 21 months of patients with typical secretory myeloma (Smith et al 1982). The features of non-secretory myeloma in this study included a high incidence of neurologic features at presentation, minimal lytic bone disease, and a lower median percentage of plasma cells in the marrow, plus a lower incidence of hypogammaglobulinemia. The medan survival of non-secretors with minimal lytic bone disease was remarkably iong at 74 months, compared to 21 months for those with extensive bone disease. The superior survival of the non-secretors is attributed to the earlier presentation, possibly as a result of the tendency to form symptomatic local tumors in bone. Immunoperoxidase evaluation of stored plasma cell tissue indicated that monoclonal immunoglobulin was detectable at the cellular level in all but one instance.

The overall assessment is that non-secretory myeloma basically has a similar cellular biology to secretory myeloma. The major clinical exception is that patients (certainly at large treatment centers), tend to present earlier, with lower tumor burden, therefore have a better survival duration from the time of diagnosis.

PRIMARY SYSTEMIC AMYLOIDOSIS

Systemic amyloidosis can be divided into two categories, both of which are diseases in which the amyloid deposition results from immunoglobulin derived fragments, usually light chain (Durie 1987a). In first category, primary systemic amyloidosis occurs in the absence of features of overt multiple myeloma. In this instance, the associated disease essentially has an MGUS pattern. In the second category, primary systemic amyloidosis occurs in association with otherwise typical multiple myeloma. Both types have been evaluated as part of an extensive review conducted at the Mayo Clinic (Kyle et al 1986). Some of the major prognostic factors are detailed in Table 16.7. The most negative prognostic factor was the presence of congestive

Table 16.7   Effect of individual variables on survival curves*

During first year		After first year	
Variable	P(log-rank)	Variable	P(log-rank)
Congestive heart failure	0.0001	Hemoglobin	0.0022
Urinary light chain	0.0001	Serum creatinine	0.0023
Hepatomegaly	0.0002	Myeloma	0.0037
Weight loss (amount)	0.0055	Monoclonal serum protein	0.0370
Electrophoretic pattern of albumin in urine	0.0108	Urinary light chain	0.0540
Elevated serum creatinine (>2.0 mg/dl)	0.0270		
Sex	0.0320		
Myeloma	0.0420		

* Reproduced with permission from Kyle et al 1986.

heart failure associated with cardiac involvement at the time of presentation. This occurred in approximately 25% patients at the time of diagnosis, and was associated with a median survival time of four months. Using sophisticated multi-variate regression analysis techniques, it was possible to evaluate the predictors of survival for both the first year and subsequent years. Obviously congestive heart failure was a dominant factor within the first year; beyond the first year important prognostic factors contributing to poor survival, were the severity of the anemia, the degree of renal insufficiency, and the presence or absence of overt multiple myeloma. In patients without overt multiple myeloma, treatment is extremely difficult in that only a small percentage of patients respond to melphalan, prednisone or related regimens which are used to treat multiple myeloma. However, since occasional patients can have significant benefit, this approach should at least be considered for all patients when first seen. Conversely for patients with additional overt myeloma, rather surprisingly, the prognosis can be significantly better and very similar to the survival, which can be anticipated with multiple myeloma with a similar disease stage at presentation (Fielder & Durie 1986). Therefore similar approaches to treatment are recommended and dramatic resolution of associated amyloid can occur in association with myeloma response.

Several recent reports have evaluated the diagnostic approach for cardiac amyloidosis (Sekiya et al 1984, Wahlin et al 1984, Gertz et al 1987). Techniques which have been utilized and proposed, include cross-sectional echocardiographic computed tomography, MRI scanning and technetium 99 paraphosphate bone scanning. Although all can show features of cardiac amyloidosis, computed tomography and NMR scanning may be useful in difficult cases. Interesting recent reports document the response of primary hepatic amyloidosis to melphalan and prednisone, as well as resolution of acquired Factor X deficiency on treatment of amyloidosis with melphalan and prednisone therapy (Camoriano et al 1987, Gertz & Kyle 1986). A recent report documents the utility of abdominal fat aspiration in the diagnosis of amyloidosis (Duston et al 1987).

MACROGLOBULINEMIA

Unfortunately, since earlier reports (MacKenzie & Fudenberg 1972, Durie 1987a), there are few new data to report concerning macroglobulinemia. However, one important review evaluated the spectrum of IgM monoclonal gammopathy in 430 patients (Kyle & Garton 1987). The important point was that the IgM monoclonal gammopathy can occur in the presence of a variety of B cell processes, including what is traditionally known as Waldenstrom's macroglobulinemia, but in addition, in association with non-Hodgkin's lymphomas, chronic lymphocytic leukemia and other B cell malignancies. Other recent reports included a careful review of the bone marrow histology in Waldenstrom's macroglobulinemia (Bartl et al 1983), plus an assessment of detectable circulating monoclonal B lymphocytes in the peripheral blood in patients with Waldenstrom's macroglobulinemia, correlating with the disease status (Smith et al 1983). There was also a useful review of the details of the peripheral neuropathy, which occur in Waldenstrom's macroglobulinemia with a correlation between the clinical manifestations and the detailed immunology (Dellagi et al 1983).

Table 16.8   Summary of important new observations in myeloma*

Biology
— Immunoglobulin genes: normal function and pathology
— Cellular immunology of T/B cells and monocytes
— Availability of lymphokines: IL 1–6; especially IL-6 (plasma cell growth/differentiation factor) and TNFβ (lymphotoxin, a powerful OAF)
— Knowledge of anti idiotypic myeloma protein specificity
— Information on occupations/exposures associated with myeloma

Therapy
— Use of BU-1 labelling index method
— Use of nuclear magnetic resonance imaging
— Identification of CALLA positive myeloma (poor prognosis)
— Introduction of β_2 microglobulin staging systems
— Introduction of VAD (infusion) chemotherapy
— Introduction of high-dose chemotherapy with BMT
— Benefit of α_{2b} interferon in induction and maintenance

* See discussion in appropriate subsections

MISCELLANEOUS ASSOCIATIONS WITH MONOCLONAL GAMMOPATHIES

Three recent reports document the effect of monoclonal paraproteins upon the coagulation system, including a monoclonal paraprotein with specificity for platelet glycoprotein IIIa (DiMinno et al 1986), and an IgA protein which inhibited factor VIII von Willebrand factor (Gralnick et al 1985), and a myeloma protein which had spontaneous anti-thrombin activity (Gabriel et al 1987). Other recent publications of interest included: an association between multiple myeloma and Kaposi's sarcoma (Geerling 1984); the characterization of monoclonal cryo IgG (Podell et al 1987); the association of fibrosis in the bone marrow in some patients with plasma cell dyscrasia (Vandermolen et al 1985), and cytogenetic abnormalities in four cases of alpha chain disease (Berger et al 1986).

CONCLUSIONS

Within the last five years or so, there has been considerable progress both in understanding the plasma cell disorders and applying new information to improve treatment. Table 16.8 summarizes some of the major new points. The details of these various aspects are discussed within the text. Hopefully within the next five years there will be even more dramatic breakthroughs in understanding with associated development of more effective therapy.

REFERENCES

Alberts S R, Lanier A P 1987 JNCI 78: 831–837
Alexanian R, Barlogie B, Dixon D 1986 Ann Intern Med 105: 8–11
Arnold A, Cassman J, Bakhshi A, Jaffe E S, Waldmann T A, Korsmeyer 1983 N Engl Med 309: 1593–1599
Barletta C, Pelicci P G, Kenyon L C, Smith S D, Dalla-Favera R 1987 Science 235: 1064–1967
Barlogie B, Smith L, Alexanian R 1984 N Engl Med 310: 1353–1356
Barlogie B, Hall R, Zander A et al 1986 Blood 67: 1298–1301
Barlogie B, Alexanian R, Dicke K et al 1987 Blood 70: 869–872
Barlogie B, Alexanian R, Fritsche H 1988 JCO Proce 7: 230
Bartl R, Frisch B, Burkhardt R et al 1982 Br J Haematol 51: 1–15
Bartl R, Frisch B, Mahl G et al 1983 Scand J Haematol 31: 359–375
Barton C H, Vaziri N D D 1984 J Arti Organs 7: 317–318
Bataille R 1982 Clin in Haematol 11: 113–122
Bataille R, Sany J 1981 Cancer 48: 845–851
Bataille R, Tenoudji-Cohen M, Rossi J-F 1981 Delmans & Meunier. Correspond 170
Bataille R, Magub M, Grenier J et al 1982 Eur J Cancer Clin Oncol 18: 59–66
Bataille R, Durie B G M, Grenier J 1983 Br J Haematol 55: 439–447
Bataille R, Grenier J, Sany J 1984 Blood 63: 486–476
Bataille R, Durie B G M, Grenier J, Sany J 1986 JCO 4: 80–87
Bauer S R, Piechaczyk M, Marcu K B, Nordan R P, Potter M, Mushinski J F 1986 Curr topics in Microbio Immunol 132: 339–344
Belch A, Palmer M, Hanson J 1987 (abstract), 70: 826
Berger R, Bernheim A, Tsapis A, Brouet J C, Seligmann M 1986 Cancer Genet Cytogenet 322: 219–223
Binstock M L, Mundy G R 1980 Annals of Int Med 93: 269–272
Birgens H S, Epersen F, Hertz J B, Pedersen F K, Drivsholm A 1983 Scand J Haematol 30: 324–330
Blattner W A 1980 Progress in Myeloma 1–65 (Amsterdam)
Blattner W A, Blair M A, Mason T J 1981 Cancer 48: 2547–2554
Boccadoro K M, Gavarotti P, Fossati G et al 1984 Br J Haematol 48: 689–696
Bourguet C, Grufferman S, Delzell E, DeLong E, Cohen H 1976 Soc Epidemiol Res (abstract), p 483
Boyce N W, Holdsworth S R, Thomson N M, Atkins R C 1984 Aust NZ J Med 14: 676–677
Brenning G, Simonsson B, Kallander C, Ahre A 1986 Br J Haematol 62: 85–93
Briefel G R, Spees E K, Humphrey R L, Hill G S, Saral R, Zachary J B 1983 Surgery 574–585, April
Buzaid A C, Durie B G M 1988 JCO 6: 889–1085
Camoriano J K, Griepp P R, Bayer G K, Bowie E J 1987 N Engl J Med 316: 1133–1135
Child J A, Kushwaha MRS 1984 Hematol Oncol 2: 391–401
Child J A, Crawford S M, Norfolk D R et al 1983 Br J Cancer 47: 111–114
Cohen H M, Bernstein R J, Grufferman S 1987 Am J Hematol 24: 119–126
Cooke A 1986 Plasma Ther Transfus Technol 6: 161–170
Cooper R M, Welander C H 1986 Sem in Oncol 13: 334–340
Costanzi J J, Cooper R, Scarffe J H 1985 JCO 3: 654–659
Croghan M, Durie B G M, Vela E et al 1988 (in press)
Cuzick J, Velez R, Doll R 1983 Int J Cancer 32: 13–19
Cuzick J, Cooper E H, McLennan I C M 1985 Br J Cancer 52: 1–6
Davidson A, Preud'Homme J L, Solomon A, Chang M D Y, Beebe S, Diamond B 1987 J Immunol 138: 1515–1518
Dellagi K, Dupouey P, Brouet J C et al 1983 Blood 62: 280–285
Dewald G W, Kyle R A, Hicks G A, Greipp P R 1985 Blood 66: 380–386
DiMinno G, Coraggio F, Cerbonne A M et al 1986 J Clin Invest 77: 157–164
Dreicer R, Alexanian R 1982 Am J Hematol 13: 313–318

Durie B G M 1986 Sem in Onc 13: 300–309
Durie B G M 1987a Curr Hematol 3: 239–285
Durie B G M 1987b Mayo Clin Proc 62: 1057–1058
Durie B G M, Dalton W S 1988 Br J Haematol 68: 203–206
Durie B G M, Grogan T M 1985 Blood 66: 229–232
Durie B G M, Salmon S E, Moon T E 1980 Blood 55: 364
Durie B G M, Young L A, Salmon S E 1983 Blood 61: 929–934
Durie B G M, Vela E, Baum V et al 1985 Blood 66: 548–555
Durie B G M, Baum V E, Vela E, Mundy G R 1986a (abstract), Blood 68: 710
Durie B G M, Dixon D O, Carter et al 1986b JCO 4: 1227–1237
Durie G B M, Grogan T M, Speir C et al 1988 (in press)
Duston M A, Skinner M, Shirahama T, Cohen A S 1987 Am J Med 82: 412–414
Epstein J, Barlogie B, Katxmann J, Alexanian R 1988 Blood 71: 861–856
Espersen F, Birgens H S, Hertz J B, Drivsholm A 1984 Scand J Infect Dis 16: 169–173
Fielder K, Durie B G M 1986 Am J Med 80: 413–418
Foucar K, Raber M, Foucar E, Barlogie B, Sandler C M, Alexanian R 1983 Cancer 51: 166–174
Fritz E, Ludwig H, Kundi M 1984 Blood 63: 1072–1079
Fruehwald F X J, Tscholakoff D, Schwaighofer B et al 1988 Invest Radiol 23: 193–199
Gabriel D A, Carr M E, Cook L, Roberts H R 1987 Am J Hematol 25: 85–93
Gahrton G, Tura S, Flesch M et al 1987 Blood 69: 1262–1264
Gallagher R P, Spinelli J J, Elwood J M, Skippen D H 1983 Br J Cancer 48: 853–857
Garewal H, Durie B G M, Kyle R A et al 1984 J Clin Oncol 2: 51–57
Garrett R, Durie B G M, Nedwin G et al 1987 New Engl J Med 526–532
Gazdar A F, Oie H K, Kirsch I R, Hollis G F 1986 Blood 67: 1542–1549
Geerling S 1984 S Med J 77: 931–932
Gertz M S, Kyle R A 1986 Mayo Clin Proc 61: 218–223
Gertz M A, Brown M L, Hauser M F, Kyle R A 1987 Arch Intern Med 147: 1039–1044
Gordon J, Guy G R 1987 Immunol Today 8: 339–344
Gore M E, Selby P H, Millar B, Maitland J, McElwain T J 1988 ASCO abstract 882, Proc 7: 228
Gorzillo G V, Cooper M D, Kubagawa H, Landay A, Burrows P D 1987 J Immunol 139: 1326–1335
Gould J, Alexanian R, Goodacre A, Pathak S, Hecht B, Barlogie B 1988 Blood 71: 453–456
Grace L C, Ong S, Keath E J, Piccoli S P, Cole M D 1982 Cell 31: 443–452
Gralnick H R, Flaum M A, Kessler C M, Zimbler H, Coller B S 1985 Br J Haematol 59: 149–158
Greenberg P, Parker R G, Fu Y S, Abemayor E 1987 Am J Clin Oncol 10: 199–204
Gregor P D, Morrison S L 1986 Mol Cell Biol 6: 1903–1916
Greipp P R, Kyle R A 1983 Blood 62: 166–171
Greipp P R, Raymond N M, Kyle R A, O'Fallon W M 1985 Blood 65: 305
Greipp P R, Witzig T E, Gonchoroff N J et al 1987 Mayo Clin Proc 62: 969–977
Grogan T M, Durie G G M, Lomen C et al 1987 Blood 70: 932–942
Grogan T M, Durie B G M, Spier C M, Richter L, Vela E 1988 (in press)
Guidotti S, Wright W E, Peters J M 1982 Am J Int Med 3: 169–171
Hahn T J 1986 Hosp Prac, Aug 15
Harley J B, Pajak T F, McIntyre O R et al 1979 Blood 54: 13–22
Husain M M, Metzner W S, Binet E F 1987 Neurosurg 20: 617–623
Jernberg H, Nilsson K, Zeck L, Lutz D, Nowotny H, Scheirer W 1987 Blood 69: 1605–1612
Jerne N K 1987 Ann Immunol (Paris) 125C: 373
Kantarjian H, Dreicer R, Barlogie B et al 1984 Eur J Cancer Clin Oncol 20: 227–231
Kapadia S B, Desai U M A, Cheng V S 1982 Medicine 61: 317–329
Kawano M, Hirano T, Matsuda T et al 1988 Nature 332: 83–85
Kehrl J H, Alvarez-Mon M, Delsing G A, Fauci A S 1987 Science 238: 1144–1146
Knowling M A, Harwood A R, Bergasagel D E 1983 JCO 4: 255–262
Koeppler H, Pflueger H, Knap W, Havemann 1987 Br J Haem 65: 405–409
Korsmeyer S J, Walkmann T A 1984 J Clin Immunol 4: 1–11
Kosmo M A, Gale R P 1987 Sem in Hematol 24: 202–208
Kyle R A 1987 Am J Med 64: 814
Kyle R A, Garton J R 1987 Mayo Clin Proc 62: 719–731
Kyle R A, Greipp P R 1980 N Engl J Med 302: 1347
Kyle R A, Greipp P R 1982 N Engl J Med 306: 564
Kyle R A, Greipp P R 1983 Cancer 51: 735–739
Kyle R A, Greipp P R, O'Fallon W M 1986 Blood 68: 220–224
Latreille J, Barlogie B, Johnston D, Drewinko B, Alexanian R 1982 Blood 59: 43
Leech S H, Bryan C F, Elston R C, Rainey J, Bickers J N, Pelias M Z 1983 Cancer 51: 1408–1411

Leech S H, Brown R, Schanfield M S 1985 Cancer 55: 1473–1476
Lenhard R E, Oken M M, Barnes J M et al 1984 Cancer 53: 156–1460
Lewis J P, MacKenzie M 1984 Hematol Oncol 2: 307–317
Linet M S, Harlow S D, McLaughlin J K 1987 Cancer Res 47: 2978–2981
Loh H S 1984 Br J Oral & Maxillofacial Surg 22: 216–224
Lokhourst H M, Boom S E, Bast B J E G et al 1987 J Clin Invest 79: 1401–1411
Ludwig H, Fruchwald F, Tscholakoff D, Neuhold A, Rasoul S, Fritz E 1987 Lancet ii: 364–366
Mandell F, Tribalto M, Catonetti M et al 1987 (abstract), 70: 842
McElwain T J, Powles R L 1983 Lancet 2: 822–824
MacKenzie M R, Fudenberg H H 1972 Blood 39: 874–889
MacLennan I, Kelly K, Crockson R A et al Blenheim Palace Myeloma Workshop Proc 1988 Hemat Oncology (in press)
Mellsted H, Holm G, Bjorkholm M 1984 Adv Cancer Res 41: 257–289
Monconduit M, Bauters F, Najman A 1986a Blood 68: 240a
Monconduit M, LeLoet X, Bernard J F et al 1986b Br J Haematol 63: 599–601
Montecucco C, Riccardi A, Merlini G, Ascari E 1986 Br J Haematol 62: 525–527
Mundy G R, Bertolini D R 1986 Sem Onc 13: 291–299
Nandakumar A, Armstrong B K, DeKlerk N H 1986 Int J Cancer 37: 223–226
Newcott E P 1987 J Am Podia Med Assoc 77: 187–190
Norfold D, Child J A, Cooper E H et al 1979 Br J Cancer 39: 510–515
Noring E O L, Hast R, Kjellin K G, Knutsson E, Siden A 1982 Br J Haematol 51: 531–539
O'Garra A, Umland S, De France T, Christiansen J 1988 Immunol Today 9: 45–54
Oken M M, Kyle R A, Greipp P R, Kay N E, Tsiatis A, O'Connell M J 1988 ASCO Proc 7: 225
Oldstone M B A 1987 Cell 50: 819–820
Osserman E F, DiRe L B, DiRe J et al 1982 Acta Haematol (Basel) 68: 215–223
Ozer H, Han T, Nussbaum-Blumenson A et al (in press)
Paladini G, Tonazzi C 1982 Acta Haemat 68: 256–260
Parham P 1988 Immol Today 68
Pearce N E, Smith A H, Fisher D O 1985 Am J Epidem 121: 225–237
Perren T J, Selby P J, Biddle E K et al 1986 Proc Am Soc Clin Oncol (abstract), 5: 158
Picard D, Schaffer 1984 Embo J 3: 3031–3035
Pilarski L M, Mant M J, Ruether B A, Belch A 1984 J Clin Invest 74: 1301–1306
Pilarski L M, Mant M J, Ruether B A 1985a Blood 66: 416–422
Pilarski L M, Ruehter B, Mant M J 1985b J Clin Invest 75: 2024–2029
Pillot J, Creau-Goldberg N, Gonzales Y 1976 J Immunol 117: 2042–2044
Podell D N, Packman C H, Maniloff J, Abraham G N 1987 Blood 69: 677–681
Potter M 1973 Multiple Myeloma and Related Disorders 1: 153–194
Potter M, Wax J, Mushinski E et al 1986 Curr Topics in Microbiol Immunol 132: 40–43
Potter M, Mushinski J F, Mushinski E B 1987 Reports 787 Feb
Przepiorka G, Baylin S B, McBride W O, Testa J R, Bustros A D, Neikin B D 1984 Biochem Biophys Res Commun 120: 493–499
Quesada J R, Alexanian R, Hawkins M et al 1986 Blood 67: 275–278
Raychaudhuri S, Saeki Y, Chen J J, Kohler H 1987 J Immunol 139: 3902–3910
Rossi J F, Durie B G M, Duperray C 1988 Cancer Res 48: 1213–1216
Rota S, Mougenot B, Baudouin B et al 1987 Medicine 66: 126–137
Rubio-Felix D, Giralt M, Giraldo M P et al 1987 Cancer 59: 1847–1852
Ryzen E, Martodam R R, Troxell M et al 1985 Arch Inter Med 145: 449–452
Salmon S E, Haut A, Bonnet J et al 1983 JCO 1: 453–461
Schreiman J S, McLeod R A, Kyle R A, Beabout J W 1985 Radiology 154: 483–496
Sekiya T, Foster C J, Isherwood I, Lucas S B, Kahn M K, Miller J P 1984 Br Heart J 51: 519–522
Selby P J, McElwain T J, Nandi A C et al 1987 Br J Haematol 66: 55–62
Shapiro R, Carter A 1986 Cancer 58: 206–209
Sheehan T, Judge M, Parker A C 1986 Scan J Haematol 37: 425–428
Shoenfeld Y, Shaklai M, Berlinerk S et al 1982 Post Med J 58: 12–16
Shoenfeld Y, Ben-Yehuda O, Naparstek Y et al 1986 J Clin Immunol 6: 195–204
Sidani M S, Campos M M, Joseph J I 1983 Am Soc Colon & Rectal Surg 26: 182–187
Smith B R, Robert N J, Ault K A 1983 Blood 61: 911–914
Smith D B, Harris M, Gowland E, Chang J, Scarffe J H 1986 Hematol Oncol 4: 307–313
Solomon A, Rahamani R, Seligsohn U, Ben-Artzi F 1984 Skeletal Radiol 11: 258–261
Spier C, Durie B G M, Grogan T M 1988 (in press)
Sporn J R, McIntyre R O Sem in Oncol 13: 218–325
Tonegawa S 1983 Nature 14: 575–580
Tosato G, Seamon K B, Godman N D et al 1987 Science 239: 502–504

Turesson I, Zettervall O, Cuzick J, Waldenstrom J G, Velez R 1984 N Engl J Med 310: 7, 421–424
Vandermolen L, Rice L, Lynch E C 1985 Am J Med 79: 297–302
Wahlin A, Olofsson B-O, Eriksson A, Backman C 1984 Acta Med Scand 215: 189–192
Wearne A, Joshua D E, Kronenberg H 1985a Australian and NZ J Med 15: 629–633
Wearne A, Joshua D E, Kronenberg H 1985b Br J Haematol 54: 485–489
Wearne A, Joshua D E, Brown R D Kronenberg 1987 Br J Haematol 67: 39–44
Wiltshaw E 1987 Cancer Chemother Pharmacol 1: 167–175
Witte R S, Koeller J, David T E et al 1987 Arch Inter Med 147: 937–939
Witzig T E, Gonchoroff N J, Katzmann J A, Therneau T M, Kyle R A, Greipp P R 1988 JCO 6: 1041–1046
Woodruff R 1981 Cancer Treatment Reviews 8: 225–270
Yancopoulos G D, Alt F W 1986 Ann Rev Immunol 4: 339–368
Zouali M, Fine J M, Eyquem A 1984 Eur J Immunol 14: 1085–1089

Index

ABCM regimen, 312, 313
ABL proto-oncogene, 132, 134, 135
ABVD regimen, 220, 221, 222, 223
Acquired immunodeficiency syndrome (AIDS)
  GM-CSF trial, 13, 238, 298
  therapeutic agents, 301–302
  see also HIV
Activated protein C (APC), 275, 278, 279–280
Acute lymphoblastic leukaemia (ALL), 134–135
  bone marrow transplantation, 164–166, 173
  de-regulated tyrosine kinase, 36–37
  ras genes, 39
Acute myeloblastic leukaemia (AML), 113–114,
  115, 134–135
  bone marrow transplanation, 163–164, 173
  de-regulated tyrosine kinase, 36–37
  ras genes, 38
Acylated plasminogen-streptokinase activator
  complex (Apsac), 267, 268–269, 271
Adult T cell leukaemia/lymphoma, 109, 185, 186,
  194
Allopurinol, 199
Aluminium toxicity, 93
Anaemias, aquired transfusion-dependent, 85, 87,
  89
Angioimmunoblastic lymphadenopathy, 112
Antibody diversity generation, 99–100
α_2-Antiplasmin, 266
Ataxia-telangiectasia, 118, 126–127, 128
Autografting in CML, 131, 139
3'3'-Azidothymidine (AZT), 301

BACOP regimen, 232
B-ALL (acute lymphoblastic leukaemia), 124
B cell antigen receptor, 99
  antibody diversity generation, 99–100
  Ig gene rearrangements, 100–101
B cell development, 186–188
bcl-1, 124, 194
bcl-2, 123–124, 194
B-CLL (chronic lymphoblastic leukaemia),
  111–112, 124, 182, 194
BCR gene, 133, 134, 135
Blood products, HIV and, 299–301
Bone marrow transplantation
  antibody dependent cell mediated cytotoxicity
  recovery, 159
  antigen presenting cell recovery, 159, 160
  autologous, 169–173, 223–224, 235–237
  B cell recovery, 159, 160
  GM-CSF and, 12, 13, 14

Bone marrow transplantation (*contd*)
  graft failure, 148–150, 157–158
  Hodgkin's disease, 223–224, 235–237
  IL2 deficiency, 159, 162–163
  leukaemia, 136–137, 141–150, 153–157,
  163–167, 169–173
  MHC matched unrelated donors, 148, 168–169
  mismatched family donors, 167–168
  multiple myeloma, 314, 315
  natural killer cell regeneration, 159, 160
  non-Hodgkin's lymphoma, 230–231
  post-transplant humoral immunity, 161–162
  post-transplant immunosuppression, 155–156
  T cell recovery, 158–159, 160
  T lymphocyte depletion, 144–146, 156–157,
  159–161
  thalassaemia, 67
  timing, 142–144, 154, 155
B-prolymphocytic leukaemia (B-PL), 184
Burkitt's lymphoma, 39, 116, 122–123, 234
Busulphan, 136, 137, 138, 140, 142, 148, 157, 164,
  169, 200

c-fms genes, 8, 9
c-fos proto-oncogenes, 23, 28, 30
Chelators, 67, 75–79, 83–88
  clinical applications, 93–95
  clinical trials, 88–89
  iron metabolism and, 79–83
  natural, 76
  oral, 67, 75, 89–93, 94, 95
  synthetic, 76–77, 78–79
Chlorambucil, 199, 200, 201, 202, 205–206, 230
Cholyhydroxamic acid, 88
CHOP regimen, 230, 232, 234
Chorion villus sampling, 66
Chromosomal translocations, 116–118, 132–133,
  192–193, 316
  B cell neoplasia, 122–124
  T cell neoplasia, 124–129
Chronic granulocytic leukaemia (CGL)
  blast crisis, ras genes and, 39
  bone marrow transplantation, 167
  de-regulated tyrosine kinase, 35–36
  Philadelphia chromosome, 35, 36
Chronic lymphocytic leukaemia (CLL), 179–206
  animal models, 195
  autoimmunity, 190
  B cell differentiation, 187–188
  chromosome abnormalities, 192–193
  classification, 182–186

Chromic lymphocytic leukaemia (*contd*)
de-regulated tyrosine kinase, 36–37
hypogammaglobulinaemia, 190, 198
immune features, 179–182, 188–190
natural killer cells, 189–190
oncogenes, 193–194
pathogenesis, 195–196
staging, 196–198
T lymphocytes, 189–190
transformation, 191–192
treatments, 198, 199–205
viruses and, 194–195
Chronic myeloid leukaemia (CML), 116, 131–150
accelerated phase, 132, 140–141, 143
blastic transformation, 131–132, 140–141, 143
bone marrow transplantation, 136–137, 141–150
chronic phase, 131, 136–140, 143
complete remission, 135–136
molecular biology, 132–135
pregnancy and, 139–140
Chronic T cell malignancies, 109–110
Chronic T-gamma-lymphoproliferative disease, 185, 186
Clodronate, 318
Clotting cascade, 251, 252
C-MOPP regimen, 229
c-myc proto-oncogenes, 23, 28, 29, 39, 117, 122–123, 126
COP regimen, 229
COPBLAM regimens, 232
Corticosteroids, 198, 199, 200
Cutaneous T cell lymphoma, 109, 185, 186, 205
crk oncogenes, 21, 23
Cyclophosphamide, 142, 148, 157, 164, 165, 166, 167, 200, 201, 202
Cyclosporin A, 155–156, 157, 163
Cytosine arabinoside, 166, 167
Cytoskeleton, 25
Cytoxan, 167, 169

Danazol, 285
Deletion 5q⁻, 7–8
Desferrioxamine, 78–79, 81, 83, 84, 89
aluminium toxicity, 93
acquired transfusion dependent anaemias, 85, 87
malaria, 95
side effects, 87–88
thalassaemia major, 81, 84, 85–87
Diacylglycerol (DAG), 21, 23
Diamond Black Fan syndrome, 85
Diethylenetriaminepentaacetic acid (DTPA), 78, 83, 88, 89, 93
2,3-Dihydroxybenzoic acid (2,3-DHB), 78, 82, 83, 88
1,2-Dimethyl-3-hydroxypyrid-4-one (L1), 75, 78, 79, 80, 81, 82, 83, 84, 92, 95
clinical studies, 89
pharmacology, 90–91
toxicity, 90
Disseminated intravascular coagulation, 283–284

Doxorubicin, 201

Eclampic syndromes, 284
Editronate, 318
Electroportation, 68
Endothelial cell growth factor, 7
Epidermal growth factor (EGF), 19
receptor, 20, 24
Erythropoietin, 2, 3, 5–6, 8, 10, 26, 31–32
clinical trials, 14
Ethyl maltol, 91
Ethylenediamine-N,N′-bis-(2-hydroxyphenylacetic acid) (EDHPA), 83, 88
Ethylenediaminetriacetic acid (EDTA), 78, 88
Extramedullary plasmacytomata, 320

Factor VIII
de novo mutations, 248
DNA polymorphisms, 248–249
gene deletions, 245
gene structures, 243–244
LI repetitive element insertions, 245–246
single nucleotide mutations, 247
Factor IX, 251
gene deletions, 256–259
gene structure, 252–254
inhibitor patients, 256–259
point mutations, 254–256
polymorphic gene probe, 260–262
protein engineering, 259–260
protein structure, 252–254
Fanconi anaemia, 85
Ferritin, 79–81
Fetal blood sampling, 65
Fibrinolytic system, 265–267
Fibronectin, 2
Fludarabine monophosphate, 200
Follicular lymphoma, 123–124
Free radical formation, chelators and, 93, 94

G proteins, 21, 27
Globin genes, 43–47
Graft versus host disease, 144–146, 154–157
Graft versus leukaemia phenomenon, 146–147, 156, 157
Granulocyte colony stimulating factor (G-CSF), 1, 2, 3, 4, 7, 8, 10, 11, 13, 26, 30, 31
therapeutic applications, 14, 238
Granulocyte-macrophage colony stimulating factor (GM-CSF), 2, 3, 6–7, 8, 9–10, 11, 12–13, 15, 26, 30, 31
clinical trials, 13, 238, 298
Growth signal transduction
fibroblasts, 19–25
lymphocytes, 25–29

Haemoglobin Bart's hydrops fetalis, 48, 51, 52
Haemoglobin H disease, 48, 51, 52
acquired, 52–53
Haemonectin, 2
Haemophilia A, 143–149
see also Factor VIII

Haemophilia B, 251–263
    carrier/antenatal diagnosis, 260–262
    gene therapy, 262–263
    see also Factor IX
Haemopoietic growth factors, 1–15
    biological activity, 10–11
    clinical trials, 13, 14, 15, 238, 298
    gene localisation, 7–8
    in vivo effects, 11–14
    membrane receptors, 8–9
    molecular biology, 3–7
Haemosiderin, 80, 81
Hairy cell leukaemia, 185, 186, 194, 205
Hereditary persistence of fetal haemoglobin
        (HPFH), 47, 61–62
    deletion forms, 62–63
    non-deletion forms, 63–64
HIV
    AIDS, see Acquired immunodeficiency
        syndrome
    biology, 291–294
    blood products and, 299–301
    CD4 receptor, 292–293
    epidemiology, 294–296
    haematological manifestations, 296–299
    transmission, 293, 294–295, 299
    vaccines, 301
HIV-2, 291, 292, 301
Hodgkin's disease, 113, 211–225
    autologous bone marrow transplanation, 223–224
    chemotherapy, 219–221, 222–223
    combined modality treatments, 221–222
    histological classification, 214–215
    prognostic factors, 215–217
    radiotherapy, 217–219
    staging, 211–214
4-hydroxyperoxycyclophosphamide (4-HC), 170
8-hydroxyquinoline, 94, 95
Hydroxyurea, 136, 138, 140, 141

Ig gene rearrangements, 100–101, 122, 123, 129
    haematological neoplasms, 111, 112, 113
    lymphoproliferative disorders, 114–116
Indolent myeloma, 309
Inositol lipid turnover, 20–23, 27, 37–38
Inositol trisphosphate (IP$_3$), 21, 23, 27
Interferon therapy, 136, 137, 138–139, 204–205,
        238, 315
    toxicity, 139
Interleukin 1 (IL-1), 3, 10
Interleukin 2 (IL-2), 26, 159, 162–163
    non-Hodgkin's lymphoma treatment, 238
    receptor, 25, 29
Interleukin 3 (IL-3), 2, 3, 6–7, 9, 10, 11, 26, 31
    in vivo effects, 11–12, 15
    non-Hodgkin's lymphoma treatment, 238
    receptors, 8, 30
Interleukin 4 (IL-4), 3, 26
Interleukin 5 (IL-5), 3
Iron deficiency anaemia, 95
Iron overload, 79

Kaposi's sarcoma, 296, 323
α-ketohydroxypyridines (α-KHPs), 75, 76, 78, 82,
        89–93, 94, 95
    clinical investigations, 89–90
    toxicity, 90
Ki1$^+$ lymphoma, 112

Lactoferrin, 82
Lennert's lymphoma, 112
Leukaemia, 32–39
    activated oncogenes, transformation and, 34–35
    de-regulated tyrosine kinase and, 34, 35–37
    M-CSF receptor/gene, 37
    proliferation regulation mechanisms, 32
    ras gene activation, 37–39
Leukapheresis, 137, 140, 203
LICAM (C), 82, 93
Lupus anticoagulants, 284
Lymphomatoid papulosis, 110–111
Lymphosarcoma cell leukaemia, 184–185

MACOP-B regimen, 234
Macroglobulinaemia, 323
Macrophage colony stimulating factor (M-CSF), 2,
        3, 4–5, 7, 8–9, 10, 11, 26
    receptor gene in leukaemia, 37
    receptors, 8, 15, 29–30
Mafosfamide, 170, 171
Malaria, 65, 94–95
Maltol, 91, 92, 95
M-BACOD regimen, 230, 232
Melphalan, 314, 315, 321, 322
Methotrexate, 155, 163, 164
MIME regimen, 235
Mimosine, 91, 93
Mithramycin, 141
Monoclonal antibody therapy, 203–204, 237–238
Monoclonal gammopathy of undetermined
        significance (MGUS), 305, 308–309
MOPP regimen, 219, 220, 221, 222
Multiple myeloma, 305
    aetiology, 305–306, 307–308
    bone disease and, 317–318
    genetics, 315–316
    high dose chemotherapy, 314–315
    immunology, 316–317
    induction therapy, 311–313
    infections, 318
    neurologic complications, 319
    pathogenesis, 306–307
    pretreatment evaluation, 309–311
    renal disease, 318–319
    serum β_2 microglobulin, 310–311
Myelodysplasia, 13
Myocardial infarction, thrombolysis and, 269–271

Nephrotic syndrome, 284
N,N'-ethylenebis (2-hydroxyphenylglycine)
        (EHPG), 88
Non-B, non-T acute lymphoblastic leukaemia, 111
Non-Hodgkin's lymphoma, 112, 225–238
    advanced disease, 232–234

Non-Hodgkin's lymphoma (*contd*)
anatomical staging, 227–228
autologous bone marrow transplantation, 223–224, 235–237
chemotherapy, 235, 238
chromosomal translocations, 227
CNS prophylaxis, 234–235
histological classification, 225–227
indolent disease, 229–231
localised disease, 231–232
prognostic variables, 229
serotherapy, 237–238
Non-secreting myeloma, 321

Omadine, 91, 94, 95

PAI-1, 275, 278, 279–280
Pentostatin (2′-deoxycoformycin), 201, 205
Philadelphia chromosome, 35, 36, 121, 131
see also Chronic myelogenous leukaemia
Phosphatidyl-inositol bisphosphate phosphodiesterase (PIP$_2$-PDE), 21, 27, 30, 37, 38
Plasma cell leukaemia, 320–321
Plasmin, 265, 267
Plasminogen, 265
activators, 265–266
Plasminogen activator inhibitor-1, 267
Platelet-derived growth factor (PDGF), 19, 23–24
receptor, 7, 19–20, 24
Platelet-derived growth factor-stimulated tyrosine protein kinase, 19, 20, 21, 23, 24–25
Plutonium chelation, 93
Porphyria cutanea tarda, 94
Prednisone, 200, 201, 202, 205, 206
Prenatal diagnosis
haemophilia B, 260–262
thalassaemia, 65–67
Primary systemic amyloidosis, 321–322
Prolymphocytic leukaemia, 182, 184, 193
ProMACE-MOPP regimen, 230, 232, 234
Protein C
acquired deficiency, 283–284
deficiency treatment, 284–285
haemostasis and, 279–280
hereditary deficiency, 281–283
normal levels, 280–281
regulation of activity, 277–279
structural aspects, 276
Protein C inhibitor (PCI), 277, 278, 279
disseminated intravascular coagulation and, 284
normal levels, 281
Protein S, 276, 277, 278
C4b binding, 278
deficiency treatment, 284
disseminated intravascular coagulation and, 284
haemostasis and, 279, 280
hereditary deficiency, 283
normal levels, 281
Pyridoxal isonicotinoyl hydrazone (PIH), 75, 78, 80, 82, 83, 84, 89

Radiopharmaceuticals chelation, 94
ras oncogenes, 21, 37–39
Retrovirus-mediated gene transfer, 68–69
Rhodotorulic acid, 83, 88
Richter syndrome, 191

Serum β_2 microglobulin, 310–311
Sickle cell anaemia, 85
Sideroblastic anaemia, 85
Siderophores, 78
Single-chain urokinase-type plasminogen activator (scu-PA), 266, 267, 268, 271, 272
Smoldering myeloma, 308–309
Stanazolol, 285
Streptokinase, 265–266, 267–268, 269

Targeted gene modification, 69–70
T cell acute lymphoblastic leukaemia (T-ALL), 107–109, 118, 126
T cell chronic lymphocytic leukaemia (T-CLL), 109, 118, 126, 185, 193
T cell leukaemia/lymphoma, 110, 118
molecular genetics, 124–126, 128–129
T cell polymorphic leukaemia (T-PLL), 109, 126
T cell prolymphocytic leukaemia (T-PL), 109, 185, 186, 194
T cell receptor gene rearrangements
chromosomal translocations and, 116–118
haematological neoplasms, 106, 107–114
lymphoproliferative disorders, 114–116
T cell receptor genes (TcR), 25, 27, 101, 124
activation, 27–28
cloning, 102
IL2 and, 29
organisation, 103–104, 105–106
proto-oncogenes expression, 28–29
recombination, 106
tcl-1, 127
tcl-2, 128
tcl-3, 128
Thalassaemias
α, 48–53, 65
acquired with myeloproliferative disorders and mental retardation, 52–53
classification, 48
clinical phenotypes, 51–52
deletion forms, 48–50
non-deletion forms, 50–51
β, 53–57, 65
deletion forms, 53, 55
non-deletion forms, 55–57
silent carrier, 57, 60
δβ
deletion forms, 62–63
notation/classification, 61–62
γδβ, 63
notation, 61
bone marrow transplantation, 67
cholyhydroxamic acid therapy, 88
desferrioxamine therapy, 81, 84, 85–86
2,3-DHB therapy, 88
EHPG/EDHPA therapy, 88

Thalassaemias (*contd*)
  forms, 47–48
  intermedia, 57–61, 62, 63
  malaria and, 64
  population genetics, 64–65
  prenatal diagnosis, 65–67
  rhodotorulic acid therapy, 88
  specific gene therapy, 67–71
  symptomatic treatment, 67
6-thioguanine, 137, 138
Thrombolytic therapy, 265–272
  acute myocardial infarction, 269–271, 272
  fibrin specific thrombolysis and, 267
  synergism between agents, 271–272
Thrombomodulin, 275, 277–278, 280
Tissue-type plasminogen activator (tPA), 266, 267, 268, 270, 271, 272

Transferrin, 79, 81–82, 93
Transgenic studies, 70–71
Tropolone, 91
Tumour necrosis factor, 10
Tyrosine protein kinases, 19, 20, 30
  de-regulated in leukaemia, 34, 35–37
  inositol lipid cycle and, 21

Urokinase, 265, 266, 267, 268, 271, 272

VAD regimen, 313–314
v-fms genes, 9, 29, 30
Vincristine, 201, 202
VMCP/VBAP, regimen, 312, 313

Waldenstrom's macroglobulinaemia, 184, 323
Wilm's tumor, 117